D1593501

Progress in Pain Research and Management
Volume 29

Psychological Methods of Pain Control: Basic Science and Clinical Perspectives

Mission Statement of IASP Press®

The International Association for the Study of Pain (IASP) is a nonprofit, interdisciplinary organization devoted to understanding the mechanisms of pain and improving the care of patients with pain through research, education, and communication. The organization includes scientists and health care professionals dedicated to these goals. The IASP sponsors scientific meetings and publishes newsletters, technical bulletins, the journal *Pain*, and books.

The goal of IASP Press is to provide the IASP membership with timely, high-quality, attractive, low-cost publications relevant to the problem of pain. These publications are also intended to appeal to a wider audience of scientists and clinicians interested in the problem of pain.

Progress in Pain Research and Management
Volume 29

Psychological Methods of Pain Control: Basic Science and Clinical Perspectives

Editors

Donald D. Price, PhD

*Departments of Oral and Maxillofacial Surgery and Neuroscience,
McKnight Brain Institute, University of Florida,
Gainesville, Florida, USA*

M. Catherine Bushnell, PhD

*Centre for Research on Pain and Departments
of Anesthesia and Dentistry, McGill University,
Montreal, Quebec, Canada*

IASP PRESS® • SEATTLE

Library of Congress Cataloging-in-Publication Data

Psychological methods of pain control : basic science and clinical perspectives / editors,
    Donald D. Price, M. Catherine Bushnell.
        p. ; cm. -- (Progress in pain research and management ; v. 29)
    Includes bibliographical references and index.
    ISBN 0-931092-52-3 (alk. paper)
      1. Pain--Psychosomatic aspects. 2. Chronic pain--Alternative treatment. 3. Analgesia.
    4. Placebo (Medicine) I. Price, Donald D. II. Bushnell, M. Catherine, 1949- III. Series.
        [DNLM: 1. Pain--psychology. 2. Pain--therapy. WL 704 P97332 2004]
    RB127.P835 2004
    616'.0472--dc22

                                                                    2004048277

Published by:

IASP Press
International Association for the Study of Pain
909 NE 43rd Street, Suite 306
Seattle, WA 98105-6020 USA
Fax: 206-547-1703
www.iasp-pain.org
www.painbooks.org

Printed in the United States of America

Contents

v

Contributing Authors

Joseph Barber, PhD *Department of Rehabilitation Medicine, University of Washington School of Medicine, Seattle, Washington, USA*

Fabrizio Benedetti, MD *Department of Neuroscience, Clinical and Applied Physiology Program, University of Turin Medical School, Turin, Italy*

M. Catherine Bushnell, PhD *Centre for Research on Pain and Departments of Anesthesia and Dentistry, McGill University, Montreal, Quebec, Canada*

Luana Colloca, MD *Department of Neuroscience, Clinical and Applied Physiology Program, University of Turin Medical School, Turin, Italy*

Lauren A. Dade, PhD *Department of Anaesthesia, The University of Toronto, Toronto, Ontario, Canada*

Gary H. Duncan, DDS, PhD *Faculty of Dental Medicine, University of Montreal, Montreal, Quebec, Canada*

Steven J. Linton, PhD *Department of Occupational and Environmental Medicine, Örebro University Hospital; and Department of Behavioral, Social, and Legal Sciences, Örebro University, Örebro, Sweden*

Barton H. Manning, PhD *Department of Neuroscience, Amgen Inc., Thousand Oaks, California, USA*

Patricia A. McGrath, PhD *Chronic Pain Program, Departments of Anaesthesia and Psychology, The Hospital for Sick Children, and the Brain and Behavior Program, Research Institute at The Hospital for Sick Children, Toronto, Ontario, Canada*

Antonella Pollo, MD *Department of Neuroscience, Clinical and Applied Physiology Program, University of Turin Medical School, Turin, Italy*

Donald D. Price, PhD *Departments of Oral Surgery and Neuroscience, University of Florida, Gainesville, Florida, USA*

Pierre Rainville, PhD *Department of Stomatology, Faculty of Dental Medicine, University of Montreal, Montreal, Quebec, Canada*

Joseph L. Riley III, PhD *Division of Public Health Service and Research, College of Dentistry, University of Florida, Gainesville, Florida, USA;*

Michael E. Robinson, PhD *Department of Clinical and Health Psychology, University of Florida, Gainesville, Florida, USA*

Lene Vase, MS *Department of Psychology, University of Aarhus, Aarhus, Denmark*

G. Nicholas Verne, MD *Department of Gastroenterology, Veterans Administration Hospital, Gainesville, Florida, USA*

Chantal Villemure, PhD *Centre for Research on Pain, McGill University, Montreal, Quebec, Canada*

James B. Wade, PhD *Department of Psychiatry, Medical College of Virginia, Richmond, Virginia, USA*

Foreword

Since its inception, the International Association for the Study of Pain (IASP) has promoted the concept that pain is a multidimensional phenomenon that is a function of sensory, emotional, motivational, and evaluative processes. Within this theoretical framework, it is not surprising that neuroscientists and psychologists have been able to inspire one another and collaborate in endeavors such as the creation of this book.

Recent years have seen a considerable growth of interest in the placebo effect and in psychological factors related to this phenomenon. With the use of sophisticated psychophysical methodologies and human brain imaging, scientists are now able to examine the neural underpinnings of psychological influences on pain. The recent spate of placebo-related articles in top international journals and the high standard of scientists involved speak for themselves. IASP has been at the forefront of scientific interest in the study of the placebo effect and of the more general influence of psychological state on pain. It is within this atmosphere that the Special Interest Group on Placebo was founded in 1996 at the 8th World Congress on Pain in Vancouver. Interest grew rapidly, as was expressed at the 9th World Congress on Pain in Vienna, which included a session on placebo that featured talks by Donald D. Price, Fabrizio Benedetti, and Patrick D. Wall. The session caused intense interest and excitement, and from this meeting emerged the idea of writing a book that would integrate the ideas of both clinicians and scientists to better reveal how psychological factors can influence pain.

Dr. Price and his coeditor, M. Catherine Bushnell, have brought together an international team of scientists and clinicians to synthesize the most recent research on psychological aspects of pain perception and pain treatment. The historical perspective surrounding this book is unusual; in only a few years our understanding of such phenomena as hypnotic and placebo analgesia and the role of psychological factors in pain has expanded rapidly, so that we are beginning to understand for the first time the neural mechanisms underlying these phenomena.

This book discusses the influence of placebo, hypnosis, expectation, attention, emotions, and suggestions in a structured manner that gives nurturance and direction to further developments in the field. The content, meaning, and style come together in a manner that will stimulate and inspire the reader.

ROEL GAYMANS, MD, PhD (RETIRED CLINICIAN)
Pain Clinic, Amphia Hospital
Breda, The Netherlands

GIDEON B. HEKSTER, PhD
Pain Clinic, Erasmus University Hospital, Rotterdam
Pain Clinic, St. Antonius Hospital, Nieuwegein, The Netherlands

Preface

The past decade has seen remarkable developments in studies of psychological factors that influence pain, including attention, emotions, and suggestions, and improved developments of psychological methods of pain control, such as hypnosis. These developments have several sources, including improved designs of both experimental and clinical studies and the interface of brain imaging with thoughtful questions. Yet this new information comes at a time of some skepticism about the role of psychological influences on pain, such as the insistence that placebo analgesic effects are nothing beyond the changes seen in natural history.

This skepticism is surprising, because it has been known since antiquity that psychological factors and interventions can powerfully modulate the experience of pain. Recently we have learned that pain can be influenced by factors as straightforward as giving the patient one or two simple suggestions or as subtle as changing the clinical or experimental context. What are these factors or interventions that modify pain, and how do they work? And if they do work, could understanding of their mechanisms facilitate their use in clinical contexts? With these types of questions in mind, in editing this book we had two overall objectives. The first is to explain some of the fundamental principles by which pain is modulated by psychological factors, such as suggestion, expectations, attention, emotions, and cognitive reframing. The second is to show how these principles can be applied to the treatment of patients who have acute or chronic pain.

The book is divided into four sections; each section contains chapters that analyze pain modulation from clinical or basic science perspectives or both. The first section is about the general mechanisms of psychological control of pain. The chapters of this section are written from the perspective that pain is multidimensional and that pain experience can be modified at different neural levels and within specific dimensions (e.g., sensory, immediate affective, secondary affective). The second section is about general psychological factors that modulate pain, such as attention, emotions, and environmental factors. The third section is about placebo analgesia, a topic currently of intense and productive investigation. The final section is about hypnotic analgesia and contains a chapter written by cognitive neuroscientists and a chapter written by a psychologist who has had extensive clinical experience using hypnosis to control pain. The topics of this book by no means include all psychological methods of pain control, yet they are chosen to reflect how understanding of underlying mechanisms can contribute to the way in which clinical practice is conducted.

This book, inspired and organized in part by the IASP Special Interest Group on placebo, is intended to reflect basic science and clinical knowledge about how pain can be psychologically modulated by factors that occur naturally in clinical and experimental contexts and by explicit therapeutic interventions. Although the book can serve partly as a practical guide to the clinical use of psychological factors such as expectation, attention, and emotions in pain treatment, it does not include a definitive "how to" manual for psychological interventions. For such details, readers are referred to other sources.

The editors are grateful for the editorial assistance of Elizabeth Endres and others at IASP Press and for the timely efforts of our authors.

DONALD D. PRICE, PhD
M. CATHERINE BUSHNELL, PhD

Part I

General Mechanisms of Pain Modulation

Psychological Methods of Pain Control: Basic Science and Clinical Perspectives, Progress in Pain Research and Management, Vol. 29, edited by Donald D. Price and M. Catherine Bushnell, IASP Press, Seattle, © 2004.

1

Overview of Pain Dimensions and Their Psychological Modulation

Donald D. Price[a] and M. Catherine Bushnell[b]

[a]Departments of Oral Surgery and Neuroscience, University of Florida, Gainesville, Florida, USA; [b]Centre for Research on Pain and Departments of Anesthesia and Dentistry, McGill University, Montreal, Quebec, Canada

Milton Erickson, a world-renowned practitioner of medical hypnosis during the last century, was known to powerfully alter symptoms through the use of well-designed indirect suggestions (Haley 1967). An example was that of a patient, "Joe," who was terminally ill and in unremitting pain. Erickson spent several sessions with Joe talking about a tomato flower, interspersing suggestions such as "You have seen movies of flowers *slowly, slowly* opening, giving one *a sense of peace, a sense of comfort.*" Joe's outward demeanor gradually changed from distress to serenity, his behavior suggestive of severe pain subsided, and although he was still terminally ill, gradual improvements were noted in his physical condition. This dramatic example of pain reduction by hypnotic intervention is as mysterious as it is inspiring. What was in Joe's experience that accompanied changes in pain? What dimensions of pain were altered by this intervention? Did Joe still experience the same burning, piercing, or aching sensations or was there just a profound alteration in the meanings of these sensations? Did Joe become "dissociated" from his body or did he experience his body in a radically different manner? Similar questions can be asked about situational factors that alter pain or pain behavior. Beecher's battleground observations at the landing at Anzio point to the critical influence of context and meaning in pain (Beecher 1959). He found that soldiers wounded in battle complained much less and requested much less pain medication than civilians similarly injured in street accidents. What was different about their pain experience? Did the meanings associated with these two contexts bring about differences in perceived sensory intensity, in emotional dimensions, or only in pain-related behavior?

Clearly, psychological factors can sometimes influence pain in powerful ways, yet the myriad questions about how this takes place need not remain forever mysterious or unanswerable. The purpose of this book is to review evidence concerning the mechanisms by which psychological factors modulate pain both in clinical and experimental contexts. These reviews should be helpful for pain researchers who seek a scientific understanding of psychological modulation of pain as well as for clinicians who wish to optimize the influence of psychological factors in their treatment of pain patients.

The examples described above serve to remind us that the experience of pain is never an isolated sensory event and that it never occurs without the influence of context and meaning. Pain is influenced by beliefs, attention, expectations, and emotions, regardless of whether it occurs during the most controlled laboratory circumstances or during circumstances of physical trauma or emotional distress. The chapters in this book explore the mechanisms and the consequences of psychological modulation of pain from both clinical and experimental perspectives. In order to provide a preliminary foundation for these discussions, the first part of this chapter provides very general and somewhat simplified psychological and neurophysiological overviews of pain-processing mechanisms. The remaining chapters explore these mechanisms in greater detail and precision. As a starting point for discussion, one can think of pain modulatory mechanisms as those that can intervene in the pathways outlined in Figs. 1 and 2.

PSYCHOLOGICAL STAGES OF PAIN PROCESSING

Pain contains both sensory and emotional dimensions and is often accompanied by desires to terminate, reduce, or escape its presence (Hardy et al. 1952; Buytendyck 1961; Melzack and Wall 1965; Melzack and Casey 1968). By definition, pain has both unique sensory qualities and involves unpleasantness and sometimes other emotional feelings, largely due to the fact that the sensory qualities of physical pain dispose us to feel unpleasantness in most contexts. Thus, sensory qualities associated with pain are usually unpleasant for the same reasons that nausea and air hunger are perceived as unpleasant, as indicated by the path from nociceptive sensations to immediate unpleasantness in Fig. 1. In addition, however, there are parallel contributions to pain unpleasantness because the meaning of these sensory qualities is shaped by context and by a person's ongoing anticipations and attitudes. These contextual and cognitive factors are partly the result of the fact that pain often occurs within a situation that is threatening, such as during physical trauma or disease. Part of the affective dimension of pain is

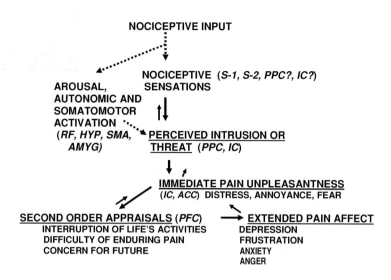

Fig. 1. A schematic used to illustrate interactions between pain sensation, pain unpleasantness, and secondary pain affect (solid arrows). Neural structures likely to have a role in these dimensions are shown by abbreviations in adjacent parentheses. HYP = hypothalamus; IC = insular cortex; PFC = prefrontal cortex; PPC = posterior parietal complex; RF = reticular formation; S1, S2 = first and second somatosensory cortical areas; SMA = supplemental motor area. Dashed arrows indicate nociceptive or endogenous physiological factors that influence pain sensation and unpleasantness.

its moment-by-moment unpleasantness, comprising emotional feelings that pertain to the present or short-term future, such as annoyance, fear, or distress. This component of pain-related emotional feeling will be referred to as *immediate pain unpleasantness* both in this chapter and Chapter 2. Immediate pain unpleasantness is often—although not always—closely linked to both the intensity and the unique qualities of the painful sensation. Another component of pain affect, *extended pain affect*, includes emotional feelings directed toward the long-term implications of having pain (e.g., "suffering"), as shown in Fig. 1 by the path extending from immediate pain unpleasantness to extended pain affect.

PSYCHOLOGICAL INTERRELATIONSHIPS BETWEEN SENSORY AND EMOTIONAL DIMENSIONS OF PAIN

Multiple factors contribute to immediate pain unpleasantness. Several sensory attributes of pain tend to create unpleasant emotional feelings. The foremost among these is that sensations of pain are often more intense than other types of somatic sensations. It is commonly accepted that perceived

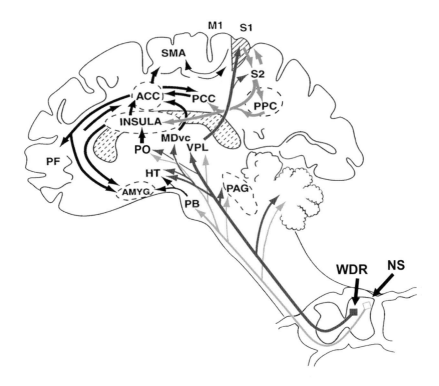

Fig. 2. A schematic of ascending pathways, subcortical structures, and cerebral cortical structures involved in processing pain. ACC = anterior cingulate cortex; PO = posterior nuclear complex; AMYG = amygdala; HT = hypothalamus; M1 = primary motor area; MDvc = ventrocaudal part of the medial dorsal nucleus; NS = nociceptive specific; PAG = periaqueductal grey; PB = parabrachial nucleus of the dorsolateral pons; PCC = posterior cingulate cortex; PF = prefrontal cortex; PPC = posterior parietal complex; S1, S2 = first and second somatosensory cortical areas; SMA = supplementary motor area; VPL = ventroposterior lateral nucleus; WDR = wide dynamic range.

intensity is a salient factor that contributes to the unpleasantness of pain, and this may be the reason that very loud sounds and bright lights are sometimes metaphorically referred to as "painful." In addition, pain presents character-istics of slow adaptation (i.e., persistence), temporal summation (increased sensation as a function of stimulus repetition for some types of pain), spatial spread of sensation at suprathreshold levels (i.e., radiation), spatial summa-tion (increased sensation as a function of the size of the affected area), and unique sensory qualities, as implied by words such as stinging, burning, and aching (Price 1999, 2000). Qualities of sensations evoked by tissue-damag-ing stimuli or by stimuli that would produce tissue damage if maintained (i.e., *nociceptive* stimuli) dispose us to perceive pain as invasive and intru-sive for both the body and consciousness (Buytendyck 1961). Both neural and psychological processes related to sensory qualities of pain can be conceived as important causal links in the production of pain-related emotional disturbance. The persistence of these sensory qualities over time enhances unpleasantness. Thus, there exists a serial interaction between pain sensation intensity and immediate pain unpleasantness (Fig. 1).

Perhaps the most direct demonstration of this serial interaction is a study by Rainville et al. (1999). These investigators found that hypnotic suggestions targeted toward unpleasantness could selectively decrease or enhance ratings of immediate unpleasantness of a 47°C stimulus without changing pain sensation intensity. In contrast, when suggestions were directed *only* toward changing pain sensation intensity, both pain sensation intensity and pain unpleasantness ratings changed in parallel. The combination of these two sets of results helps to establish that pain sensation intensity is a cause of pain unpleasantness and not vice versa. These results also have neurophysiological correlates, as will be described in Chapter 11.

Immediate pain unpleasantness, in turn, causes extended emotions related to pain because it can provide an immediate cue for the meanings related to pain-related negative emotions once these meanings have been established over time (Barber and Adrian 1982; Price 1999). For example, the sudden exacerbation of pain in a cancer patient serves as an instant reminder of the progress of the disease with its implications for deterioration and death. In addition, the difficulty of having to endure immediate pain unpleasantness over long periods of time (days, weeks, months) can lead to pain-related negative emotions because this difficulty provokes reflection and meanings related to suffering. Parallel influences on extended pain-related emotions also can occur because unpleasantness and extended negative emotions can be enhanced or diminished by arousal, contextual meanings, and other psychological factors that are present.

Nociceptive, exteroceptive (e.g., sight, sound), and interoceptive sensory processes (e.g., startle, increased visceral responses) may provide parallel contributions to pain affect (Price 1999). Pain itself can be conceptualized as both an exteroceptive and interoceptive phenomenon depending on the type of tissue that is stimulated and the types of sensory qualities that are present during pain. Consistent with Damasio's (1994) neurological view of the mechanisms of emotion, pain unpleasantness reflects the contribution of several sources, including pain sensory qualities, arousal, and visceral and somatomotor responses. Thus, these psychophysiological sources of input, in combination with appraisal of the context in which they occur, give rise to a felt meaning of what is happening to the body and self, often not necessarily accompanied by specific thoughts. This felt meaning derives largely from the experience of the body and constitutes the immediate unpleasantness of pain. For Damasio, "the essence of feeling an emotion is the experience of such changes in juxtaposition to the mental images that initiated the cycle" (Damasio 1994, p. 145). In the case of pain, the mental image is that of a physically intrusive and qualitatively unique somatic perception.

Psychophysical studies demonstrate that pain sensation and pain unpleasantness represent two distinct dimensions of pain that demonstrate reliably different relationships to nociceptive stimulus intensity and are separately influenced by various psychological factors. Pain unpleasantness can be selectively influenced by emotions; by changes in meaning of the pain; and by factors related to the predictability, controllability, and duration of pain (Buytendyck 1961 ; Melzack and Casey 1968). Pain unpleasantness also often leads to and sustains pain-related emotions that are based on cognitive appraisals that are more reflective than those which support pain unpleasantness. We term these latter pain-related emotional feelings *extended pain affect*. Unlike pain unpleasantness, extended pain affect is based on more elaborate reflection related to that which one remembers or imagines. Such reflection involves meanings such as perceived interference with one's life, difficulties of enduring pain over time, and implications for the future (Buytendyck 1961; Price 1999). Pain is often experienced as a threat not only to the present state of one's body, comfort, or activity, but also to one's future well-being and quality of life in general. The perceived implications that pain-related distress or annoyance holds for future well-being and functioning support the link between pain unpleasantness and extended pain affect, as illustrated in Fig. 1. Studies of pain patients show the distinction between immediate pain unpleasantness and extended pain affect and their sequential interactions, a topic that will be covered in detail in Chapter 2.

Different circumstances and meanings give rise to different levels of extended pain affect in proportion to pain unpleasantness. For example, a cancer patient who experiences a new abdominal pain may associate the pain with increased growth of a tumor and consequently may experience anxiety, dread, or depression in relation to the unpleasant qualities of pain. On the other hand, a woman in the pushing stage of labor would be likely to experience less extended pain affect, particularly if she associates the pain with the impending birth of the baby (Price 1999).

OVERVIEW OF NEUROPHYSIOLOGICAL PROCESSING OF PAIN

The stages of pain processing just described are also related to our present understanding of the neurophysiology of pain. Underlying neural mechanisms of sensory as well as primary and secondary affective dimensions of pain include multiple ascending spinal pathways to the brain and both serial and parallel processing in the brain. The neural representation of the experience of pain is likely to be related to a distributed network of brain structures that participate in the different dimensions of pain, such as arousal, identification of unique sensory qualities and their intensity, response selection, emotional feelings, and finally, emotional expression and motivation. This network of brain circuitry is itself controlled by inhibitory and facilitatory interactions within the brain, and is subject to descending inhibitory and facilitatory control within brain-to-spinal cord pathways (Basbaum and Fields 1984; Fields and Price 1997; Rainville et al. 1997, 1999; Price 2000). Thus, pain can be enhanced or reduced by interactions that take place at any one of several points in the schematics shown in Figs. 2 and 3. A major pathway for pain modulation, known since the 1970s, is that of a brainstem-to-spinal cord pathway that utilizes endogenous opioids (Fig. 3). Both intracortical and brain-to-spinal cord mechanisms will be discussed in Chapters 3, 5, 6, 8, and 11 in association with the topics of general mechanisms of pain modulation, placebo analgesia, and hypnotic analgesia. Explanation of pain processing in terms of multiple ascending pathways and a distributed brain network has gradually emerged in the last 15 years and it has replaced the classic textbook view of one or two ascending pathways and single discrete "pain centers" in the brain.

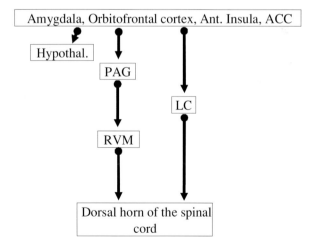

Fig. 3. A schematic, modified from Basbaum and Fields (1984), used to illustrate pathways and mechanisms that modulate pain. ACC = anterior cingulate cortex; LC = locus ceruleus; PAG = periaqueductal gray; RVM = rostroventral medial medulla.

ASCENDING NERVOUS SYSTEM PATHWAYS FOR PAIN

The main ascending pathways for pain originate in specialized receptors in body tissues, called nociceptors. These receptors are specialized to respond to stimuli to tissues that either cause damage or would cause damage if they were maintained for a sufficient length of time. Nociceptors are connected to primary afferent neuron axons that synapse onto dorsal horn neurons (Figs. 2 and 3). The dorsal horn of the spinal cord receives somatosensory information from most of the body, and the dorsal horn of the medulla oblongata receives input from the orofacial area via the trigeminal nerve. There are different classes of primary nociceptive afferent neurons that innervate different types of tissues, such as skin, muscle, joints, and viscera. Dorsal horn neurons that receive input from primary nociceptive neurons are at the origin of ascending pathways to the brain that have different functional roles in pain processing. The main somatosensory pathway is that of the spinothalamic tract that originates in the dorsal horn and projects to a ventroposterior lateral thalamic nucleus (VPL), some medial thalamic nuclei, and nuclei just posterior and inferior to the VPL. The VPL (and the ventroposterior medial nucleus [VPM] in the case of the trigeminal system) projects to the somatosensory cortices (S1 and S2), whereas the medial and posterior thalamic nuclei primarily project to limbic cortical areas (Fig. 2). The pathway to the VPL and VPM is critical for sensory qualities of pain and appreciation of its perceived sensory intensity. In addition to this major pathway, there are pathways that proceed from the dorsal horn directly to reticular formation nuclei of the medulla and midbrain and to the hypothalamus. There also is a pathway that ascends to the amygdala by way of a synapse in the pons (Bernard et al. 1996). These various target structures are involved in pain because they participate in such functions as arousal and diffuse cortical activation (reticular formation nuclei), body regulation (hypothalamus), and affective states such as fear (amygdala). The central nucleus of the amygdala has been strongly implicated in fear, emotional memory and behavior, and autonomic and somatomotor responses to threatening stimuli (Bernard et al. 1996). Various hypothalamic nuclei have also been implicated in these functions. Based largely on their central targets, all of these pathways are very likely to participate in the affective dimension of pain. Thus, some pathways directly activate cortical and subcortical limbic structures, and the pathway to the VPL/VPM and somatosensory cortex activates these same limbic structures through a ventrally directed route, as shown in Fig. 2. This latter pathway reflects the serial interaction between the sensory qualities and intensity of pain and its unpleasantness. Thus, direct and indirect activation of emotion-related limbic structures is consistent with the pathways shown in the schematic of Fig. 1.

Emotions related to pain are a consequence of sensations related to pain (i.e., serial interrelationships) as well as other psychophysiological and contextual factors (i.e., parallel interrelationships). Some aspects of pain-related emotions may occur automatically as a result of direct input to subcortical limbic areas such as the amygdala, a structure implicated in fear.

NEURONS WITHIN ASCENDING PATHWAYS

Dorsal horn neurons whose axons form ascending pathways for pain are classified as either wide dynamic range (WDR) neurons or nociceptive-specific (NS) neurons. These two types of neurons have functional significance for processing the different dimensions and stages of pain. WDR neurons respond differentially over a broad range of stimulus intensity, extending from very gentle to distinctly painful levels of stimulation. However, their output is controlled not only by input from nociceptive afferent impulses but also by interactions between non-nociceptive and nociceptive afferent impulses and by descending influences (both inhibitory and facilitatory) from the brain itself. In a general sense, these various types of interactions form the basis of the gate control theory proposed by Melzack and Wall in 1965. On the other hand, NS neurons respond predominantly to nociceptive stimuli.

Both WDR and NS neurons receive synaptic input from primary nociceptive afferent neurons innervating cutaneous, visceral, muscular, or other tissues. However, WDR but not NS neurons also receive synaptic convergence from Aβ primary afferent neurons that supply sensitive mechanoreceptors in the skin. These Aβ afferent neurons also activate inhibitory interneurons that inhibit WDR neurons. Thus, a brief tactile stimulus will result in an initial excitation and a subsequent inhibition within WDR neurons. The inhibitory effects of repetitive stimulation of "touch" receptors on pain have their parallels in the inhibition of WDR neurons by similar types of stimulation.

Both WDR and NS neurons can undergo sensitization as a result of facilitation mechanisms within the dorsal horn. This facilitation is evoked by repetitive impulse input from primary nociceptive afferents, particularly C-fiber nociceptive afferents (Price 1999). Repetitive or tonic impulse input from C fibers produces slow temporal summation of WDR and NS neuron responses to C-fiber input, termed "wind-up" (Price 1999). Wind-up leads to increased responsiveness of these central dorsal horn neurons to both innocuous and nociceptive stimuli, termed *central sensitization.* This mechanism provides at least part of the underlying basis for the hyperalgesia and allodynia observed during some types of persistent pain conditions.

The input-output relationships between primary afferent neurons and dorsal horn sensory transmission neurons are controlled by inhibition evoked by large-fiber mechanoreceptive input and facilitation evoked by tonic nociceptive input. Whether pain is perceived or not is controlled to an extent by a balance between these two factors. The responses of dorsal horn nociceptive neurons to somatic stimuli also can be inhibited or facilitated by descending pathways from the brain, and this bidirectional control is integral to psychological mechanisms of pain modulation. Psychological mechanisms of placebo analgesia and nocebo hyperalgesia may utilize these descending pathways, as will be discussed in Chapters 8 and 9.

CENTRAL PROJECTIONS OF DORSAL HORN NOCICEPTIVE NEURONS

The physiological characteristics of WDR and NS neurons and the differences between them are found at all central levels, including the dorsal horn, the VPL, and the somatosensory cortices. Although WDR neurons are more prevalent within the spinothalamic pathway to VPL and somatosensory cortices, NS and WDR neurons are intermingled at these levels, suggesting that they function in concert to encode the sensory discriminative features of nociceptive stimuli. NS neurons predominate in ascending pathways to the amygdala and the posterior/medial thalamic nuclei. Nociceptive neurons within the medial and posterior thalamic nuclei are highly modifiable by attentional and motivational state (Chapter 5). They may be somewhat more directly involved in affective motivational components of pain. On the other hand, WDR and NS neurons within the ascending pathway to the VPL and somatosensory cortices participate in the emotional dimension of pain because there is a serial pathway from the somatosensory cortices to limbic-related brain areas (Fig. 2).

BRAIN PATHWAYS AND REGIONS INTERRELATING SENSORY AND AFFECTIVE DIMENSIONS OF PAIN

Once impulses in ascending pathways from the dorsal horn reach different targets within the brain, both serial and parallel circuitry is activated. The serial interconnections are established by the pathway to VPL and to somatosensory cortices that is anatomically interconnected with a ventrally directed corticolimbic pathway that integrates somatosensory input with other sensory modalities such as vision and audition and with learning and memory (Friedman et al. 1986). This pathway proceeds from primary and secondary somatosensory cortices to posterior parietal cortical areas and to the insular cortex (IC) and from the latter to subcortical limbic structures such as the amygdala, perirhinal cortex, and hippocampus. This corticolimbic soma-tosensory pathway, which is critical for pain affect (Friedman et al. 1986), ultimately converges on the same limbic and subcortical structures that may be more directly accessed by other ascending spinal pathways. This dual convergence reflects both parallel and serial processing and may be related to a mechanism whereby multiple neural sources, including somatosensory cortices S1 and S2, contribute to pain affect. This corticolimbic serial path-way directly implies that somatosensory cortices contribute to pain affect. This implication is consistent with psychophysical studies showing that pain unpleasantness is the result of pain sensation intensity and with studies showing deficits in both pain sensation and pain unpleasantness as a result of somatosensory cortical lesions (see references in Price 1999, 2000).

THE PIVOTAL ROLE OF THE ANTERIOR CINGULATE CORTEX IN PAIN AFFECT

As illustrated in Fig. 2, the anterior cingulate cortex (ACC) receives anatomical projections from several sources, including the insular cortex. The ACC, in turn, is part of the brain's attentional and motivational network because it projects to prefrontal cortical areas involved in executive functions and to the supplementary motor area, which is involved in response selection (Devinsky et al. 1995). Parts of the ACC are consistently activated during pain, and in fact the ACC is the region most consistently activated in brain-imaging studies of pain (Casey and Bushnell 2000). Such studies show that ACC is more directly involved in pain affect than in appreciating the sensory qualities of pain (Chapter 11). These studies suggest that the ACC may be more important to the production of pain affect than somatosensory cortical areas (Chapters 5, 11). However, the latter also contribute to pain affect by virtue of their interconnections to the insular cortex and hence the ACC.

As shown in Fig. 2, the ACC receives inputs from multiple sources, including the thalamus, insular cortex, posterior cingulate cortex (PCC), and prefrontal cortex. Convergence of these inputs at the level of the ACC would be consistent with a mechanism in which somatic perceptual and cognitive features of pain would be integrated with attentional and rudimen-tary emotion mechanisms. Neurological evidence indicates that the ACC may have a complex pivotal role in interrelating attentional and evaluative functions with the task of establishing emotional valence and response pri-orities (Devinsky et al. 1995). Response priorities would be closely related to premotor functions that are integrally related to motivation and emotions and may be associated with immediate efforts to cope with, escape, or avoid the pain and the pain-evoking situation. For example, the projection of the ACC to the supplementary premotor area (Fig. 2) may reflect the "motor" side of an overall affective-motivational dimension of pain. In this view, cortical areas controlling sensory, attentional, premotor, and affective functions of pain are part of a distributed network, one that has both serial and parallel connections. This network has implications for psychological modulation of pain because each of these connections represents a stage of pain processing that can in principle be modified by psychological factors.

Response priorities change over an extended period of time. Pain unpleasantness endured over time engages prefrontal cortical areas involved in reflection and rumination about the future implications of a persistent pain condition. The ACC may serve this function by coordinating somatosensory features of pain with prefrontal cerebral mechanisms involved in attaching significance and long-term implications to pain, a function associated with secondary pain affect (Devinsky et al. 1995; Apkarian et al. 2001; Verne et al. 2003). Thus, ACC may be a region that coordinates inputs from parietal areas involved in perception of bodily threat with frontal cortical areas involved in plans and response priorities for pain-related behavior. Both functions would help explain observations in patients with prefrontal lobotomy and in patients with pain asymbolia as a result of insular cortical lesions (Price 1999). The former have deficits in spontaneous concern or rumination about their pain but can experience the immediate threat of pain once it is brought to their attention. In contrast, asymbolia patients appear incapable of perceiving the threat of nociceptive stimuli under any circumstances. The role of medial prefrontal cortical areas in secondary pain affect is also supported by recent brain imaging studies. These studies show increased prefrontal neural activity in clinical pain patients likely to have high levels of secondary pain affect (Apkarian et al. 2001; Verne et al. 2003).

TOP-DOWN MODULATION OF PAIN SENSATION AND AFFECT BY COGNITIVE FACTORS

The schematic of Fig. 2 refers to ascending pathways and afferent circuitry involved in pain processing. Absent from this model are neural circuits that provide top-down modulation of the pain experience. Central neural mechanisms associated with such phenomena as placebo/nocebo, hypnotic suggestion, attention, distraction, and ongoing emotions are now thought to modulate pain by decreasing or increasing neural activity within many of the brain structures shown in Fig. 2. This modulation includes endogenous pain-inhibitory and pain-facilitatory pathways that descend to the spinal dorsal horn, the origin of ascending spinal pathways for pain (Basbaum and Fields 1977). Recent brain-imaging studies have begun to reveal the cortical areas involved in pain modulation (Rainville et al. 1997; Hofbauer et al. 2001; Koeppe and Stohler 2001; Petrovic et al. 2001; Zubieta et al. 2001; Chapter 8 of this volume).

The modulation of pain by endogenous opioid systems by cortical and subcortical networks is consistent with other types of brain-imaging experiments that show that anticipation of pain affects cortical nociceptive regions (Chapter 5). Interestingly, these brain regions are the same ones that are directly activated during pain itself. Thus, the cortical networks shown in Fig. 2 may be directly influenced by cognitive factors. These are likely to include not only anticipation of the presence of pain, but also anticipation of its reduction, as in the case of placebo or hypnotic analgesia. The modulatory mechanisms are likely to be diverse, extending from those which are confined only to neural interactions within the brain to those involving activation of brain-to-spinal cord circuits long known to potently reduce or enhance pain, as represented in Fig. 3 (Basbaum and Fields 1977). The remaining chapters will focus on different aspects of these modulatory mechanisms and on their various roles during clinical treatments for pain.

CONCLUDING REMARKS

The combination of anatomical, neurophysiological, and psychological approaches to understanding the mechanisms underlying sensory and affective dimensions of pain has led to a vastly improved ability to answer questions that only 10 years ago were relatively impenetrable. In particular, studies that combine brain imaging with psychophysical methods and sophisticated experimental designs have led to the possibility of understanding complex mechanisms by which sensory and affective dimensions of pain are interrelated. They have also led to an understanding of how these dimensions can be modulated by cognitive factors and by treatments that are commonly given for pain. The brain networks for these mechanisms are extensive and involve both serial and parallel circuitry that is itself under dynamic control from several brain regions. This view is radically different from classical models that present central pain pathways as two parallel lines, one for affect and the other for sensation, or that propose one or two discrete pain centers of the brain. The remaining chapters will review knowledge about psychological modulation of pain obtained from both clinical and basic science studies and perspectives and thereby attempt to address several questions.

The first section will address questions about general factors that modulate pain concerning how personality and demographic factors influence the stages and dimensions of pain (Chapter 2), how environmental factors interact with neural mechanisms during pain modulation (Chapter 3), and how psychological factors modulate pain in clinical settings (Chapter 4). The second section will deal with specific psychological factors that modulate pain. These factors include attention (Chapter 5), emotions (Chapter 6), and environmental and behavioral factors that influence chronic pain (Chapter 7). Placebo analgesia is the topic of the third section, which will present discussions of biological mechanisms (Chapter 8), psychological mechanisms (Chapter 9), and the basis for understanding and enhancing placebo responses in clinical contexts (Chapter 10). The final section presents the topic of hypnotic analgesia, from both a research laboratory (Chapter 11) and a clinical (Chapter 12) perspective. All sections reflect an integration of basic science and clinical approaches to understanding the psychological modulation of pain.

REFERENCES

Apkarian, AV, Thomas PS, Krauss BR, Szeverenyi NM. Prefrontal cortical hyperactivity in patients with sympathetically mediated pain. *Neurosci Lett* 2001; 311(3):193–197.

Barber J, Adrian C. *Psychological Approaches to the Management of Pain.* New York: Brunner/Mazel, 1982.

Basbaum AI, Fields HL. Endogenous pain control systems: brainstem pathways and endorphin circuitry. *Annu Rev Neurosci* 1984; 7:309–338.

Beecher HK. *Measurement of Subjective Responses: Quantitative Effects of Drugs.* New York: Oxford University Press, 1959.

Bernard et al. Involvement of the spino-parabrachial amygdaloid and hypothalamic pathways in the autonomic and affective emotional aspects of pain. *Prog Brain Res* 1996; 107:243–255.

Buytendyck FJJ. *Pain.* London: Hutchinson, 1961.

Casey KL, Bushnell MC (Eds). *Pain Imaging,* Progress in Pain Research and Management, Vol. 18. Seattle: IASP Press, 2000.

Damasio, A. *Descartes Error.* New York: Avon Books, 1994.

Devinsky O, Morrell M J, Vogt BA. Contributions of anterior cingulate cortex to behavior. *Brain* 1995; 118(Pt 1):279–306.

Fields HL, Price DD. Toward a neurobiology of placebo analgesia. In: Harrington A (Ed). *The Placebo Effect.* Boston: Harvard University Press, 1997.

Friedman DP, Murray EA, O'Neill JR. Cortical connections of the somatosensory fields of the lateral sulcus of macaques: evidence for a corticolimbic pathway for touch. *J Comp Neurol* 1986; 252(3):323–347.

Haley J (Ed). *Advanced Techniques of Hypnosis and Therapy: Selected Papers of Milton H. Erickson, M.D.* New York: Grune & Stratton, 1967.

Hardy JD, Wolff HG, Goodell H. *Pain Sensations and Reactions.* Baltimore: Williams and Wilkins, 1952.

Hofbauer RK, Rainville P, Duncan GH, Bushnell MC. Cognitive modulation of pain sensation alters activity in human cerebral cortex. *J Neurophysiol* 2001; 86(1):402–411.

Koeppe RA, Stohler CS. Regional mu opioid receptor regulation of sensory and affective dimensions of pain. *Science* 2001; 293(5528):311–315.

Melzack R, Casey KL. Sensory, motivational, and central control determinants of pain. In: Kenshalo D (Ed). *The Skin Senses.* Springfield: CC Thomas, 1968, pp 423–443.

Melzack R, Wall PD. Pain mechanisms: a new theory. *Science* 1965; 150:971–979.

Petrovic P, Kalso E, Petersson KM, Ingvar M. Placebo and opioid analgesia—imaging a shared neuronal network. *Science* 2001; 295(5560):1737–1740.

Price DD. *Psychological Mechanisms of Pain and Analgesia,* Progress in Pain Research and Management, Vol. 15. Seattle: IASP Press, 1999.

Price DD. Psychological and neural mechanisms of the affective dimension of pain. *Science* 2000; 288:1769–1772.

Rainville P, Duncan GH, Price DD, Carrier B, Bushnell MC. Pain affect encoded in human anterior cingulate but not somatosensory cortex. *Science* 1997; 277:968–971.

Rainville P, Carrier B, Hofbauer R, et al. Dissociation of sensory and affective dimensions of pain using hypnotic modulation. *Pain* 1999; 82(2):159–171.

Verne GN, Himes NC, Robinson ME, et al. Central representation of visceral and cutaneous hypersensitivity in the irritable bowel syndrome. *Pain* 2003; 103(1–2):99–110.

Zubieta JK, Smith YR, Bueller JA, et al. Regional mu opioid receptor regulation of sensory and affective dimensions of pain. *Science* 2001; 293:311–315.

Correspondence to: Donald D. Price, PhD, Department of Oral and Maxillofacial Surgery, University of Florida, P.O. Box 100416, Gainesville, FL 32610-0416, USA. Email: dprice@dental.ufl.edu.

Psychological Methods of Pain Control: Basic Science and Clinical Perspectives, Progress in Pain Research and Management, Vol. 29, edited by Donald D. Price and M. Catherine Bushnell, IASP Press, Seattle, © 2004.

2

Psychological and Demographic Factors that Modulate the Different Stages and Dimensions of Pain

Joseph L. Riley III[a] and James B. Wade[b]

[a]Division of Public Health Service and Research, College of Dentistry, University of Florida, Gainesville, Florida, USA; [b]Department of Psychiatry, Medical College of Virginia, Richmond, Virginia, USA

Since the early work of Melzack and Casey (1968), the experience of pain has been conceptualized as multidimensional, rather than as a unitary construct. Therefore, in addition to temporal and spatial factors, other important components of the pain experience include initial sensory-discriminative input (intensity), negative affective response generated by higher levels of central processing (unpleasantness), longer-term reflective or cognitive processes that relate to the meanings or implications of pain (extended negative affect), and behavioral response to pain (activity modification). The gate control theory of pain has provided a perceptual mechanism that links these dimensions and suggests that pain is modulated (facilitated and inhibited) at spinal levels by a host of behavioral and psychological factors. These could range from culturally related beliefs about the nature of a painful symptom to expectations related to outcome or emotions associated with loss of important role functioning. Although the gate control theory acknowledges interrelationships between these dimensions, it does not specifically propose temporal sequencing in how they are processed.

FOUR-STAGE MODEL OF PAIN PROCESSING

A conceptual model that lends itself to the study of the processing of pain is the four-stage model proposed by Wade et al. (1992b, 1996) and Price (1999). This model (Fig. 1) consists of an initial sensory-discriminative stage,

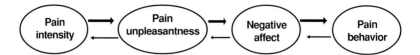

Fig. 1. Four-stage model of pain processing. The recursive arrows acknowledge that although the earlier stages give rise to later stages over time, there is a reciprocal effect in that past and current levels of later stages can influence future levels of earlier stages.

of which the major component is the perceived intensity of the pain sensation. This stage is related to immediate appraisals associated with the sensory features of the pain, autonomic and somatomotor activation, and perception of the immediate context surrounding the pain. This is the dimension typically assessed in primary care medical settings and epidemiological studies. The second stage of pain processing, termed *immediate unpleasantness,* reflects an individual's immediate affective response and involves limited cognitive processing. This stage is fueled by the first stage and yet is additionally related to reflection about the immediate implications of having pain. It comprises the moment-by-moment unpleasantness, distress, and possible annoyance often closely linked with the intensity of the painful sensation and its accompanying arousal.

The third stage of pain processing involves longer-term reflective or cognitive processes that relate to the meanings or implications that pain holds for one's life and is manifested by an extended affective response related to pain (Price 1999). This stage has previously been termed "the secondary stage of pain affect" (Price 1999), referring to pain unpleasantness as the primary affective stage. We have replaced this previous term with *extended pain affect* so as to avoid confusion when discussing the four-stage model. Extended pain affect may be conceptualized in simple terms as suffering, which might include experiencing depression, frustration, anxiety, and anger. Indeed, it reflects the experiential side of suffering, as opposed to its overt behavioral manifestations. Consistent with Damasio's (1994) view of extended consciousness, it is largely autobiographical and is directed toward the long-term past and long-term future. It is influenced by expectations, beliefs, and meanings, such as hope for alleviation, belief in one's ability to endure the pain, and perceived control over reducing the pain intensity. Thus, an individual's attitudes, beliefs, and memories about the real or imagined long-term consequences of having pain influence his or her adaptation to this stage. Consequently, these are the mediators that are the focus of cognitive-behavioral interventions and may explain differing levels of adaptation. A final component of this model is that of the overt behavioral expression of pain, such as moaning, lying down during the day, and declining to participate in daily responsibilities. Few studies have explicitly examined this stage, and it would be useful to broaden the operational definition of this stage to include behaviors to manage or reduce pain, such as taking medications. In the context of this model, the four stages refer to different levels of processing of the experience of pain, which could all be occurring at one time; however, the earlier stages also give rise to later stages over time.

The four-stage model of pain processing is consistent with the neural mechanisms of the sensory and affective dimensions of pain presented in Chapter 1, which emphasize serial processing but also include parallel processing of pain-related information. For example, serial interactions between pain sensation, immediate pain unpleasantness, and extended pain-related affect are respectively associated with serial interactions between somatosensory cortices, insular and cingulate cortices, and prefrontal and temporal cortical areas. The model is also consistent with both clinical and experimental studies of pain modulation, as described in Chapters 1 and 11.

MODERATORS AND MEDIATORS OF THE FOUR STAGES OF PAIN PROCESSING

Evidence supporting the four-stage model comes from clinical studies that show how exogenous variables moderate and mediate selective stages and the relationships among the stages, consistent with the sequential nature of the theory. Moderators are qualitative variables that are associated with changes in the direction or strength of the relationship between two variables (Baron and Kenny 1986). In the context of clinical pain, important moderating variables are the clinical diagnosis, the race and ethnicity of the patient, and various personality characteristics. This chapter focuses on several studies that have tested hypotheses related to the influence of moderating variables using the four-stage model of pain processing. Clinical and experimental pain studies that have demonstrated differences across groups of subjects or patients have typically documented differences in the early stages of pain processing while failing to test for linkages with pain-related negative emotions or behavioral manifestations of pain, thus relying on overly simplistic models of pain.

When studies demonstrate group differences, they are seldom able to differentiate between effects of biological factors and psychosocial influences that mediate the particular pain-related outcome that is observed. Mediators are exogenous variables that change as a function of an antecedent variable and account for the relationship between the predictor and the outcome of interest and can be thought of as the mechanism of change (Baron and Kenny 1986). For an excellent discussion of the mediators associated with this theory, see Price (1999). In this context, moderators and mediators are not likely to operate independently. Whereas moderator variables specify when certain effects will hold, mediators speak to how or why such effects occur. For example, take sex differences in pain report. A mediation process may be stronger for one group (e.g., males) than for another (e.g., females), and so differences in the effects of the mediator explain the moderation effect. Therefore, in presenting the following studies, we will discuss various mediators that may in part account for the group differences reported.

CRITERIA FOR PAIN MEASUREMENT

Neuropsychological and pain assessments have two things in common. First, both require evaluation of several distinct domains. Neuropsychological assessment requires evaluation of cognitive processes (e.g., intelligence, language skills, visual spatial analysis, attention, memory, and learning), sensory processes (tactile, visual, and auditory channels), and motor processes. Neglecting any one of these domains limits the power of the examination. Likewise, comprehensive pain assessment involves separate assessment of sensory/discriminative, affective/motivational, and behavioral dimensions. Second, interpretation of pain and neuropsychological data requires the explicit recognition that sociocultural and demographic factors must be accounted for. Age, years of education completed, and sex influence neuropsychological performance. For example, if an 18-year-old and an 88-year-old take the same memory test and obtain identical scores (e.g., 6 out of 10 items correct), the clinician might conclude that the elderly subject did well, but the young adult did poorly. Age affects memory performance. Similarly, pain assessment requires the recognition that demographic variables may influence the patient's data. Take the example of two women with the same degree of pain sensation intensity. The first woman is suffering because she has end-stage renal cancer. The second woman, with identical pain intensity, is in the active stage of labor. Although both women experience the same pain intensity, their medical diagnoses differ. Thus, individuals' understanding of the meaning or context for the pain shapes their pain experience. As shown by Price (1988), patients in pain manifest differing levels of anxiety, frustration, fear, depression, and anger depending on the meanings and implications they attach to the pain situation. Since the writings of the ancient Greek scholars Aurelius (translation 1980) and Sophocles

(Greene 1957), nonpathological factors such as age, gender, ethnicity, and medical diagnosis have been thought to influence pain processing.

Clinicians have speculated that in complex regional pain syndrome (CRPS), pain sensation intensity seems more severe than expected based on the degree of tissue damage alone (Blumberg et al. 1990). These observations, along with the presence of significant psychiatric comorbidity in CRPS patients (Haddox 1990; Lynch 1992), suggested that suffering and illness behavior are disproportionately higher in such patients. Indeed, some have speculated that underlying psychopathology in these patients could predispose an individual to develop this painful medical condition (De Vilder 1980). The use of multivariate (LISREL) analysis in examining the potential for differences in pain processing between diagnostic groups could provide additional evidence for the validity and cogency of the four-stage model of pain processing offered in this chapter, and could yield normative clinical data. Standardizing clinical norms in a large sample of chronic pain sufferers would allow for control of potential moderating factors such as age, gender, ethnicity, and medical diagnosis in interpreting each patient's pain profile. This process would facilitate the development of an individualized comprehensive treatment plan.

To accomplish this goal, Wade and Price (2000) studied a large population of chronic pain patients ($n = 1,434$) and examined the extent to which medical diagnosis influenced the four stages of pain processing. Methodology was similar to that of their previous study (Wade et al. 1996). LISREL was used to assess the causal interrelationships between the four stages of pain processing in three chronic pain conditions (CRPS, myofascial pain dysfunction, and failed back surgery syndrome). The investigators found that a visual analogue scale (VAS) could be used to assess pain sensation intensity, immediate pain unpleasantness, and extended negative affect, and determined that a structured interview could assess overt pain-related behavior. The model's overall goodness of fit supported the four-stage model of pain processing. No pain-processing differences at any of the four pain stages emerged for medical diagnosis.

RACE AND ETHNICITY DIFFERENCES IN PAIN STAGES

Some evidence suggests that the experience of clinical pain varies across racial and ethnic groups (Breitbart et al. 1996; Creamer et al. 1999), but not all studies find differences (Jordan et al. 1998). Race differences in pain report vary according to the site of pain (Sheffield et al. 2000; Riley et al. 2002a), with African Americans reporting more pain only at some locations

(Moore and Brodsgaard 1999). Some studies have shown variations in racial and ethnic differences according to pain measure, such as intensity, unpleasantness, or verbal descriptor. Recent experimental pain studies have found that African-American subjects had lower tolerance for thermal pain and rated painful stimuli as more unpleasant in comparison to white subjects (Edwards and Fillingim 1999; Sheffield et al. 2000). Similarly, studies of childbirth pain found few differences in pain intensity across racial and ethnic groups, whereas pain descriptors and pain behaviors varied by ethnicity (Lee and Essoka 1998; Moore et al. 1998). Finally, Greenwald (1991) found no racial and ethnic differences in pain sensation, but noted differences in the affective words used to describe cancer pain.

There is less evidence for racial and ethnic differences in the later stages of pain processing. Among patients with chronic orofacial pain, Lipton and Marbach (1984) found that ethnic group differences were most apparent across measures of emotionality in response to pain and measures of interference with daily functioning attributed to pain. Sanders and colleagues (1992) found important cross-cultural differences in self-perceived level of dysfunction among patients with chronic low back pain, even though pain intensity levels were similar. Finally, a recent community-based study of individuals experiencing orofacial pain found that African Americans were nearly twice as likely to describe orofacial pain as severe enough to affect their behavior than were white respondents (Riley et al. 2002a).

As we have reviewed above, some evidence suggests racial and ethnicity group differences across the stages of the four-stage model, particularly the later stages. To our knowledge, our recent study is the only one that has examined racial and ethnic differences across the whole model (Riley et al. 2002b). In this study, we used the four-stage model of pain processing to examine differences between African Americans and whites in a sample of 1,557 chronic pain patients. We found that relative to white patients, African-American patients reported significantly higher levels of pain unpleasantness, higher levels of extended negative affect, and more pain behavior (Fig. 2). There were no differences in pain intensity, the first stage of pain processing. The greatest differences were found for the emotion measures, particularly depression and fear, where groups differed by approximately 1.0 VAS units. Group differences of this magnitude may well be clinically significant. There were also differences in linear associations between pain measures, with African Americans showing a stronger link between extended pain affect and pain behavior.

Our finding of racial and ethnic differences in pain unpleasantness, but not in pain intensity, is consistent with previous research with experimental pain (Edwards and Fillingim 1999; Sheffield et al. 2000), headache (Stewart

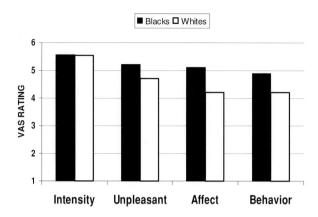

Fig. 2. Mean visual analogue scale (VAS) ratings of pain intensity, immediate pain unpleasantness, extended negative affect, and overt pain behaviors for black and white chronic pain patients (data from Riley et al. 2002b).

et al. 1996), and cancer pain (Greenwald 1991) and supports the sequencing of the first two stages of the model. The model suggests that the perception of pain intensity is less influenced by psychosocial factors than is pain unpleasantness (Price 1999). Previously documented racial differences in psychosocial factors that would mediate between the stages, such as attitudes toward care, attributions for pain, and coping styles, may therefore contribute to our findings. Other mediators that could differ across racial and ethnic groups may include cognitive factors such as "locus of control" beliefs about pain (Bates and Rankin-Hill 1994) and interpretations of pain.

Racial and ethnic differences in negative affect or behavioral responses to pain may derive from potential differences in the meaning of pain and its intrusiveness in patients' role functioning. For example, we may speculate that pain that intrudes on the ability to maintain employment might be particularly salient and distressing for those individuals in lower income brackets, as is more often the case for African Americans, or for those who face racial discrimination in workplace hiring and promotion practices (McGuire and Reskin 1993). Evidence for potential race differences in the consequences of role intrusion comes from studies showing that participation in the labor force has in some cases been associated with racially differentiated health-protective effects favoring African Americans over whites (Waldron and Jacobs 1989; Rushing et al. 1992).

Several studies have described racial and ethnic differences in coping with pain (Bates and Rankin-Hill 1994; Jordan et al. 1998; Jordan 1999) and also in dysfunction associated with pain (Bates and Edwards 1992).

Demonstration of differences in pain behaviors may be suggestive of decreased functioning, secondary gain from pain demonstration, or some combination thereof. Research has shown that African-American patients with
acute chest pain report lower functioning as measured by the Short Form-36
of the Medical Outcomes Study than do Caucasian patients (Johnson et al.
1995). The higher incidence of negative emotion in general in African Americans may play a role in such report. Studies have shown that pain patients
with negative emotion experience lower rates of functioning due to lethargy,
fatigue, and lowered motivation related to mood (e.g., Banks and Kerns
1996).

Overall, the increased suffering and pain behavior by African-American
pain patients, as well as a stronger association between extended negative
affect and pain behaviors, suggest that treatment *targeting both affect and
pain behavior* may be particularly important for these patients. Historically,
African Americans have been undertreated for depression, with estimates of
as high as 50% of diagnoses of depression going undetected (Sussman et al.
1987). This guidance should not be interpreted as applying to individual
patients, because there is considerable intragroup variability among racial/
ethnic groups, and stereotyping of patients according to race or other characteristics is to be avoided.

AGE COHORT DIFFERENCES IN PAIN STAGES

Consistent with the pain and ethnicity literature, studies examining the
relationship between pain and age have focused primarily on the first stage
of pain processing, that of pain sensation intensity, and have yielded contradictory findings (Woodrow et al. 1972; Harkins et al. 1986; McMillan 1989;
Sorkin et al. 1990; Edwards et al. 2003). With the limitations of most previous demographic studies of pain in mind, Riley et al. (2000) examined the
extent to which age influenced the magnitude of the various stages of pain
processing 1,712 chronic pain patients.

No effects of age were found for pain intensity ratings or immediate
unpleasantness ratings. Thus, no age effects were observed for the first two
stages of pain processing. However, age had large (>1.5 VAS units) and
selective effects on the stages of extended negative affect and illness behavior, with the oldest group reporting less emotional distress and pain behavior
than the youngest or middle-aged cohorts (Fig. 3). Older pain patients had
considerably lower ratings of anxiety, frustration, anger, and fear, but no
differences were found for depression. These patients also had significantly
lower composite ratings of these five pain-related emotional feelings. Harkins

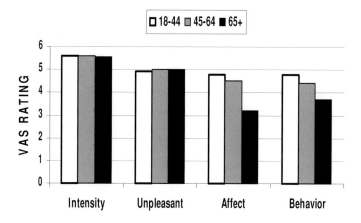

Fig. 3. Mean VAS ratings of pain intensity, immediate pain unpleasantness, extended negative affect, and overt pain behaviors for younger, middle-aged, and older adult chronic pain patients (data from Riley et al. 2000).

and Price (2001) also observed a large and selective effect of age on the extended negative affective stage of pain processing. In addition, the linear association between these two stages was also different, with the middle-aged group demonstrating the highest association between their emotional response to pain and pain behavior and the elderly group demonstrating the least association.

In comparison to the youngest and middle-aged groups, older adults in this sample appear to suffer less emotional distress related to pain. Because individuals interpret pain in the context of their lives, attitudes toward aging are likely to contribute to the emotional response to pain (Leventhal and Prohaska 1986). For example, the attribution of medical symptoms to the aging process is greater for older than for younger medical patients and is associated with reduced emotional response to these symptoms (Prohaska et al. 1987). Therefore, the elderly may accept pain-related losses as an aging-related natural reduction in overall health and thus experience less negative emotion related to their symptoms. It is also possible that middle age is the time that marks the beginning of the aches and pains of aging, which makes the symptoms of chronic pain more difficult to accept (Thomas and Roy 1999).

There has been little research into age-related differences in behavioral expression of pain. The behavioral domain in this study included pain behaviors manifested by the patient, degree of social reinforcement for pain behavior, and the impact of pain on daily activity. Some researchers have suggested that elderly individuals may overemphasize pain to hide functional impairment from cognitive deficits or other causes (McIntosh 1990). On the other hand, if the elderly dismiss pain as normal aging, they may reduce pain behavior because of their acceptance of pain and their desire to minimize the behavioral communication of the need for invasive treatment (Clinton and Eland 1990). Our data are consistent with the second hypothesis.

Overall, our data support the four stages of pain processing. It seems logical that younger adults report more pain-related negative affect and greater lifestyle disruption due to pain. These later stages of pain processing are more dependent on an individual's perception of the meaning and anticipated impact that pain will have on satisfying one's needs and expectations (Price 1999). Differences in developmental life stage imply different life challenges. The inability to maintain full-time employment because of chronic pain may have different meaning and be related to more emotional distress (i.e., feeling frustrated and angered by pain) for those in the younger and middle-aged years. These individuals perceive the problem to be more disabling and report more illness behavior.

No age-related differences were found in the linear association between pain and extended affective response to pain. This finding is consistent with the extensive literature examining the association between chronic pain and negative emotion (Robinson and Riley 1998). An individual's emotional response to pain may be linked to the perceived effectiveness of one's ability to control pain (DeGood and Shutty 2001). Therefore the link between pain and pain-related emotions should be mediated by the ability to cope with pain. Although some studies have suggested that the elderly use more externally mediated coping (i.e., hoping and praying), most studies have not found age-related differences in perceived ability to control pain or in ratings of the effectiveness of coping strategies (Keefe and Williams 1990; McCracken and Gross 1993).

An important contribution of this study to the pain and aging literature is the finding of age-related differences in the linear association between affective response to pain (third stage) and pain behavior (fourth stage). Older adults were found to be less likely to manifest signs of illness behavior to family and friends (moaning or asking for help with things they would normally be able to do themselves) as a function of emotional response to pain. It is possible that the elderly have different environmentally related contingencies reinforcing pain behavior than do those in younger age groups. For example, older individuals may be less likely to have access to immediate social support. Cross-sectional research suggests that environmental influences, such as social support (Gil et al. 1987; Kerns et al. 1990), are likely to play a complex role in moderating the expression of pain for all individuals.

The findings that middle-aged adults have a stronger link between their negative affect and pain behavior and that their overall level of emotional distress is greater than older adults have clinical implications for both age ranges. The multidisciplinary treatment of chronic pain conditions is often designed to address multiple aspects of this complex syndrome. However, these data suggest that different treatment foci might be indicated based on the age of the patient. For younger and middle-aged patients, the impact of loss of income or changes in family and work identities may be a greater focus for cognitive-behavioral interventions because they are likely to be major contributors to the pain and negative affect cycle. Therefore, the middle-aged group may benefit more from pharmacological interventions aimed at managing affective distress. In contrast, the older group may need a relatively greater emphasis on behavioral interventions aimed at increasing function, with a lesser focus on affective distress. Older patients, for whom pain relief is the primary goal, may be expected to have lesser affective contribution and fewer complications to limit analgesic effectiveness. Middle-aged patients, with higher levels of extended negative affect, may not respond to typical analgesic medications with the same efficacy. These suggestions are speculative at present and need confirmation from further controlled studies before the causal links we have suggested should be accepted. The data once again suggest the importance of assessing the multidimensional nature of the chronic pain experience and demonstrate the potential from such assessment for the tailoring of treatment.

SEX DIFFERENCES IN PAIN STAGES

Most studies addressing the relationship between sex and pain sensitivity have suggested that women have a lower pain threshold and tolerance than men (Fillingim and Maixner 1995; Riley et al. 1998). The experimentally induced pain has typically taken the form of heat, cold, pressure application, or electric shock, with most studies targeting the sensory-discriminative dimension (intensity) of pain. One criticism of experimental pain has been its inability to duplicate the responses that characterize clinical pain; this limitation applies to studies demonstrating sex differences in ratings of induced pain. In contrast to studies of experimental pain, there is less evidence that males and females differ in clinical pain sensitivity. For example, a multi-sample study of clinical patients did not find sex differences in numerical ratings or in several self-report questionnaires for pain intensity or unpleasantness (Robinson et al. 1998). Certainly one weakness of these data is the bias of patients in pain clinics toward seeking clinical care.

The concept of sex-specific relationships between pain and affect is supported by the pain-processing model. This concept is suggested by several studies in pain clinic samples that have not found significant sex differences in pain ratings (Robinson et al. 1998). That women report more psychological distress in the general population than men (Nolen-Hoeksema 1990) may contribute to sex differences in the experience of pain, but not until later stages of the pain-processing model. For example, evidence suggests that females with pain would continue to be more likely to experience pain related-negative affect than males. Haley et al. (1985) reported sex-related patterns in pain and mood, with depression significantly related to pain for females, whereas for males, depression was associated with reduced activity but not pain. This would suggest sex differences in links between later stages of the four-stage model. Dowdy et al. (1996) directly tested whether psychological adjustment could be explained by differences in sex, over and above the variance associated with pain, coping strategies, and emotional support. Sex-related differences were most marked for measures of depression and weakest for scores more closely associated with anxiety, suggesting that the emotional component on which sexes differ the most is depression. Evers et al. (1997) studied patients with rheumatoid arthritis over the course of the first year following diagnosis and examined the determinants of psychological distress. Women reported higher mean levels of anxiety and depression than men at initial diagnosis. One year after diagnosis, disease severity and female sex continued to be related to psychological distress.

Building on the literature described above, we performed a study that systematically examined sex differences in dimensions of pain across multiple pain-related emotions (Riley et al. 2001). This study used simultaneous regression methodology to test for sex differences in dimensions of pain processing with data collected from a sample of 680 males and 967 females experiencing chronic pain. This approach partials out the shared component of negative mood involved in suffering (e.g., multicollinearity) to reveal the unique contribution of each emotion. We tested the hypothesis that sex differences may help to determine which pain-related emotions are most highly associated with pain intensity and unpleasantness. Further, we tested for differences in regression parameters, hypothesizing that relative to males, female subjects would report higher levels of extended pain-related emotions and would have greater associations between pain intensity or unpleasantness and these emotions. Finally, consistent with the sequential processing of the four-stage model of pain, we hypothesized that the relationship between immediate pain unpleasantness and extended pain-related emotions would be reflected in higher values than would the relationship between pain intensity and extended pain affect.

We found that male and female chronic pain patients experienced different emotional responses to chronic pain. Of the five negative emotions assessed (depression, anxiety, anger, fear, and frustration), frustration best characterized the emotional response to pain for females, whereas anxiety best characterized the emotional response for males. Univariate analyses indicated that females experienced statistically higher fear and frustration than males. Our results also suggest that the more important sex differences in pain-related emotional suffering may not be manifested as large group differences in mean levels of these emotions, but as differences in the linear relationships between pain and emotions. In contrast to our hypothesis based on previous research, the magnitude of the associations between pain and the pain-related emotions was higher in males than in females. Specifically, males demonstrated a higher linear association between pain unpleasantness and extended negative affect associated with pain than did females. It is possible that the contrast between the current results and those obtained previously is explained by the fact that the earlier studies focused on depression, without looking at important sex differences in the relationships between pain and other emotional responses to pain.

There is a clear clinical rationale for examining patients' variability in pain intensity and pain-related unpleasantness ratings (i.e., lowest, usual, highest) in order to understand the course of their symptoms and their subjective experience of pain. The data from Riley et al. (2001) provide further justification for distinguishing among fluctuating pain levels and for recognizing the associated emotional responses. The findings regarding frustration have additional important clinical implications, given that psychological and psychotropic interventions for pain generally focus on ameliorating depression and anxiety. Our results suggest that frustration represents a pain-related emotion warranting targeted treatment. In a different patient sample, Wade et al. (1990) also found frustration to be significantly associated with pain unpleasantness. The consistent result across patient samples reinforces the finding that frustration is a critical concomitant of immediate pain-related unpleasantness. Furthermore, the reliability of these findings across studies supports the validity of associations between an individual's immediate affective response to pain unpleasantness and specific extended pain-related emotions of the sequential pain-processing model.

PERSONALITY AND PAIN STAGES

This section reviews the impact of personality factors, primarily neuroticism and extraversion, on the multistage model of pain processing. When discussing the impact of personality on pain it is important to draw a distinction between normal personality and psychopathology. Both terms describe aspects of personality, but psychopathology has its roots in a disease-based model. An assessment is made regarding the presence or absence of psychopathology. Its presence is always problematic and implies maladaptation. The Minnesota Multiphasic Personality Inventory-2 (MMPI-2) is a widely used measure of psychopathology (Piotrowski and Lubin 1990). Psychopathology can remit with or without treatment. In contrast, the concept of normal personality has its derivation in personality trait theory. It represents a comprehensive framework for the description of individual differences. The fundamental underpinning of personality theory is that an individual's interpersonal, experiential, and enduring emotional world consists of a set of basic dimensions. These dimensions represent universal and enduring factors in all individuals, regardless of demographic or cultural differences. An individual's score on these domains is not affected by stressful life events, changes in development life stage, or prior experience (McCrae 1993).

It follows that both psychopathology and normal personality traits may influence the meaning and perceived context for pain. Pain-related suffering and illness behavior are the culmination of processes that include pain sensation intensity, somatomotor and autonomic activation, and private reflection concerning the long-term implications or meanings of the persistent pain problem. This private interpretation will impact on desires, goals, and expectations for the future. This dynamic process influences emotions and ideas that culminate in suffering and illness behavior. Correlation studies have shown an association between pain-related illness beliefs and measures of physical function (Strong et al. 1990, 1992; Slater et al. 1991; Flor et al. 1993; Rainville et al. 1993; Anderson et al. 1995; Vlaeyen et al. 1995), psychological function (Boston et al. 1990; Gil et al. 1990; Vlaeyen et al. 1990; Herr et al. 1993; Williams et al. 1994), and behavioral function (Boston et al. 1990; Jacob et al. 1993; Buckelew et al. 1994). Although several studies have explored the relationship between personality and pain, most have focused largely on one or two of the four pain stages. Lauver and Johnson (1997) specifically assessed the relationship between neuroticism and illness behavior in an older group of patients with chronic pain with a mean age of 65 years. They controlled for the amount of social support the patients received by using multiple regression. Neuroticism was a significant predictor of observable pain behavior. High neuroticism scores were associated with a quantitative increase in illness behavior.

In this chapter we have emphasized that it is critical to characterize pain as represented by four unique stages. Doing so allows the clinician to clarify at which point in the pain-processing schema personality factors and therapeutic interventions exert their influence. Unfortunately, few studies have systematically characterized the influence of personality on each pain-processing stage. One of the few studies to do so (Harkins et al. 1989) found that neuroticism was unrelated to the sensory-intensive dimension for both experimental and clinical pain among myofascial pain patients. Neuroticism exerted a small but statistically reliable enhancement of pain unpleasantness for both experimental and clinical pain within this group of patients. In contrast with its small or negligible effects for the first two stages of the pain, neuroticism exerted a large enhancement of extended pain affect and illness behavior in these patients.

Confirmation of these types of selective influences was attained in a replication study conducted by Wade et al. (1992b), which used canonical correlation to control for pain sensation intensity in evaluating the dimensions of pain and to control for neuroticism and extraversion in assessing the effects of other personality variables on the pain stages. Consistent with the findings of Harkins et al. (1989), neither neuroticism nor extraversion was related to pain sensation intensity. Neuroticism alone was related to immediate pain-related unpleasantness. Neuroticism, not extraversion, exerted its greatest influence on extended pain affect.

Although several studies (Harkins et al. 1989; Wade et al. 1992a; BenDebba et al. 1997) have suggested that extraversion is related to suffering, its relationship is weaker than that of neuroticism. In the Wade et al. (1992a) study, assertiveness, a facet score of extraversion, was the most important predictor of pain suffering. Both assertiveness and activity level were the only extraversion facet scores associated with illness behavior. The relationship between extraversion and behavior is complicated. It appears that highly assertive patients manifest more pain behavior at home and during clinical interviews when they are unobtrusively observed. In contrast, they also report less lifestyle disruption (i.e., sickness impact) and fewer incidents of solicitous behavior from family members. Several reports (Eysenck 1967; Gordon and Hitchcock 1983; Harkins et al. 1989) provide support for the finding that extraverts express their suffering more frequently than do introverts.

In summary, the literature suggests that personality factors have their greatest influence on extended pain affect and illness behavior. This finding reinforces the uniqueness of these later stages of pain processing. Although the literature provides evidence of an association between measures of normal personality (mainly neuroticism and extraversion) and pain-related suffering, it does not clearly assign a causal relationship between these variables. One possibility is that chronic anxiety and lifelong depression contribute to a pattern of catastrophizing, which exacerbates emotional disturbance in chronic pain patients. Alternatively, lifestyle disruption resulting from pain leads to an intensification of catastrophizing or psychopathology and subsequent suffering. A neuroplastic hypothesis posits that cortical changes associated with the sensory/discriminative pain stage can affect structures associated with emotional processes, leading to dynamic changes in brain structure and function. These resulting alterations include cognitive impairment and increased levels of suffering.

NEUROPLASTICITY AND PAIN STAGES

In this section we explore the relationship between cortical processes associated with chronic pain and their influence on the four pain stages. Sensory-discriminative and affective-motivational components of pain appear to be processed both in series and in parallel by different parts of the nociceptive system (Vogt et al. 1996; Price 1999; Treede et al. 1999; Peyron et al. 2000). Recently, studies have begun to shed light on which specific brain regions are most closely associated with the different stages of pain processing (see Chapters 1 and 11).

While studies of activation of the anterior cingulate cortex (ACC) have often interpreted this area as being integral for affective processing (Treede et al. 1999), this region has also been implicated in cognition (MacLeod and MacDonald 2000). Indeed, functional magnetic resonance imaging (fMRI) studies suggest that, while the ACC's rostral-ventral region is associated with affective processes, the dorsal region plays a critical role in cognition (Devinsky et al. 1995; Bush et al. 2000). Recent studies suggest that the ACC participates in executive function by facilitating sustained attention and gating irrelevant, distracting stimuli (Pardo et al. 1990; Belger et al. 1995; MacLeod and MacDonald 2000; Ochsner et al. 2001). This hypothesis is supported by findings of increased ACC activation in anticipation of performing cognitive tasks (Murtha et al. 1996; Ploghaus et al. 1999). Derbyshire et al. (1998) investigated the specificity of regional ACC activation using three-dimensional positron emission tomography (PET) imaging under multiple conditions. Their data revealed substantial overlap of ACC regional activation during performance of an attentional task and during noxious pain stimulation. These data support the notion that the ACC partially mediates both attentional mechanisms and affective processes. A greater degree of pain-related suffering may limit the reserve capacity of the ACC to support attention.

Following up on this notion, Wade and Hart (2002a) evaluated attention in a sample of 736 pain patients consecutively evaluated at a university-based pain center. The multidimensional aspects of pain were evaluated according to the four-stage model of pain processing. Patients completed VASs of pain sensation intensity, immediate pain unpleasantness, extended pain-related emotions, and negative illness beliefs associated with suffering. A structured pain interview was used to assess illness behavior. Stepwise multiple regression analyses were completed using measures of each pain stage as predictors and Digit Span, a subtest of the Wechsler Adult Intelligence Scale-Revised (Wechsler 1981), as the criterion. A final regression analysis using only those predictor variables reliably related to attention (Digit Span subtest) indicated that measures of pain-related depression, perceived lifestyle interference, and the degree of social reinforcement for pain-related behavior were uniquely related to attention. Attentional performance was not related to pain sensation intensity or immediate pain-related unpleasantness. These data support the notion that extended pain affect and, to a lesser extent, illness behavior are associated with attentional problems in chronic pain patients.

In a second study (Wade and Hart 2002b), a measure of verbal learning (e.g., the Verbal Paired Associate Learning subtest from the Wechsler Memory Scale-Revised) was administered to 274 pain patients. Similar analyses that controlled for pain sensation intensity revealed that deficits in verbal learning were associated with pain-related anxiety. Like neuroticism, the attentional impairment and verbal learning difficulties seen in this pain population were uniquely associated with the later stages of pain processing. These findings are consistent with the notion that mechanisms related to competitive demand on resources, interference effects, or reciprocal suppression between the affective and cognitive subdivisions of the ACC may underlie the disruption of cognitive function in pain patients. Dysfunction is enhanced by the reciprocal relationship between immediate affective response (pain unpleasantness) and cognitive impairment in these patients. Pain-related suffering contributes to reduced cognitive function, which in turn influences expectations regarding the longer-term impact of one's illness on quality of life, which serves to increase suffering and further affects cognition.

Considerable evidence indicates that dysregulation of the hypothalamic-pituitary-adrenocortical (HPA) axis is associated with chronic pain (Drolet et al. 2001; Crofford 2002; Korszun et al. 2002). Dysregulation of the HPA axis in pain patients may affect neuronal plasticity. McEwen (1999) reviewed animal and human research that supports a link between stress and neuronal plasticity at the hippocampus. This neural structure plays a critical role in learning and memory. Repeated stress suppresses neurogenesis of dentate gyrus neurons and produces atrophy of dendrites. Dendritic atrophy appears to be the result of excitatory amino acid (glutamate) release during repeated stress, which is facilitated by circulating adrenal steroids. Stress and elevated adrenal steroids are associated with signs of brain atrophy (McEwen 1999). The hippocampus is particularly sensitive to the neurotoxic effect of adrenal steroids and is a primary target for them. An increase in glutamate production and release in response to HPA activation has been implicated in reduced hippocampal volume in patients suffering from anxiety and depressive disorders (Duman et al. 1999; Shelton 2000). In patients who are depressed, volume loss in the hippocampus correlates with volume loss in the core nuclei of the amygdala, where glutamatergic pyramidal cells predominate. Sheline et al. (1999) have suggested that overexcitation in one structure can produce damage in the other through their reciprocal connections. This explanation would seem consistent with evidence of reduced brain volume in patients high in trait neuroticism who tend to experience more life events as stressful and are more susceptible to psychological distress. In a recent study of healthy subjects (Knutson et al. 2001), neuroticism (measured using the Revised NEO Personality Inventory) showed a negative association with the ratio of the brain to the remainder of intracranial volume. Specifically, the tendency to experience anxiety and negative emotions was related to reductions in brain volume. The relationship between reduced brain volume and neuroticism may be important in light of Wade et al.'s (1992a) observation that 20% of patients with chronic pain from a multidisciplinary pain program had elevated scores on the same measure of neuroticism.

The four-stage model of pain processing specifically addresses the fact that psychological factors, demographics, and cortical structures selectively influence these stages. Therefore, in evaluating a person with chronic pain it is critical to understand what the individual "brings" to the pain situation. This task involves evaluating the individual's normal personality structure as well as assessing for psychopathology. The goal of the assessment process should be to establish a treatment plan that incorporates the individual's social and cultural background, pain stage data, and personality functioning. Periodic reassessment using a subset of the original test battery facilitates an evaluation of treatment efficacy.

The data previously presented suggest that personality and age influence extended pain affect (the third stage of pain processing). In addition, extended pain affect and personality may influence cognition. Personality traits such as neuroticism appear to enhance anxiety associated with chronic pain. Increased levels of suffering may reduce the reserve capacity of brain structures such as the ACC to allocate attentional resources. Attention and memory processes may be disrupted by pain-related suffering. Psychotherapy targeting negative illness beliefs and encouraging the development of healthy outlets for negative emotion may reduce suffering and improve cognitive function in pain patients. When a strictly antinociceptive treatment is given to a patient it may not eliminate the pain sensation. Therefore, psychological factors may continue to perpetuate the later stages of pain processing. We need to direct our efforts at therapies to reduce the pain sensation intensity and immediate pain unpleasantness, and develop approaches that will selectively reduce extended pain affect and illness behavior. Future directions in pharmacotherapy may be directed at altering glutamatergic and GABAergic axis activation, reducing cognitive inefficiency associated with pain and emotional distress, and thus mitigating the associated stress-related cortical changes in structure and function.

SUMMARY

Studies conceptualizing pain as a multidimensional experience are scarce, yet the studies reviewed in detail in this chapter (Riley et al. 2000, 2001, 2002b) provide preliminary evidence that the manner in which the four pain stages are processed is similar across various demographics (diagnosis, ethnicity, and gender), with perhaps the exception being age. It appears that older subjects cope better with their pain and suffer less. In summary, these data provide additional support for the four-stage model of pain processing (Wade et al. 1990, 1992b, 1996; Price 1999; Riley et al. 2000, 2001; Wade and Price 2000), the validity of measures used to assess these stages, and the universality of pain processing.

REFERENCES

Anderson KO, Dowds BN, Pelletz RE, Edwards WT, Peeters-Asdourian C. Development and initial validation of a scale to measure self-efficacy beliefs in patients with chronic pain. *Pain* 1995; 63:77–84.

Aurelius M. *Meditations 7:16* (Long G, Trans). In: Eliot CW (Ed). The Harvard Classics. Danbury, CT: Grolier, 1980.

Banks SM, Kerns RD. Explaining high rates of depression in chronic pain: a diathesis-stress framework. *Psychol Bull* 1996; 119:95–110.

Baron RM, Kenny DA. The moderator-mediator variable distinction in social psychological research: conceptual, strategic, and statistical considerations. *J Pers Soc Psychol* 1986; 51(6):1173–1182.

Bates MS, Edwards WT. Ethnic variations in the chronic pain experience. *Ethn Dis* 1992; 2:63–83.

Bates MS, Rankin-Hill L. Control, culture and chronic pain. *Soc Sci Med* 1994; 39:629–645.

Belger A, McCarthy G, Gore J, et al. Evaluation of frontal and parietal association cortex contributions to attention using FMRI. *Schizophr Res* 1995; 15(1):76.

BenDebba M, Torgerson WS, Long DM. Personality traits, pain duration and severity, functional impairment, and psychological distress in patients with persistent low back pain. *Pain* 1997; 72:115–125.

Blumberg H, Griesser HJ, Hornyak M. New viewpoints on the clinical picture, diagnosis and pathology of reflex sympathetic dystrophy. *Unfallchirurgie* 1990; 16:95–106.

Boston K, Pearce SA, Richardson PH. The pain cognitions questionnaire. *J Psychosom Res* 1990; 34:103–109.

Breitbart W, McDonald MV, Rosenfeld B, et al. Pain in ambulatory AIDS patients. I: Pain characteristics and medical correlates. *Pain* 1996; 68:315–321.

Buckelew SP, Parker JC, Keefe FJ, et al. Self-efficacy and pain behavior among subjects with fibromyalgia. *Pain* 1994; 59:377–384.

Bush G, Luu P, Posner MI. Cognitive and emotional influences in anterior cingulate cortex. *Trends Cogn Sci* 2000; 4(10):215–222.

Clinton P, Eland J. Pain. In: Mass M, Buckwalter K (Eds). *Nursing Diagnoses and Interventions for the Elderly.* Reading, MA: Addison-Wesley, 1990, pp 348–368.

Creamer P, Lethbridge-Cejku M, Hochberg MC. Determinants of pain severity in knee osteoarthritis: effect of demographic and psychosocial variables using 3 pain measures. *J Rheumatol* 1999; 26:1785–1792.

Crofford LJ. The hypothalamic-pituitary-adrenal axis in the pathogenesis of rheumatic diseases. *Endocrinol Metab Clin North Am* 2002; 31:1–13.

Damasio A. *Descartes' Error.* New York: Avon Books, 1994.

DeGood DE, Shutty MS. Assessment of pain beliefs, coping and self-efficacy. In: Turk DC, Melzack R (Eds). *Handbook of Pain Assessment,* 2nd ed. New York: Guilford Press, 2001.

Derbyshire SWG, Vogt BA, Jones AKP. Pain and Stroop interference tasks activate separate processing modules in anterior cingulate cortex. *Exp Brain Res* 1998; 118(1):52–60.

De Vilder J. Personality of patients with Sudeck's atrophy following tibial fracture. *Acta Orthop Belg* 1980; 58:463–468.

Devinsky D, Morrell MH, Vogt BA. Contributions of anterior cingulate cortex to behavior. *Brain* 1995; 46:279–306.

Dowdy SW, Dwyer KA, Smith CA, Wallston KA. Gender and psychological well-being of persons with rheumatoid arthritis. *Arthritis Care Res* 1996; 9(6):449–456.

Drolet G, Dumont EC, Gosselin I, et al. Role of endogenous opioid system in the regulation of the stress response. *Prog Neuropsychopharmacol Psychiatry* 2001; 25:729–741.

Duman RS, Malberg J, Thome J. Neural plasticity to stress and antidepressant treatment. *Biol Psychiatry* 1999; 46:1181–1191.

Edwards RR, Fillingim RB. Ethnic differences in thermal pain responses. *Psychosom Med* 1999; 61(3):346–354.

Edwards RR, Fillingim RB, Ness TJ. Age-related differences in endogenous pain modulation: a comparison of diffuse noxious inhibitory controls in healthy older and younger adults. *Pain* 2003; 101(1–2):155–165.

Evers AW, Kraaimaat FW, Geenen R, Bijlsma JW. Determinants of psychological distress and its course in the first year after diagnosis in rheumatoid arthritis patients. *J Behav Med* 1997; 20(5):489–504.

Eysenck HJ. *Biological Basis of Personality.* Springfield, IL: Charles C. Thomas, 1967.

Fillingim RB, Maixner W. Gender differences in the responses to noxious stimuli. *Pain Forum* 1995; 4(4):209–221.

Flor H, Behle DJ, Birbaumer N. Assessment of pain-related cognitions in chronic pain patients. *Behav Res Ther* 1993; 31:63–73.

Gil KM, Keefe FJ, Crisson JE, Van Dalfsen PJ. Social support and pain behavior. *Pain* 1987; 29(2):209–217

Gil KM, Williams DA, Keefe FJ, Beckham JC. The relationship of negative thoughts to pain and psychological distress. *Behav Ther* 1990; 21:349–362.

Gordon A, Hitchcock ER. Illness behavior and personality in intractable facial pain syndromes. *Pain* 1983; 17(3):267–276.

Greene D (Trans). *Sophocles II.* Chicago: University of Chicago Press, 1957.

Greenwald HP. Interethnic differences in pain perception. *Pain* 1991; 44:157–163.

Haddox JD. Psychological aspects of reflex sympathetic dystrophy. In: Stanton-Hicks M (Ed). *Pain and the Sympathetic Nervous System.* Boston: Kluwer Academic, 1990, pp 207–224.

Haley WE, Turner JA, Romano JM. Depression in chronic pain patients: relation to pain, activity, and sex differences. *Pain* 1985; 23(4):337–343.

Harkins SW, Price DD. Assessment of pain in the elderly. In: Turk DC, Melzack R (Eds). *Handbook of Pain Assessment,* 2nd ed. New York: Guilford Press, 2001.

Harkins SW, Price DD, Martelli M. Effects of age on pain perception: thermonociception. *J Gerontol* 1986; 41(1):58–63.

Harkins SW, Price DD, Braith J. Effects of extraversion and neuroticism on experimental pain, clinical pain, and illness behavior. *Pain* 1989; 36(2):209–218.

Herr KA, Mobily PR, Smith C. Depression and the experience of chronic back pain: a study of related variables and age differences. *Clin J Pain* 1993; 9:104–114.

Jacob MC, Kerns RD, Rosenberg R, Haythornthwaite J. Chronic pain: intrusion and accommodation. *Behav Res Ther* 1993; 31:519–527.

Johnson PA, Goldman L, Orav EJ, Garcia T. Comparison of the Medical Outcomes Study Short-Form 36-item Health Survey in African American patients and Caucasian patients with acute chest pain. *Med Care* 1995; 33:145–160.

Jordan MS. Effect of race and ethnicity on outcomes and rheumatic conditions. *Curr Opin Rheumatol* 1999; 11:98–103.

Jordan MS, Lumley MA, Leisen JC. The relationships of cognitive coping and pain control beliefs to pain and adjustment among African-American and Caucasian women with rheumatoid arthritis. *Arthritis Care Res* 1998; 11:80–88.

Keefe FJ, Williams DA. A comparison of coping strategies in chronic pain patients in different age groups. *J Gerontol* 1990; 45(4):P161–165

Kerns RD, Haythornthwaite J, Southwick S, Giller EL. The role of marital interaction in chronic pain and depressive symptom severity. *J Psychosom Res* 1990; 34(4):401–408.

Knutson B, Momenan R, Rawlings RR, Fong GW, Hommer D. Negative association of neuroticism with brain volume ratio in healthy humans. *Biol Psychiatry* 2001; 50:685–690.

Korszun A, Young EA, Singer K, et al. Basal circadian cortisol secretion in women with temporomandibular disorders. *J Dent Res* 2002; 81:279–283.

Lauver SC, Johnson JL. The role of neuroticism and social support in older adults with chronic pain behavior. *Pers Individ Dif* 1997; 23(1):165–167.

Lee MC, Essoka G. Patient's perception of pain: comparison between Korean-American and Euro-American obstetric patients. *J Cult Divers* 1998; 5:29–37.

Leventhal EA, Prohaska TR. Age, symptom interpretation, and health behavior. *J Am Geriatr Soc* 1986; 34(3):185–191.

Lipton JA, Marbach JJ. Ethnicity and the pain experience. *Soc Sci Med* 1984; 19:1279–1298.

Lynch ME. Psychological aspects of reflex sympathetic dystrophy: a review of the adult and pediatric literature. *Pain* 1992; 49:337–347.

MacLeod CM, MacDonald PA. Interdimensional interference in the Stroop effect: uncovering the cognitive and neural anatomy of attention. *Trends Cogn Sci* 2000; 4(10):383–391.

McCracken LM, Gross RT. Does anxiety affect coping with chronic pain? *Clin J Pain* 1993; 9(4):253–259.

McCrae RR. Moderated analyses of longitudinal personality stability. *J Pers Soc Psychol* 1993; 65(3):577–585.

McEwen BS. Stress and hippocampal plasticity. *Annu Rev Neurosci* 1999; 22:105–122.

McGuire GM, Reskin BF. Authority hierarchies at work: the impacts of race and sex. *Gend Soc* 1993; 7:487–506.

McIntosh IB. Psychological aspects influence the threshold of pain. *Geriatric Med* 1990; 20:37–41.

McMillan SC. The relationship between age and intensity of cancer-related symptoms. *Oncol Nurs Forum* 1989; 16(2):237–241.

Melzack R, Casey KL. Sensory, motivational, and central control determinants of pain: a new conceptual model. In: Kenshalo D (Ed). *The Skin Senses.* Springfield, IL: Chas C. Thomas, 1968.

Moore R, Brodsgaard I. Cross-cultural investigations of pain. In: Crombie IK, Croft PR, Linton SJ, LeResche L, Von Korff M (Eds). *Epidemiology of Pain.* Seattle: IASP Press, 1999, pp 53–80.

Moore R, Brodsgaard I, Mao TK, Miller ML, Dworkin SF. Acute pain and use of local anesthesia: tooth drilling and childbirth labor pain beliefs among Anglo-Americans, Chinese, and Scandinavians. *Anesth Prog* 1998; 45:29–37.

Murtha S, Chertkow H, Beauregard M, Dixon R, Evans A. Anticipation causes increased blood flow in the anterior cingulate cortex. *Hum Brain Mapp* 1996; 120:103–112.

Nolen-Hoeksema S. *Sex Differences in Depression.* Stanford: Stanford University Press, 1990.

Ochsner KN, Kosslyn SM, Cosgrove GR, et al. Deficits in visual cognition and attention following bilateral anterior cingulotomy. *Neuropsychologia* 2001; 39(3):219–230.

Pardo JU, Pardo RJ, Janer KW, Raichle ME. The anterior cingulate cortex mediates processing selection in the Stroop attentional conflict paradigm. *Proc Natl Acad Sci USA* 1990; 87(1):256–259.

Peyron R, Laurent B, Garcia-Larrera L. Functional imaging of brain responses to pain: a review and meta-analysis. *Clin Neuropsychol* 2000; 30(5):263–288.

Piotrowski C, Lubin B. Assessment practices of health psychologists: survey of APA Division 38 clinicians. *Prof Psychol Res Pract* 1990; 21(2):99–106.

Ploghaus A, Tracey I, Gati JS, et al. Dissociating pain from its anticipation in the brain. *Science* 1999; 284:1979–1981.

Price DD. *Psychological and Neural Mechanisms of Pain.* New York: Raven Press; 1988.

Price DD. *Psychological Mechanisms of Pain and Analgesia,* Progress in Pain Research and Management, Vol. 15. Seattle: IASP Press, 1999.

Prohaska TR, Keller ML, Leventhal EA, Leventhal H. Impact of symptoms and aging attribution on emotions and coping. *Health Psychol* 1987; 6(6):495–514.

Rainville J, Ahern DK, Phalen L. Altering beliefs about pain and impairment in a functionally oriented treatment program for chronic low back pain. *Clin J Pain* 1993; 9:196–201.

Riley JL III, Robinson ME, Wise EA, Myers CD, Fillingim RB. Sex differences in the perception of noxious experimental stimuli: a meta-analysis. *Pain* 1998; 74(2–3):181–187.

Riley JL III, Wade JB, Robinson ME, Price DD. The stages of pain processing across the adult lifespan. *J Pain* 2000; 1:162–170.

Riley JL III, Robinson ME, Wade JB, Myers CD, Price DD. Sex differences in negative emotional response to chronic pain. *J Pain* 2001; 2:354–359.

Riley JL III, Gilbert GH, Heft MW. Orofacial pain: racial and sex differences among older adults. *J Public Health Dent* 2002a; 62(3):132–139.

Riley JL III, Wade JB, Myers CD, et al. Racial/ethnic differences in the experience of chronic pain. *Pain* 2002b; 100(3):291–298.

Robinson ME, Riley JL III. Role of negative emotions in pain. In Gatchel RJ, Turk DC. *Psychosocial Factors in Pain: Critical Perspectives.* New York: Guilford Press, 1998.

Rushing B, Ritter C, Burton RPD. Race differences in the effects of multiple roles on health: longitudinal evidence from a national sample of older men. *J Health Soc Behav* 1992; 33:126–139.

Sanders SH, Brena SF, Spier CJ, et al. Chronic low back pain patients around the world: cross-cultural similarities and differences. *Clin J Pain* 1992; 8(4):317–323.

Sheffield D, Biles PL, Orom H, Maixner W, Sheps DS. Race and sex differences in cutaneous pain perception. *Psychosom Med* 2000; 62:517–523.

Sheline YI, Shanghavi M, Mintun MA, Gado MH. Depression duration but not age predicts hippocampal volume loss in medically healthy women with recurrent major depression. *J Neurosci* 1999; 19:5034–5043.

Shelton RC. Cellular mechanisms in the vulnerability to depression and responses to antidepressants. *Psychiatr Clin North Am* 2000; 23:713–729.

Slater MA, Hall HF, Atkinson JH, Garfin SR. Pain and impairment beliefs in chronic low back pain: validation of the Pain and Impairment Relationship Scale (PAIRS). *Pain* 1991; 44:51–56.

Sorkin BA, Rudy TE, Hanlon RB, Turk DC, Stieg RL. Chronic pain in old and young patients: differences appear less important than similarities. *J Gerontol* 1990; 45(2):P64–68.

Stewart WF, Lipton RB, Liberman J. Variation in migraine prevalence by race. *Neurology* 1996; 47:52–59.

Strong J, Ashton R, Cramond T, Chant D. Pain intensity, attitude and function in back pain patients. *Aust Occup Ther J* 1990; 37:179–183.

Strong J, Ashton R, Chant D. The measurement of attitudes towards beliefs about pain. *Pain* 1992; 48:227–236.

Sussman LK, Robins LN, Earls F. Treatment-seeking for depression by African American and Caucasian Americans. *Soc Sci Med* 1987; 24:187–196.

Thomas MR, Roy R. *The Changing Nature of Pain Complaints over the Lifespan.* New York: Plenum Press, 1999.

Treede RD, Kenshalo DR, Gracely RH, Jones AK. The cortical representation of pain. *Pain* 1999; 79:105–111.

Vlaeyen JWS, Geurts SM, Kole-Snijders AMJ, et al. What do chronic pain patients think of their pain? Towards a pain cognition questionnaire. *Br J Clin Psychol* 1990; 29:383–394.

Vlaeyen JWS, Kole-Snijders AMJ, Rotteveel A, Ruesink R, Heuts PHT. The role of fear of movement/(re)injury in pain disability. *J Occup Rehab* 1995; 5:235–252.

Vogt BA, Derbyshire S, Jones AK. Pain processing in four regions of human cingulate cortex localized with co-registered PET and MR imaging. *Eur J Neurosci* 1996; 8:1461–1473.

Wade JB, Hart RP. Attention and the stages of pain processing. *Pain Med* 2002a; 3:30–38.

Wade JB, Hart RP. Impact of emotional suffering on learning in chronic pain. *Pain* 2002b; 3:33.

Wade JB, Price DD. Nonpathologic factors in chronic pain: implications for assessment and treatment. In: Gatschall RJ, Weisberg JN (Eds). *Personality Characteristics of Patients with Pain.* Washington, DC: American Psychological Association, 2000, pp 89–109.

Wade JB, Price DD, Hamer RM, Schwartz SM, Hart RP. An emotional component analysis of chronic pain. *Pain* 1990; 40(3):303–310.

Wade JB, Dougherty LM, Hart RP, Cook DB. Patterns of normal personality structure among chronic pain patients. *Pain* 1992a; 48:37–43.

Wade JB, Dougherty LM, Hart RP, Rafii A, Price DD. A canonical correlation analysis of the influence of neuroticism and extraversion on chronic pain, suffering, and pain behavior. *Pain* 1992b; 51(1):67–73.

Wade JB, Dougherty LM, Archer CR, Price DD. Assessing the stages of pain processing: a multivariate analytical approach. *Pain* 1996; 68:157–167.

Waldron I, Jacobs JA. Effects of multiple roles on women's health: evidence from a national longitudinal study. *Women Health* 1989; 15:3–19.

Wechsler D. *Wechsler Adult Intelligence Scale-Revised Manual.* San Antonio: Harcourt Brace Jovanovich, 1981.

Williams DA, Robinson ME, Geisser ME. Pain beliefs: assessment and utility. *Pain* 1994; 59:71–78.

Woodrow KM, Friedman GD, Siegelaub AB, Collen MF. Pain tolerance: differences according to age, sex and race. *Psychosom Med* 1972; 34(6):548–556.

Correspondence to: Joseph L. Riley III, PhD, Division of Public Health Service and Research, College of Dentistry, University of Florida, 1600 Archer Rd, P.O. Box 100404, Gainesville, FL 32610-0404, USA.

Psychological Methods of Pain Control: Basic Science and Clinical Perspectives, Progress in Pain Research and Management, Vol. 29, edited by Donald D. Price and M. Catherine Bushnell, IASP Press, Seattle, © 2004.

3

Preclinical Studies of Pain Modulation: Lessons Learned from Animals

Barton H. Manning

Department of Neuroscience, Amgen Inc., Thousand Oaks, California, USA

Anyone who has witnessed athletic events or come into contact with patients in hospitals knows intuitively that the magnitude of pain perception often does not follow stimulus intensity in a linear fashion. Two classes of observation support the complexity of this relationship. The first is the clinical observation that pain often is present without any *apparent* precipitating pathophysiology. The second is the common observation that sometimes the perception of pain is not experienced despite the presence of factors that normally produce it. That is, under a variety of circumstances, partial or total analgesia may occur in the absence of any exogenous analgesic drugs. Indeed, early theoretical models of pain recognized these concepts despite the lack of direct supporting evidence (Irwin et al. 1951; Noordenbos 1959; Melzack and Wall 1965). Thus, the concept that the central nervous system (CNS) contains intrinsic pain-inhibitory mechanisms was theorized when only indirect evidence was available.

A great deal of progress has been made in the past 40 years in identifying and characterizing neural circuitry that contributes to the modulation of pain transmission and pain perception. It is known that many of the brain's ascending pain-related pathways terminate within cortical and subcortical structures that represent origins of efferent pain-modulatory pathways, such as the amygdala, hypothalamus, and midbrain periaqueductal gray (PAG). Three areas of psychology and neuroscience under active investigation are relevant to our understanding of pain modulation. These include learning and memory; environmental, threat-elicited defensive behavior; and neural mechanisms relating directly to pain modulation itself. Environmental threat and modulation of pain are interrelated during the production of anxiety and of unconditioned and conditioned fear (Fanselow 1984, 1991; Vidal and Jacob 1986; Helmstetter and Tershner 1994; Rhudy and Meagher 2003).

Furthermore, our knowledge of the circuitry underlying each of these three general phenomena is growing. These areas, in turn, relate to questions about general neural mechanisms of pain modulation. First, under what psychological and environmental circumstances do endogenous analgesia and hyperalgesia systems operate? That is, what phenomena trigger changes (either increases or decreases) in pain threshold or in the manner in which ongoing pain is tolerated? Second, once this environmental, psychological, and neural stage has been set, what are the mechanisms by which these changes are produced?

This chapter outlines a theoretical and mechanistic foundation for explaining both simple and complex changes in human pain perception elicited by psychological state. This goal will be approached for the most part by examining data collected in animal studies. Thus, this chapter is mainly concerned with the general neural mechanisms of pain modulation and the biological conditions under which changes in pain threshold are triggered in animals.

ANIMAL STUDIES OF PAIN MODULATION
RELATED TO LEARNING

Activation of endogenous analgesia or hyperalgesia mechanisms (i.e., in the absence of exogenous drugs) in human patients primarily involves external environmental cues or conditions. For example, cues associated with past relief of pain (analgesia) may be visual (a type of pill or syringe), auditory (a nurse's voice), or tactile (the prick of the needle associated with intravenously administered morphine). These cues may be effective for evoking analgesia or hyperalgesia mechanisms because they were present during treatments for pain that were previously effective or because they have symbolic meaning. For example, if the phrase "this is a very strong painkiller" accompanies an intravenous injection, analgesia may occur or be enhanced as a result of the meaning inherent in this statement. The potential neurobiology underlying something as elusive as symbolic meaning is much more problematic than that of simple forms of learning, such as classical conditioning.

Nevertheless, animal models of learning as they relate to analgesia and hyperalgesia are useful and have some relevance even to changes in pain threshold evoked by complex meanings. Conditioned antinociceptive responses in animals can be robust and can be elicited in ways that have relevance to analgesia in humans, particularly placebo analgesia. The most extensively studied form of conditioned antinociception is that related to fear-evoked defense responses. In studies of this phenomenon, rats or mice are subjected to an inescapable noxious stimulus (e.g., mild electric shock) leading to stress and apparent antinociception (Watkins and Mayer 1982b; Watkins et al. 1983; Fanselow 1984, 1991; Helmstetter and Tershner 1994). This acute fear-induced antinociception subsides, but when the rats are later returned to the apparatus in which the noxious stimulus was administered, the environmental context alone is sufficient to produce an antinociceptive effect. The antinociception associated with this kind of conditioning can be blocked by the opioid antagonist naloxone or by lesions of a specific neural circuit implicated in the production of defense behaviors in response to threat (Helmstetter 1992; Helmstetter and Tershner 1994). Over 20 years ago, Watkins and Mayer (1982a) proposed this type of conditioned antinoci-ception as a general model for placebo analgesia in humans.

Specific CNS circuitry has been implicated in these forms of conditioned antinociception in animals. Therefore, these animal models of learned analgesia are relevant to *psychologically* mediated changes in pain perception in humans. In humans, the extent to which both "basic" psychological states (e.g., fear, anxiety) and more complicated learning phenomena contribute to changes in pain perception is of particular interest; these factors are likely to contribute to placebo analgesia, to analgesia due to threatening circumstances, and to hyperalgesia due to anticipation of an adverse event. The following discussion will focus on endogenous pain-modulatory circuitry in animal models of antinociception and hypernociception associated with learning. At the end of this chapter, I will briefly draw some parallels between the animal data and observations on pain modulation in humans. The chapters that follow will allude to this discussion in order to link neurobiological and psychological explanations of pain modulation.

ENDOGENOUS OPIOID PAIN-MODULATORY SYSTEMS IN ANIMALS

It is clear that information about tissue damage is not passively received by the nervous system. Rather, it is modulated even at the first synapse within the spinal dorsal horn by complex inhibitory and facilitatory control systems (Fields et al. 1991). The discovery of these systems inspired the notion that the CNS contains endogenous substances that possess analgesic properties virtually identical to those of opiates of plant and synthetic origin (Hughes 1975). This section examines the development of these concepts and considers opioid and non-opioid CNS pain-modulatory mechanisms activated by environmental and psychological circumstances.

The earliest work indicating that opiates produce analgesia, at least in part, by activation of endogenous pain-inhibitory systems was performed by Irwin et al. (1951). These investigators demonstrated that, in spinalized rats, systemically administered morphine was not effective in inhibiting the spinally mediated tail-flick response. They reasoned, based on this result, that morphine must activate supraspinal neural circuitry that has an output to the spinal cord and inhibits the processing of nociceptive information at the spinal level. This work was largely ignored until the early 1970s.

The first impetus for the detailed study of pain-modulatory circuitry resulted from the observation that electrical stimulation of the PAG region of the rat brain could powerfully suppress pain-related behaviors (Reynolds 1969; Mayer et al. 1971). Further investigation of brain-stimulation-produced antinociception (SPA) in rats and other species provided considerable detail about the neural circuitry involved (see Mayer and Manning 1995 for a detailed review of this topic). Significantly, at that time, several similarities were recognized between these observations and information emerging from a concomitant resurgence of interest in the mechanisms of opioid antinociception (Mayer et al. 1971). Two important parallel findings resulted from these studies. First, effective loci for both microinjected opioids (Tsou and Jang 1964; Pert and Yaksh 1974) and focal brain stimulation (Mayer and Liebeskind 1974) reside within the periaqueductal and periventricular gray matter of the brainstem. Second, both opioid antinociception and SPA are mediated in part by the activation of an endogenous control system that descends from the brain and inhibits pain transmission at the level of the spinal and trigeminal dorsal horns (Mayer and Price 1976). Thus, antinociception ultimately occurs, at least in part, at initial nociceptive processing stages in the spinal cord dorsal horn and in the homologous trigeminal nucleus caudalis, as a result of selective inhibition of nociceptive neurons (Sato and Takagi 1971).

In addition to these two parallel observations, studies of SPA provided direct evidence of mechanisms in the mammalian CNS that depend upon endogenous opioids. Sub-antinociceptive doses of morphine were shown to synergize with sub-antinociceptive levels of brain stimulation to produce behavioral antinociception (Saminin and Valzelli 1971). Mayer and Hayes (1975) observed that animals developed tolerance (a phenomenon invariably associated with repeated administration of opioids) to the antinociceptive effects of brain stimulation and demonstrated cross-tolerance between the antinociceptive effects of brain stimulation and systemic opioids. Finally, focal SPA could be at least partially antagonized by naloxone (Akil et al. 1976). This last observation, in particular, could be most parsimoniously explained if focal electrical stimulation of the PAG resulted in the release of an endogenous opiate-like factor. Indeed, naloxone antagonism of SPA was a critical impetus leading eventually to the discovery of the endogenous opioid enkephalin (see below).

Coincidental with work on SPA, another discovery was of critical importance for our current concepts of endogenous analgesia systems. Several laboratories, almost simultaneously, reported the existence of stereospecific binding sites for opioids within the CNS (Hiller et al. 1973; Pert and Snyder 1973; Terenius 1973). Opiate receptor sites were subsequently shown to be localized to neuronal synaptic regions (Pert et al. 1974) and to overlap anatomically with loci involved in the neural processing of pain (Pert et al. 1975). Again, the existence of an opiate receptor suggested the likelihood of an endogenous compound with opioid properties to occupy it.

In 1975, Hughes reported the isolation from neural tissue of a factor (enkephalin) with such properties. An immense amount of subsequent work has characterized this and other neural and non-neural molecules with opioid properties. As with opioid receptors, the anatomical distribution of endogenous opioid ligands shows overlap with sites involved in pain processing (see Przewlocki and Przewlocka 2001 for a review).

NEURAL CIRCUITRY INVOLVED IN ANTINOCICEPTION PRODUCED BY EXOGENOUS OPIOIDS

Considerable data have been published concerning the sites and mechanisms involved in the inhibition of pain by the administration of exogenous opioids. Primarily, two lines of experimentation have been conducted. First, several areas in the CNS have been mapped, and specific sites have been identified at which direct application of opioids results in antinociception and the administration of opioid antagonists blocks antinociception produced by systemic opioids. Second, investigators have located specific brain areas where lesions block the antinociceptive effects of systemically administered opioids.

Opioid microinjection mapping studies determined that periaqueductal-periventricular regions of the mesencephalon and diencephalon contain critical sites at which microinjection of opioids results in antinociception (Tsou and Jang 1964; Jacquet and Lajtha 1973; Pert and Yaksh 1974; Yaksh et al. 1976). The effective sites for opioid microinjection strikingly resembled those sites that could be electrically stimulated to produce antinociception (Mayer et al. 1971). Overall, these and other studies confirmed the importance of the periaqueductal-periventricular region in opioid antinociception and provided an impetus for the examination of other brain areas.

A second brain area that has been found to be of considerable importance for opioid action is the anatomically complex region of the rostral ventromedial medulla (RVM). This region consists primarily of two distinct nuclei (Mason 2001): the medially located nucleus raphe magnus and the more laterally situated nucleus magnocellularis. Microinjection of morphine into this region results in antinociception, although some differences in sensitivity can be noted (Takagi et al. 1977; Takagi 1980; Azami et al. 1982; Llewelyn et al. 1983; Jones and Gebhart 1988; Rossi et al. 1994; Mitchell et al. 1998; Morgan and Whitney 2000). In addition, microinjection of other μ (Fang et al. 1989; Heinricher et al. 1994; Rossi et al. 1994; Hurley et al. 2003), δ (Ossipov et al. 1995; Thorat and Hammond 1997; Hurley et al. 1999; Kovelowski et al. 1999; Hurley et al. 2003), and κ (Hamann and Martin 1992; Ackley et al. 2001) opioid agonists into this region elicit antinociception in a number of behavioral pain assays.

Other brain areas that produce antinociception when microinjected with opioids include the amygdala (Rodgers 1977; Helmstetter et al. 1995; Pavlovic and Bodnar 1998; Nandigama and Borszcz 2003; Shane et al. 2003), the posterior hypothalamic area (Manning et al. 1994), the thalamic nucleus submedius (Yang et al. 2002), the ventrolateral orbital cortex (Huang et al. 2001), the nucleus of the solitary tract (Oley et al. 1982), the substantia nigra (Baumeister 1991), and the rostral agranular insular cortex (Burkey et al. 1996).

A final region of critical importance is the spinal dorsal horn. Although Tsou and Jang (1964) reported no apparent antinociception from direct spinal application of morphine, subsequent work has consistently demonstrated relatively potent effects of intrathecal morphine microinjection (Yaksh and Rudy 1976; Fairbanks and Wilcox 1997; Cahill et al. 2003). This observation is important in clinical application because direct intrathecal application of opioids produces analgesia without the concomitant psychoactive effects observed with systemic administration (Kedlaya et al. 2002).

Several distinct CNS regions thus appear to be involved in opioid antinociception, including the amygdala, hypothalamus, periaqueductal-periventricular gray matter, RVM, and spinal dorsal horn. Clearly, the antinociceptive effects of systemically administered opioids might result from action at any, all, or some combination of these distinct regions. Fortunately, microinjection of opioid antagonists has provided at least partial answers to questions as to whether activation of each of these structures is necessary or sufficient for opioid antinociception.

A number of studies have provided evidence that *supraspinal*, as opposed to spinal, sites of opioid action are important because antinociception from systemically administered opioids was antagonized by either intracerebroventricular or intracerebral microinjection of opioid antagonists (Tsou 1963; Albus et al. 1970; Jacquet and Lajtha 1974; Manning and Franklin 1998). Parallel lines of evidence, however, demonstrated that naloxone administered intrathecally (spinally) could antagonize the antinociception resulting from even relatively high doses of systemically administered opioids (Yaksh and Rudy 1977). Thus, these studies lead to the paradoxical conclusion that both supraspinal and spinal sites of opioid action are critically involved in generating antinociception.

This apparent paradox was resolved in a series of complex studies by Yeung and Rudy (1980a,b). These investigators demonstrated that simultaneous administration of various doses of morphine intrathecally (spinal cord) and intracerebroventricularly (brain) created a multiplicative dose-response function. That is, simultaneous spinal and supraspinal morphine resulted in much greater antinociception than the same total dose administered at either location alone. Similarly, the antinociceptive effects of low to moderate doses of systemically administered morphine could be antagonized *completely* either by intrathecal or intracerebroventricular naloxone. The authors took this result as further evidence of a synergistic interaction between spinal and brain sites of action for systemically administered opioids.

Another approach for dissecting the neural circuitry underlying opioid antinociception utilizes the selective destruction or reversible inactivation of neuroanatomical nuclei and pathways suspected of being involved in opioid antinociception. Opioids are administered systemically or at discrete sites in the nervous system, and the effect of particular lesions is examined. An overview of this work supports the conclusion of Yeung and Rudy (1980b). It appears that several brain areas, including the rostral agranular insular cortex (Burkey et al. 1996), central nucleus of the amygdala (Manning et al. 2001), PAG (Zambotti et al. 1982; Collins et al. 1995), and RVM (Mitchell et al. 1998) need to be intact for the full expression of systemic opioid-induced antinociception.

Evidence suggests that the central nucleus of the amygdala (CeA) is a major component of the mammalian pain-modulatory system (Manning and Mayer 1995a,b; Manning 1998; Manning et al. 2001, 2003). Neurons in the CeA appear to be necessary for systemic morphine to be fully efficacious in reducing prolonged, formalin-induced nociceptive behaviors. In both rats and nonhuman primates, bilateral excitotoxin-induced lesions of the CeA reduce morphine's ability to suppress the noxious heat-evoked tail-flick reflex (Manning and Mayer 1995b; Manning et al. 2001). Furthermore, lesions of the CeA reduce morphine's ability to suppress formalin-induced nociceptive behaviors in rats (Manning and Mayer 1995a; Manning 1998). It seems apparent that these results complement other evidence linking the amygdala to several forms of conditioned (Helmstetter 1992; Lee et al. 2001) and unconditioned (Fox and Sorenson 1994) antinociception that occur under environmental circumstances that are aversive to rats. These data have resulted in the CeA being incorporated into current models of endogenous pain control circuitry.

In totality, this endogenous pain control system appears to be organized such that it is capable of being activated by different external conditions, particularly those related to an acute threat and the concomitant fear associated with it. Thus, the connections of this system, shown in Fig. 1, show that cerebral cortical structures, as well as the amygdala, the PAG, and the hypothalamus, are connected either directly or indirectly with the RVM, which in turn projects to the spinal cord dorsal horn. The RVM, then, represents a "final pathway" that modulates nociceptive transmission. At least some of these structures, including the amygdala, hypothalamus, and PAG, receive

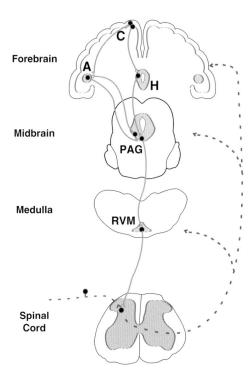

Fig. 1. A simplified schematic showing the major pain-modulating pathways in the mammalian brain. The origins of these pathways include cerebral cortical areas (C), the amygdala (A), the hypothalamus (H), the periaqueductal gray matter (PAG), and the rostral ventromedial medulla (RVM). Many of these regions also serve as the targets of ascending pain pathways. Adapted from Fields and Price (1997) and Millan (2002).

direct input from ascending pain-related pathways (Hsieh et al. 1996; Bornhovd et al. 2002; Millan 2002). Thus, the circuitry for pain modulation is, to some degree, part of a feedback loop. Stimuli that represent either a potential threat or an acute threat (e.g., painful stimuli) can produce a psychological state of fear through afferent activation of limbic, cortical, and subcortical structures. Ultimately, this afferent input results in activation of various efferent systems and the elicitation of defensive behaviors, of which antinociception can be a component. Clearly, one way in which these efferent systems could achieve antinociception is through activation of the RVM, which, through its descending projections, would reduce spinal nociceptive responsiveness.

OUTPUT NEURONS OF DESCENDING MODULATORY SYSTEMS

Fortunately, now there exists detailed knowledge of the neural mechanisms by which opioids act at these sites within the pain-modulatory circuitry. Neurons in all relevant brain areas are enriched with opioid receptors (Mansour et al. 1994; Arvidsson et al. 1995a,b,c; Schulz et al. 1998) and are densely innervated by other neurons containing endogenous opioid peptides (Atweh and Kuhar 1977; Watson et al. 1982; Delfs et al. 1994; Zadina et al. 1999). Furthermore, detailed knowledge exists of the neural mechanisms by which opioids act at some of these brain areas to produce antinociception (see Millan 2002 for review). For example, two distinct types of pain-modulating neuron have been identified in the rat RVM (Fields et al. 1991), both of which project to the spinal dorsal horn (Fields et al. 1995). One type is referred to as the ON cell. When the action potential firing frequency of these neurons is measured concurrently with application of noxious heat to the tail, the firing frequency increases dramatically just prior to reflexive tail withdrawal. ON cells are inhibited directly by opioids (Heinricher et al. 1994), and their activation appears to have a facilitatory influence on spinal nociceptive transmission and withdrawal reflexes (Bederson et al. 1990; Kaplan and Fields 1991). The second class of RVM pain-modulating neuron is the OFF cell. The firing frequency of this cell type decreases dramatically just prior to reflexive tail withdrawal from noxious heat. Interestingly, after systemic administration of analgesic doses of opioid receptor agonists, OFF cells discharge continuously, rather than in bursts (Fields et al. 1983). Given that OFF cells are not affected directly by opioids (Heinricher et al. 1994), their activation under these circumstances must result from a process of disinhibition; that is, opioids "release" OFF cells from the inhibitory effects of another cell type by inhibiting that cell type. The identity of this cell type remains to be determined. It is unlikely to be the ON cell, because ON cell

activity can be inhibited with glutamatergic antagonists without changing
the firing characteristics of OFF cells (Heinricher and McGaraughty 1998).
Regardless, the increase in OFF cell discharge is associated with
antinociception (as indicated by concomitant tail-flick suppression), which
has been interpreted as evidence that OFF cells are the cell type whose
activation in the nucleus raphe magnus and nucleus magnocellularis leads to
an inhibitory effect on spinal nociceptive transmission.

The existence of ON cells and OFF cells within the RVM and elsewhere
within the pain-modulating system (e.g., PAG) (Heinricher et al. 1987) has
important implications for how pain is modulated by various psychological
conditions. ON cells and OFF cells, with their descending projections to the
spinal dorsal horn, provide a physiological substrate for dynamically reducing *or enhancing* the transmission of nociceptive signals from the spinal
cord to the brain. A third class of RVM neuron (not mentioned above), the
serotonergic neutral cell, may be involved in more tonic regulation of nociceptive responsiveness that depends on behavioral state (for example, sleeping or waking states) (Mason 2001). In the next section it will become clear
that different psychological factors can bidirectionally modulate pain perception in a manner resulting in either analgesia or hyperalgesia as environmental circumstances warrant.

THE PHYSIOLOGICAL ACTIVATION OF ENDOGENOUS
PAIN-MODULATORY SYSTEMS

The demonstration that exogenous opioids activate a well-defined pain-
inhibitory system capable of potently blocking nociceptive transmission
suggests, but by no means proves, that the normal function of this particular
system (i.e., in the absence of exogenous drugs) is to reduce the perceived
intensity of painful stimuli. If, in fact, this system has such a physiological
role, one might expect that the level of activity within the system would
increase under certain psychological circumstances. The identification of
such circumstances that produce analgesia would give credibility to the idea
that invasive procedures, such as brain stimulation or exogenous opioid
drugs, inhibit pain by mimicking the natural activity within these neural
pathways.

Hayes et al. (1978a,b) initiated the first systematic search for "drug-
free" conditions that activate endogenous pain inhibitory systems in animals. They observed that, in rats, potent antinociception could be produced
by such diverse stimuli as brief footshock, centrifugal rotation, and intra-
peritoneal injection of hypertonic saline. Subsequent research from many
different laboratories catalogued numerous types of external/environmental

manipulations that evoke behavioral antinociception in animals (see Mayer and Manning 1995 for review). Importantly, these experiments revealed that opioid antagonists, such as naloxone, block some, but not all, forms of environmentally induced antinociception (Hayes et al. 1978a,b). Therefore, it appears that *non-opioid* endogenous pain control systems must exist in addition to the system or systems involving endogenous opioid peptides.

Another important discovery that has arisen from this line of investigation is that of environmentally induced *hypernociception,* in which certain environmental manipulations can enhance or heighten nociceptive responsiveness. This phenomenon became evident in early studies that demonstrated that certain forms of moderate, non-nociceptive stress (e.g., certain forms of restraint or exposure to a novel environment) could result in enhanced nociceptive responsiveness in rats (Vidal and Jacob 1982, 1986). Later, Meagher, Grau, and colleagues systematically investigated a range of shock parameters for their effects on nociception (King et al. 1999; Meagher et al. 2001). For example, brief, moderate shocks (3 shocks, 0.75 s, 1.0 mA) lowered vocalization thresholds to noxious heat (indicating hypernociception), while shocks of greater severity (3 shocks, 25 s, 1.0 mA; or 3 shocks, 2 s, 3.0 mA) increased vocalization thresholds to noxious heat (indicating antinociception). The data seemed to indicate that brief, moderate shock enhances, while severe shock decreases, the "aversiveness" of heat pain. As mentioned in the previous section, the neuronal cell type in the RVM referred to as the ON cell provides a potential physiological substrate for the generation of environmentally induced hypernociception.

Of considerable interest is the fact that some forms of antinociception or hypernociception produced by environmental manipulations can be classically conditioned. For example, in rats, repeated pairings of certain cues with foot-shock leads to conditioned antinociception. That is, the cues by themselves acquire the ability to evoke antinociception (Hayes et al. 1978a; Watkins et al. 1982a; Watkins and Mayer 1982b). This conditioning activates an opioid antinociceptive system because conditioned antinociception is eliminated by systemic or intrathecal spinal naloxone, morphine tolerance, or lesions of descending pathways of the endogenous pain-modulatory circuit (Watkins et al. 1982b). In addition, as would be expected, higher structures are involved in the conditioned antinociception because it is eliminated by decerebration, or more specifically by lesions of the amygdala (Helmstetter 1992) or PAG (Watkins et al. 1982a).

A point that should be emphasized is that the involvement in these processes of other neurotransmitters or neuromodulators at the spinal cord level may be complex. For example, cholecystokinin (CCK) appears to modulate endogenous opioid systems. In rats, intrathecal application of CCK

antagonizes antinociception induced either by exogenous opioids or by activation of endogenous opioids (Faris et al. 1983; Watkins et al. 1984). Also,
CCK-receptor antagonists applied intrathecally potentiate these forms of
antinociception and reverse opioid tolerance (Watkins et al. 1984). These
findings support the notion that other transmitters and/or modulators interact
with opioids to form complex circuits. The circuits relate, in turn, to the
complexity of psychological factors that regulate pain and antinociception.
For example, stimuli that signal safety *reduce* the antinociceptive effects of
morphine in rats (Wiertelak et al. 1992). Furthermore, this anti-opioid effect
occurs because the safety signal leads to the release of CCK in the spinal
cord. Interestingly, this general schema appears to have a human correlate—
placebo analgesia can be potentiated by the CCK-receptor antagonist
proglumide (Benedetti and Amanzio 1997), an agent that can also reduce the
"nocebo" response (Benedetti et al. 1997). The nocebo response essentially
is the opposite of the placebo response. An experimental volunteer, informed that a manipulation will increase the perceived intensity of a painful
stimulus, reports that indeed this is the case, despite the fact that in reality
the treatment (e.g., i.v. saline solution) is not hyperalgesic.

PAIN MODULATION IN CHRONIC PAIN STATES

The experiments discussed above relate to modulation of nociceptive
thresholds in the absence of injury or other pathophysiology (i.e., in the
normal animal). It is also of interest to examine whether the endogenous
pain-modulatory circuitry described above contributes to the development
and/or maintenance of neuropathic pain.

In 1988, Bennett and Xie published an article describing their development of an animal model of painful peripheral mononeuropathy. Since the
publication of this article, other animal models of chronic neuropathic pain
have been developed (Seltzer et al. 1990; Kim and Chung 1992; Kupers et
al. 1998; Decosterd and Woolf 2000). These models have revealed that
pathophysiology in a number of categories contributes to the development
and maintenance of the spontaneous pain, allodynia, and hyperalgesia that
accompany neuropathic pain states. These categories are inclusive of both
peripheral and central mechanisms. Peripheral events include sensitization
of Aδ and C fibers, phenotypic switch of Aβ fibers, and awakening of
"silent" nociceptors, all of which could contribute to abnormal ectopic discharges of affected dorsal root ganglia (DRGs). Regarding the CNS, efforts
have focused mainly on the spinal cord. Central mechanisms include loss of
Aβ-mediated inhibition in the spinal dorsal horn (e.g., deafferentation hypersensitivity of spinal neurons), central sensitization (i.e., enhancement of

previously existing synaptic connections between large myelinated afferents and nociceptive-specific [NS] neurons in the spinal cord), and sprouting of mechanoreceptive fibers in the dorsal horn (i.e., novel synaptic contacts between the central terminals of mechanoreceptive fibers with nociceptive neurons). With regard to both central and peripheral contributors to neuropathic pain, a wide array of molecules and mechanisms have been implicated. A discussion of these molecules is outside the scope of this chapter, but they include abnormally distributed ion channels (e.g., Na^+ channels); neurotrophins (e.g., nerve growth factor) and cytokines (e.g., tumor necrosis factor α) in the periphery; various intracellular signaling cascades in spinal neurons mediated by protein kinases (e.g., protein kinase C) leading to immediate early gene induction; and widespread changes in protein synthesis, which generally underlie neuroplastic changes (see Millan 1999 and Zimmermann 2001 for reviews of this topic).

Given the contribution of plastic changes in the spinal cord to neuropathic pain, several investigators have directed attention toward the possibility that descending circuitry might play a modulatory role in these processes. Indeed, it seems clear that intra-PAG microinjection of morphine can reduce tactile allodynia in the rat spinal nerve ligation (SNL) model of neuropathic pain (Pertovaara and Wei 2003), perhaps more effectively than systemically administered morphine. It is the potential contribution of descending pain-*facilitatory* systems that may be more interesting with respect to neuropathic pain, however. Although injury-induced discharges may drive the *initiation* of a neuropathic pain state, the *maintenance* of the state appears to depend, at least in part, on the pain-facilitatory system descending from the RVM (Ossipov et al. 2000; Porreca et al. 2001; Burgess et al. 2002). Microinjection of lidocaine into the RVM apparently blocks neuropathic pain in the SNL model, while in normal animals this manipulation does not affect acute nociceptive withdrawal responses such as von Frey mechanical withdrawal thresholds and thermal paw and tail withdrawal thresholds (Kovelowski et al. 2000; Burgess et al. 2002). Lesions of the dorsolateral funiculus produced ipsilateral to the site of nerve injury produce a similar result (Burgess et al. 2002).

Finally, there are clues as to which class of RVM neuron is responsible for this effect. Selective destruction, with dermorphin-saporin, of μ-opioid-receptor-expressing RVM neurons produces a pattern of results similar to that for intra-RVM lidocaine or unilateral lesion of the dorsolateral funiculus (Porreca et al. 2001; Burgess et al. 2002). This last observation is particularly intriguing, given that a large proportion of μ-opioid-receptor-expressing neurons in the RVM is likely to consist of ON cells (Heinricher et al. 1994).

The timing of these effects is of great interest. When performed shortly after SNL surgery, all three manipulations fail to prevent the *onset* of SNL-induced tactile and thermal hypersensitivity, but instead reverse these signs to baseline levels beginning on post-SNL day 4–6. Animals in control experiments will continue to show hypersensitivity for several additional weeks. This finding suggests that when initial injury-induced afferent discharges subside, descending pain-enhancing systems from the RVM contribute heavily to the maintenance of the neuropathic pain state. This finding may also help to explain why systemically administered opioids are inconsistent in their ability to effectively control pain associated with postherpetic neuralgia, diabetic neuropathy, and peripheral nerve injury in humans (McCleane 2003).

IMPLICATIONS FOR UNDERSTANDING PAIN MECHANISMS

In summary, a review of the animal data provides strong evidence for the existence of endogenous pain-modulatory circuitry that can increase or decrease nociceptive responsiveness, depending on environmental circumstances. I have described some of the environmental circumstances under which this circuitry is activated and the different physiological classes of pain modulating neuron (ON cells, OFF cells) that might mediate increases or decreases in pain thresholds. The relevant environmental circumstances are largely those involving threats (either acute threats or the anticipation of such events) or aversive stimulation, including pain itself. In addition, it appears that descending pain-modulatory circuitry can bidirectionally influence the maintenance of neuropathic pain states in a manner analogous to bidirectional modulation of nociceptive thresholds in normal animals. Clearly, knowledge of this circuitry and of the conditions under which its different components are activated has important implications for understanding general principles of pain modulation in humans.

**EVIDENCE FOR ENDOGENOUS PAIN-MODULATORY
SYSTEMS IN HUMANS**

It is difficult to determine directly whether pain-modulatory circuitry similar to that characterized in animal experiments exists in humans. Nevertheless, several independent, albeit indirect, lines of evidence support the likelihood that similar systems exist in humans. First, the descending circuitry implicated in endogenous opioid antinociception is highly conserved in a variety of mammalian species, including rodents, felines (Abols and Basbaum 1981), and nonhuman primates (Manning et al. 2001). Importantly, the locations and extent of neurotransmitters, including opioid peptides, in this circuitry appears to be similar in a number of species, including humans (Zadina et al. 1999). The homogeneity of pain-modulatory circuitry across this diversity of species leaves little doubt of a corresponding system in humans. Second, opioid drugs that significantly reduce clinical pain are effective in inhibiting a variety of behaviors relating to nociceptive processing in various animal species, including nociceptive withdrawal reflexes, more integrated escape behaviors, and responses of individual nociresponsive neurons to painful stimuli (Fields et al. 1991). In these species, antinociceptive effects of opioids are exerted in part through actions upon the descending pain-modulatory circuitry that mediates acute fear-induced and conditioned antinociception. Third, recent functional neuroimaging studies in humans have suggested that the analgesic effects of μ-opioid analgesics such as fentanyl, remifentanil, and hydromorphone are correlated with activation of many of the same brain regions shown to contribute to μ-opioid-induced antinociception in animals. These regions include the brainstem (lower pons/ medulla) (Petrovic et al. 2002) and amygdala (Schlaepfer et al. 1998), as well as cortical areas such as the anterior cingulate (Adler et al. 1997; Casey et al. 2000), insular, and orbitofrontal cortices (Petrovic et al. 2002).

In addition to these indirect lines of evidence, there exists an older body of literature that relates to determinations of endogenous pain-modulatory circuitry in humans that can be considered somewhat more direct. Indeed, it is possible to draw parallels between the animal work described in the previous sections and experimental and clinical studies in humans. These parallels are important because they highlight the potential relevance of this work to the difficult problem of treating human pain syndromes. Throughout this discussion, it will be important to keep in mind the data presented earlier in this chapter indicating that several distinct modulatory systems have been identified under controlled laboratory conditions in animals. Indeed, as will become apparent later, the same can be said of humans. In the more naturalistic circumstances of clinical research, it is likely that more than one of these systems may be active at any given time, which may account for some of the variability and controversy in the clinical literature relating to pain modulation.

Broadly, at least two situations are available for study in which endogenous pain-modulatory systems may be active in humans. The first involves the basal, tonic activity within these systems and allows the experimenter to assess whether pain inhibition occurs continuously, at least to some degree. The second involves clinical manipulations that attempt to *activate* pain-inhibitory or pain-enhancing systems.

Attempts have been made to determine whether pain-modulatory systems are tonically active in humans. These studies have assumed that administration of opioid antagonists should alter the perception of pain if descending, opioidergic systems indeed are tonically active. This change in pain perception would be apparent either as a decreased pain threshold or as an increased level of ongoing pain. In this regard, naloxone generally has failed to affect pain thresholds of normal human volunteers (El-Sobsky et al. 1976; Grevert and Goldstein 1977; Stacher et al. 1988). On the other hand, Buchsbaum et al. (1977) found that naloxone lowered the thresholds of subjects with naturally high pain thresholds, yet had no effect in subjects with low pain thresholds. This observation is consistent with reports that the high pain thresholds seen in some cases of congenital insensitivity to pain can be lowered by naloxone (Dehen et al. 1977; Cesselin et al. 1984). These studies, taken together, suggest that endogenous opioid pain control circuits are not always tonically active in humans.

Naloxone appears to be more consistently effective when delivered to experimental subjects who are experiencing some level of clinical pain. In this regard, these results are consistent with the animal studies described above in which pain is an activator of endogenous antinociception systems. Thus, Levine et al. (Levine et al. 1978, 1979; Levine and Gordon 1986) and Gracely et al. (1983) reported that naloxone can increase the reported intensity of postoperative pain, although these data later proved to be somewhat controversial (see ter Riet et al. 1998). Thus, it can be concluded that, under normal circumstances, endogenous opioid pain control systems have little spontaneous activity. However, when some level of pain is present, these systems seem to be activated and can be antagonized, to some degree at least, by naloxone administration.

A second line of research on the involvement of endogenous opioids in pain modulation in humans has examined a number of external, non-drug-related manipulations that are known to have some degree of efficacy in reducing clinical and experimental pain. Many of these procedures were developed before the recent explosion of information about endogenous pain-modulatory systems. Indeed, many of them evolved from theoretical approaches that are now outdated or proven to be incorrect. Nevertheless, the procedures are efficacious and have inspired a considerable body of research aimed at determining the involvement of endogenous opioids in pain modulation.

This research has utilized two primary experimental strategies. The first strategy reasons that if a particular physiological or psychological condition induces analgesia by releasing endogenous opioids, it should be possible to antagonize this analgesia with an opioid antagonist (usually naloxone). The second strategy reasons that if endogenous opioids are involved in these forms of analgesia, then changes should be observed in the levels of these compounds in plasma or in the CNS. The rationale for these two types of tests is as follows. Endogenous opioid peptides and opioid receptors exist at CNS sites involved in pain modulation (as discussed earlier). Exogenous opioids, which potently inhibit pain in humans, are likely to act at these same endogenous opioid receptor sites. If these two assumptions are correct, there should be physiological and psychological conditions under which endogenous opioids reduce pain, and under these conditions administration of an opioid receptor antagonist should block the resultant analgesia. For similar reasons, the release of endogenous opioid peptides should be detectable during those psychological or physiological conditions that activate endogenous pain-inhibitory circuitry.

BRAIN-STIMULATION-PRODUCED ANALGESIA IN HUMANS

Perhaps the most dramatic outcome of the basic science research on endogenous opioids and pain-modulatory systems has been its rapid and effective clinical application to the treatment of chronic pain syndromes in humans. In the early 1970s, Richardson and Akil (1977a,b) began reporting on the use of focal electrical stimulation of the periaqueductal/periventricular gray matter to treat pain syndromes. Since that time many reports have evaluated this technique in the PAG and other brain areas. In a review of this early literature, Young et al. (1985) concluded that "electrical stimulation of the brain offers a safe and relatively effective method for the treatment of chronic pain in appropriately selected patients, who are unresponsive to other forms of therapy." Although use of this procedure fell out of favor to a large degree in the United States, more recent, cumulative data from other countries suggests that stimulation of structures such as the PAG, specific thalamic sensory nuclei, and the internal capsule can be very effective and safe in the long-term control of pain associated with trigeminal neuropathy and peripheral neuropathy (Kumar et al. 1997).

Interestingly, studies in recent years have shown that focal electrical stimulation of the "motor" portion of the cerebral cortex (i.e., the precentral gyrus, or primary motor cortex) is remarkably efficacious (Tsubokawa et al. 1991a,b) in treating several kinds of central and neuropathic pain states in humans, including trigeminal deafferentation pain, central pain secondary to stroke, trigeminal neuralgia, sciatic nerve injury, and phantom limb pain (see Brown and Barbaro 2003 for review). Although the exact mechanisms underlying such analgesia remain obscure, it is possible that at least part of the effectiveness of this manipulation is due to activation of descending pain-control circuits described above. Electrophysiological studies show that motor cortex stimulation reduces flexion nociceptive reflexes (R-III reflexes) in the spinal cord (Garcia-Larrea et al. 1999). Positron emission tomography (PET) studies show that analgesic motor cortex stimulation increases regional cerebral blood flow (rCBF) in the ipsilateral thalamus, the contralateral anterior cingulate, anterior insular, and orbitofrontal cortices, and the ipsilateral upper brainstem (Peyron et al. 1995; Garcia-Larrea et al. 1997, 1999). The somatosensory cortex and immediate subcortical zones apparently are not activated by motor cortex stimulation. The level of analgesia achieved appears to correlate with the increased rCBF in the anterior cingulate cortex. Interestingly, the authors speculated that activation of the PAG also might be a consequence of motor cortex stimulation.

Regarding endogenous opioids, several lines of evidence indicate a likely, but not unequivocal, role for endogenous opioids in stimulation-produced analgesia (SPA) in humans. Opioid antagonists are reported to reduce SPA elicited from the PAG (Adams 1976; Hosobuchi et al. 1977; Hosobuchi 1978), and tolerance eventually develops to SPA (Hosobuchi 1978). Somewhat controversial early literature suggested that the endogenous opioids β-endorphin (Akil et al. 1978a; Hosobuchi et al. 1979) and enkephalin (Akil et al. 1978b) are released into ventricular cerebrospinal fluid by electrical stimulation of the PAG in humans. It seems likely that endogenous opioids mediate, at least in part, the analgesia elicited by PAG stimulation in humans. The particular endogenous opioid(s) and relevant sites and mechanisms of action have not been established.

ENVIRONMENTALLY INDUCED ANALGESIA
AND HYPERALGESIA IN HUMANS

Further evidence for the existence of endogenous pain-modulatory systems in humans comes from studies of external (environmental) manipulations. Enough experimental evidence has accumulated to suggest that the bidirectional modulation of nociceptive thresholds by different environmental manipulations occurs in humans in a manner equivalent to that seen in animals. Early efforts in this area were propelled principally by the notion that the brain contains an endogenous pain-inhibitory system. Thus, investigators explored the hypothesis that stressful events *reduce* pain perception. Perhaps not surprisingly, results were mixed in this regard. Some stressful events decreased pain threshold (Bobey and Davidson 1970; Malow 1981; Willer et al. 1981; Bandura et al. 1988; Pitman et al. 1990; al Absi and Rokke 1991; Janssen and Arntz 1996), but others resulted in an apparent increase in pain threshold, or hyperalgesia (Haslam 1966; Bowers 1968;

Dougher 1979; Schumacher and Velden 1984; Weisenberg et al. 1984; Dougher et al. 1987; Cornwall and Donderi 1988; al Absi and Rokke 1991). Recently, Rhudy and Meagher (2000) attempted to reconcile these contrasting results by operationally defining and categorizing, in a more thorough manner, the experimental manipulations presented in these preceding reports. Ultimately, they proposed that these contradictory findings were obtained, in part, because the paradigms employed produced two different psychological states—fear and anxiety. The authors pointed out that fear is a psychological and physiological alarm reaction to a threat that is *present* in the environment. It is characterized by the urge to escape or avoid the threat and typically results in heightened sympathetic arousal. In contrast, anxiety is a *future*-oriented emotion characterized by negative affect and anticipation of potential threats in an apprehensive manner. The psychological state of anxiety results in hypervigilance and somatic tension (e.g., muscle tension). Fear mobilizes the organism to take action (fight/flight response), whereas anxiety leads to increased environmental scanning that facilitates the gathering of data from all senses. Related to these concepts is the common clinical experience that anxiety that occurs in anticipation of pain can enhance the perceived intensity of a painful stimulus upon application.

With this conceptual foundation as a framework, Rhudy and Meagher (2000) set about testing the hypothesis that experimentally induced fear and experimentally induced anxiety would have opposite effects on radiant heat pain thresholds. They randomly assigned 60 human subjects to one of three experimental conditions: (1) fear, produced by exposure to three brief shocks; (2) anxiety, elicited by the *threat* of shock; and (3) a "neutral," no-intervention condition. As hypothesized, the psychological state of fear produced an *increase* in radiant heat pain threshold (i.e., analgesia), while that of anxiety produced a *decrease* in pain threshold (i.e., hyperalgesia).

With respect to stress-induced analgesia in humans, recent neuroimaging studies have provided insights into the concomitant release of endogenous opioids in discrete brain areas. These studies have taken advantage of the selective μ-opioid-receptor ligand [^{11}C]carfentanil, which can be used as a radiotracer to image μ-opioid receptors using PET. A manipulation that causes a decrease in [^{11}C]-carfentanil binding in a particular brain area is taken to reflect an increase in the release of endogenous opioids, which then compete with [^{11}C]-carfentanil for binding sites. Using this sort of approach, the pain or stress associated with topical application of capsaicin or sustained, experimentally induced jaw muscle pain results in release of endogenous opioids in such areas as the contralateral ventrolateral thalamus, ipsilateral amygdala, and nucleus accumbens, which ultimately correlates with a

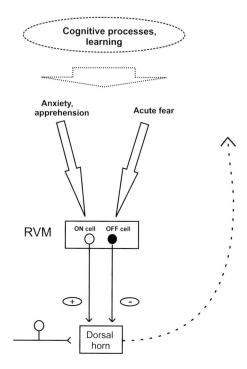

Fig. 2. An example of how psychological processes might interact with well-defined pain-modulatory circuitry. The psychological state of anxiety in humans can result in hyperalgesia and the psychological state of fear can result in analgesia. In rodents, evidence indicates that activation of ON cells in the rostral ventromedial medulla (RVM) results in hyper-responsiveness to nociceptive stimuli and that activation of OFF cells in the RVM results in antinociception. In humans, therefore, it is possible that anxiety and fear produce opposite effects on pain perception by activating the human equivalents of ON cells and OFF cells, respectively.

reduction in sensory and affective ratings of the pain experience (Zubieta et al. 2001; Bencherif et al. 2002).

Finally, Flor et al. (2002) recently showed that controlled, stress-induced analgesic responses can be classically conditioned in humans as they can be in animals. These investigators used mental arithmetic combined with white noise as an unconditioned stimulus to elicit an increase both in pain threshold and the ability to tolerate above-threshold pain. When they paired distinct auditory stimuli with the unconditioned stimulus, the auditory stimuli acquired the ability to increase pain threshold and "pain tolerance" (i.e., conditioned analgesia was observed). Interesting, these authors reported that conditioned analgesia relating to "pain tolerance" but not that relating to pain threshold, was naloxone-reversible.

Cumulatively, these results support the behavioral and physiological data collected in animals indicating the existence of a complex pain-modulatory system in the mammalian brain. In response to environmental challenges, this system is capable of bidirectionally modulating the flow of nociceptive signals through the spinal cord and into higher brain centers that process sensory, affective, and cognitive-evaluative components of pain perception. Fig. 2 provides a simple diagram suggesting how the relatively simple psychological states of anxiety and fear might exert opposing effects on nociceptive transmission; that is, through pathways and mechanisms that ultimately result in activation of RVM ON cells or OFF cells. Evidence indicating that emotional states other than fear and anxiety also modulate pain in humans is explored in detail in Chapter 6.

CONCLUSIONS

This chapter has presented a brief overview of the evidence for endogenous pain-modulatory circuitry that can be activated in all mammals under a variety of environmental, psychological, and physiological circumstances. With regard to the endogenous pain *inhibitory* system, it is likely that opioid peptides are utilized at several levels of the neuraxis to achieve analgesia in the conscious organism when warranted by environmental circumstances.

An ongoing impetus for conducting animal studies related to pain transmission and pain modulation is the notion that a thorough knowledge of the mechanisms by which pain information is processed and modulated by the peripheral and central nervous systems will lead to better treatments to combat chronic pain states in humans. Although it is clear that tremendous progress has been made in terms of the volume of data collected, the translation of this knowledge into novel or improved treatments for pain has been limited. Indeed, the predictive validity of animal pain models with respect to efficacy in humans is not always ensured (Hill 2000). Furthermore, while knowledge of the neurochemical and molecular mechanisms of afferent pain processing in normal and pathophysiological pain conditions has driven many industrial and academic drug discovery efforts, the neural circuitry relating to efferent pain *modulation* in the CNS has not always been on the conceptual "radar" of such efforts. There have been some exceptions to this generalization (e.g., Bitner et al. 1998), but knowledge of this circuitry has not yet resulted directly in the development of novel pain medications.

Nevertheless, it is apparent that humans possess powerful pain-modulatory circuits, similar to those described in animals. Furthermore, it is clear that changes in psychological states, both simple and complex, can profoundly affect the perception of sensory and affective components of pain. It follows that, in the clinical setting, psychological modulatory processes can both influence the efficacy of drug treatments and be manipulated or controlled in their own right to manage pain.

REFERENCES

Abols IA, Basbaum AI. Afferent connections of the rostral medulla of the cat: a neural substrate for midbrain-medullary interactions in the modulation of pain. *J Comp Neurol* 1981; 201; 285–297.

Ackley MA, Hurley RW, Virnich DE, Hammond DL. A cellular mechanism for the antinociceptive effect of a kappa opioid receptor agonist. *Pain* 2001; 91:377–388.

Adams JE. Naloxone reversal of analgesia produced by brain stimulation in the human. *Pain* 1976; 2:161–166.

Adler LJ, Gyulai FE, Diehl DJ, et al. Regional brain activity changes associated with fentanyl analgesia elucidated by positron emission tomography (published erratum appears in *Anesth Analg* 1997; 84:949). *Anesth Analg* 1997; 84:120–126.

Akil H, Mayer DJ, Liebeskind JC. Antagonism of stimulation-produced analgesia by naloxone, a narcotic antagonist. *Science* 1976; 191:961–962.

Akil H, Richardson DE, Barchas JD, Li CH. Appearance of beta-endorphin-like immunoreactivity in human ventricular cerebrospinal fluid upon analgesic electrical stimulation. *Proc Natl Acad Sci USA* 1978a; 75:5170–5172.

Akil H, Richardson DE, Hughes DJ, Barchas JD. Enkephalin-like material elevated in ventricular cerebrospinal fluid of patients after analgetic focal stimulation. *Science* 1978b; 201:463–465.

al Absi M, Rokke PD. Can anxiety help us tolerate pain? *Pain* 1991; 46:43–51.

Albus K, Schott M, Herz A. Interaction between morphine and morphine antagonists after systemic and intraventricular application. *Eur J Pharmacol* 1970; 12:53–64.

Arvidsson U, Dado RJ, Riedl M, et al. Delta-opioid receptor immunoreactivity: distribution in brainstem and spinal cord, and relationship to biogenic amines and enkephalin. *J Neurosci* 1995a; 15:1215–1235.

Arvidsson U, Riedl M, Chakrabarti S, et al. Distribution and targeting of a mu-opioid receptor (MOR1) in brain and spinal cord. *J Neurosci* 1995b; 15:3328–3341.

Arvidsson U, Riedl M, Chakrabarti S, et al. The kappa-opioid receptor is primarily postsynaptic: combined immunohistochemical localization of the receptor and endogenous opioids. *Proc Natl Acad Sci USA* 1995c; 92:5062–5066.

Atweh SF, Kuhar MJ. Autoradiographic localization of opiate receptors in rat brain. III. The telencephalon. *Brain Res* 1977; 134:393–405.

Azami J, Llewelyn MB, Roberts MHT. The contribution of nucleus reticularis paragigantocellularis and nucleus raphe magnus to the analgesia produced by systemically administered morphine, investigated by the microinjection technique. *Pain* 1982; 12:229–246.

Bandura A, Cioffi D, Taylor CB, Brouillard ME. Perceived self-efficacy in coping with cognitive stressors and opioid activation. *J Pers Soc Psychol* 1988; 55:479–488.

Baumeister AA. The effects of bilateral intranigral microinjection of selective opioid agonists on behavioral responses to noxious thermal stimuli. *Brain Res* 1991; 557:136–145.

Bederson JB, Fields HL, Barbaro NM. Hyperalgesia during naloxone-precipitated withdrawal from morphine is associated with increased on-cell activity in the rostral ventromedial medulla. *Somatosens Mot Res* 1990; 7:185–203.

Bencherif B, Fuchs PN, Sheth R, et al. Pain activation of human supraspinal opioid pathways as demonstrated by [¹¹C]-carfentanil and positron emission tomography (PET). *Pain* 2002; 99:589–598.

Benedetti F, Amanzio M. The neurobiology of placebo analgesia: from endogenous opioids to cholecystokinin. *Prog Neurobiol* 1997; 52:109–125.

Benedetti F, Amanzio M, Casadio C, Oliaro A, Maggi G. Blockade of nocebo hyperalgesia by the cholecystokinin antagonist proglumide. *Pain* 1997; 71:135–140.

Bennett GJ, Xie YK. A peripheral mononeuropathy in rat that produces disorders of pain sensation like those seen in man. *Pain* 1988; 33:87–107.

Bitner RS, Nikkel AL, Curzon P, et al. Role of the nucleus raphe magnus in antinociception produced by ABT- 594: immediate early gene responses possibly linked to neuronal nicotinic acetylcholine receptors on serotonergic neurons. *J Neurosci* 1998; 18:5426–5432.

Bobey MJ, Davidson PO. Psychological factors affecting pain tolerance. *J Psychosom Res* 1970; 14:371–376.

Bornhovd K, Quante M, Glauche V, et al. Painful stimuli evoke different stimulus-response functions in the amygdala, prefrontal, insula and somatosensory cortex: a single-trial fMRI study. *Brain* 2002; 125:1326–1336.

Bowers KS. Pain, anxiety, and perceived control. *J Consult Clin Psychol* 1968; 32:596–602.

Brown JA, Barbaro NM. Motor cortex stimulation for central and neuropathic pain: current status. *Pain* 2003; 104:431–435.

Buchsbaum MS, Davis GC, Bunney WE. Naloxone alters pain perception and somatosensory evoked potentials in normal subjects. *Nature* 1977; 270:620–622.

Burgess SE, Gardell LR, Ossipov MH, et al. Time-dependent descending facilitation from the rostral ventromedial medulla maintains, but does not initiate, neuropathic pain. *J Neurosci* 2002; 22:5129–5136.

Burkey AR, Carstens E, Wenniger JJ, Tang J, Jasmin L. An opioidergic cortical antinociception triggering site in the agranular insular cortex of the rat that contributes to morphine antinociception. *J Neurosci* 1966; 16:6612–6623.

Cahill CM, Dray A, Coderre TJ. Enhanced thermal antinociceptive potency and antiallodynic effects of morphine following spinal administration of endotoxin. *Brain Res* 2003; 960:209–218.

Casey KL, Svensson P, Morrow TJ, et al. Selective opiate modulation of nociceptive processing in the human brain. *J Neurophysiol* 2000; 84:525–533.

Cesselin F, Bourgoin S, Hamon M, et al. Normal CSF levels of metenkephalin-like material in a case of naloxone-reversible congenital insensitivity to pain. *Neuropeptides* 1984; 4:217–225.

Collins JJ, Berde CB, Grier HE, Nachmanoff DB, Kinney HC. Massive opioid resistance in an infant with a localized metastasis to the midbrain periaqueductal gray. *Pain* 1995; 63:271–275.

Cornwall A, Donderi DC. The effect of experimentally induced anxiety on the experience of pressure pain. *Pain* 1988; 35:105–113.

Decosterd I, Woolf CJ. Spared nerve injury: an animal model of persistent peripheral neuropathic pain. *Pain* 2000; 87:149–158.

Dehen H, Willer JC, Boureau F, Cambier J. Congenital insensitivity to pain, and endogenous morphine-like substances. *Lancet* 1977; 2:293–294.

Delfs JM, Kong H, Mestek A, et al. Expression of mu opioid receptor mRNA in rat brain: an in situ hybridization study at the single cell level. *J Comp Neurol* 1994; 345:46–68.

Dougher MJ. Sensory decision theory analysis of the effects of anxiety and experimental instructions on pain. *J Abnorm Psychol* 1979; 88:137–144.

Dougher MJ, Goldstein D, Leight KA. Induced anxiety and pain. *J Anxiety Disord* 1987; 1:259–264.

El-Sobsky A, Dostrovsky JO, Wall PD. Lack of effect of naloxone on pain perception in humans. *Nature* 1976; 263:783–784.

Fairbanks CA, Wilcox GL. Acute tolerance to spinally administered morphine compares mechanistically with chronically induced morphine tolerance. *J Pharmacol Exp Ther* 1997; 282:1408–1417.

Fang FG, Haws CM, Drasner K, Williamson A, Fields HL. Opioid peptides (DAGO-enkephalin, dynorphin A(1-13), BAM 22P) microinjected into the rat brainstem: comparison of their antinociceptive effect and their effect on neuronal firing in the rostral ventromedial medulla. *Brain Res* 1989; 501:116–128.

Fanselow MS. Shock-induced analgesia on the formalin test: effects of shock severity, naloxone, hypophysectomy and associative variables. *Behav Neurosci* 1984; 98:79–95.

Fanselow MS. The midbrain periaqueductal gray as a coordinator of action in response to fear and anxiety. In: Depaulis A, Bandler R (Eds). *The Midbrain Periaqueductal Gray Matter: Functional, Anatomical, and Neurochemical Organization.* New York: Plenum Press, 1991, pp 151–173.

Faris PL, Komisaruk BR, Watkins LR, Mayer DJ. Evidence for the neuropeptide cholecystokinin as an antagonist of opiate analgesia. *Science* 1983; 219:311–312.

Fields HL, Price DD. Toward a neurobiology of placebo analgesia. In: Harrington A (Ed). *The Placebo Effect: An Interdisciplinary Exploration.* Boston: Harvard University Press, 1997.

Fields HL, Vanegas H, Hentall ID, Zorman G. Evidence that disinhibition of brain stem neurones contributes to morphine analgesia. *Nature* 1983; 306:684–686.

Fields HL, Heinricher MM, Mason P. Neurotransmitters in nociceptive modulatory circuits. *Ann Rev Neurosci* 1991; 14:219–245.

Fields HL, Malick A, Burstein R. Dorsal horn projection targets of ON and OFF cells in the rostral ventromedial medulla. *J Neurophysiol* 1995; 74:1742–1759.

Flor H, Birbaumer N, Schulz R, Grusser SM, Mucha RF. Pavlovian conditioning of opioid and nonopioid pain inhibitory mechanisms in humans. *Eur J Pain* 2002; 6:395–402.

Fox RJ, Sorenson CA. Bilateral lesions of the amygdala attenuate analgesia induced by diverse environmental challenges. *Brain Res* 1994; 648:215–221.

Garcia-Larrea L, Peyron R, Mertens P, et al. Positron emission tomography during motor cortex stimulation for pain control. *Stereotact Funct Neurosurg* 1997; 68:141–148.

Garcia-Larrea L, Peyron R, et al. Electrical stimulation of motor cortex for pain control: a combined PET-scan and electrophysiological study. *Pain* 1999; 83:259–273.

Gracely RH, Dubner R, Wolskee PJ, Deeter WR. Placebo and naloxone can alter post-surgical pain by separate mechanisms. *Nature* 1983; 306:264–265.

Grevert P, Goldstein A. Effects of naloxone on experimentally induced ischemic pain and on mood in human subjects. *Proc Natl Acad Sci USA* 1977; 74:1291–1294.

Hamann SR, Martin WR. Opioid and nicotinic analgesic and hyperalgesic loci in the rat brain stem. *J Pharmacol Exp Ther* 1992; 261:707–715.

Haslam DR. The effect of threatened shock upon pain thresholds. *Psychol Sci* 1966; 6:309–310.

Hayes RL, Bennett GJ, Newlon PG, Mayer DJ. Behavioural and physiological studies of non-narcotic analgesia in the rat elicited by certain environmental stimuli. *Brain Res* 1978a; 155:69–90.

Hayes RL, Price DD, Bennett GJ, Wilcox GL, Mayer DJ. Differential effects of spinal cord lesions on narcotic and non-narcotic suppression of nociceptive reflexes: further evidence for the physiologic multiplicity of pain modulation. *Brain Res* 1978b; 155:91–101.

Heinricher MM, Cheng Z-F, Fields HL. Evidence for two classes of nociceptive modulating neurons in the periaqueductal gray. *J Neurosci* 1987; 7:271–278.

Heinricher MM, McGaraughty S. Analysis of excitatory amino acid transmission within the rostral ventromedial medulla: implications for circuitry. *Pain* 1998; 75:247–255.

Heinricher MM, Morgan MM, Tortorici V, Fields HL. Disinhibition of off cells and antinociception produced by an opioid action within the rostral ventromedial medulla. *Neuroscience* 1994; 63:279–288.

Helmstetter FJ. The amygdala is essential for the expression of conditional hypoalgesia. *Behav Neurosci* 1992; 106:518–528.

Helmstetter FJ, Tershner SA. Lesions of the periaqueductal gray and rostral ventromedial medulla disrupt antinociceptive but not cardiovascular aversive conditional responses. *J Neurosci* 1994; 14:7099–7108.

Helmstetter FJ, Bellgowan PSF, Poore LH. Microinfusion of *mu* but not *delta* or *kappa* opioid agonists into the basolateral amygdala results in inhibition of the tail flick reflex in pentobarbital-anesthetized rats. *J Pharmacol Exp Ther* 1995; 275:381–388.

Hill RG. NK1 (substance P) receptor antagonists—why are they not analgesic in humans? *Trends Pharmacol Sci* 2000; 21:244–246.

Hiller JM, Pearson J, Simon EJ. Distribution of stereospecific binding of the potent narcotic analgesic etorphine in the human brain: predominance in the limbic system. *Res Commun Chem Pathol Pharmacol* 1973; 6:1052–1062.

Hosobuchi Y. Tryptophan reversal of tolerance to analgesia induced by central grey stimulation. *Lancet* 1978; ii:47.

Hosobuchi Y, Adams JE, Linchitz R. Pain relief by electrical stimulation of the central gray matter in humans and its reversal by naloxone. *Science* 1977; 197:183–186.

Hosobuchi Y, Rossier J, Bloom FE, Guillemin R. Stimulation of human periaqueductal gray for pain relief increases immunoreactive beta-endorphin in ventricular fluid. *Science* 1979; 203:279–281.

Hsieh JC, Stahle-Backdahl M, Hagermark O, et al. Traumatic nociceptive pain activates the hypothalamus and the periaqueductal gray: a positron emission tomography study. *Pain* 1996; 64:303–314.

Huang X, Tang JS, Yuan B, Jia H. Morphine applied to the ventrolateral orbital cortex produces a naloxone-reversible antinociception in the rat. *Neurosci Lett* 2001; 299:189–192.

Hughes J. Isolation of an endogenous compound from the brain with pharmacological properties similar to morphine. *Brain Res* 1975; 88:295–308.

Hurley RW, Grabow TS, Tallarida RJ, Hammond DL. Interaction between medullary and spinal delta-1 and delta-2 opioid receptors in the production of antinociception in the rat. *J Pharmacol Exp Ther* 1999; 289:993–999.

Hurley RW, Banfor P, Hammond DL. Spinal pharmacology of antinociception produced by microinjection of mu or delta opioid receptor agonists in the ventromedial medulla of the rat. *Neuroscience* 2003; 118:789–796.

Irwin S, Houde RW, Bennett DR, Hendershot LC, Seevers MH. The effects of morphine, methadone and meperidine on some reflex responses of spinal animals to nociceptive stimulation. *J Pharmacol Exp Ther* 1951; 101:132–143.

Jacquet YF, Lajtha A. Morphine action at central nervous system sites in rat: analgesia or hyperalgesia depending on site and dose. *Science* 1973; 182:490–492.

Jacquet YF, Lajtha A. Paradoxical effects after microinjection of morphine in the periaqueductal gray matter in the rat. *Science* 1974; 185:1055–1057.

Janssen SA, Arntz A. Anxiety and pain: attentional and endorphinergic influences. *Pain* 1996; 66:145–150.

Jones SL, Gebhart GF. Inhibition of spinal nociceptive transmission from the midbrain, pons and medulla in the rat: activation of descending inhibition by morphine, glutamate and electrical stimulation. *Brain Res* 1988; 460:281–296.

Kaplan H, Fields HL. Hyperalgesia during acute opioid abstinence: evidence for a nociceptive facilitating function of the rostral ventromedial medulla. *J Neurosci* 1991; 11:1433–1439.

Kedlaya D, Reynolds L, Waldman S. Epidural and intrathecal analgesia for cancer pain. *Best Pract Res Clin Anaesthesiol* 2002; 16:651–665.

Kim SH, Chung JM. An experimental model for peripheral neuropathy produced by segmental spinal nerve ligation in the rat. *Pain* 1992; 50:355–363.

King TE, Crown ED, Sieve AN, et al. Shock-induced hyperalgesia: evidence forebrain systems play an essential role. *Behav Brain Res* 1999; 100:33–42.

Kovelowski CJ, Bian D, Hruby VJ, et al. Selective opioid delta agonists elicit antinociceptive suupraspinal/spinal synergy in the rat. *Brain Res* 1999; 843:12–17.

Kovelowski CJ, Ossipov MH, Sun H, et al. Supraspinal cholecystokinin may drive tonic descending facilitation mechanisms to maintain neuropathic pain in the rat. *Pain* 2000; 87:265–273.

Kumar K, Toth C, Nath RK. Deep brain stimulation for intractable pain: a 15-year experience. *Neurosurgery* 1997; 40:736–746.

Kupers R, Yu W, Persson JK, Xu XJ, Wiesenfeld-Hallin Z. Photochemically-induced ischemia of the rat sciatic nerve produces a dose-dependent and highly reproducible mechanical, heat and cold allodynia, and signs of spontaneous pain. *Pain* 1998; 76:45–59.

Lee HJ, Choi JS, Brown TH, Kim JJ. Amygdalar NMDA receptors are critical for the expression of multiple conditioned fear responses. *J Neurosci* 2001; 21:4116–4124.

Levine JD, Gordon NC. Method of administration determines the effect of naloxone on pain. *Brain Res* 1986; 365:377–378.

Levine JD, Gordon NC, Jones RT, Fields HL. The narcotic antagonist naloxone enhances clinical pain. *Nature* 1978; 272:826.

Levine JD, Gordon NC, Fields HL. Naloxone dose dependently produces analgesia and hyperalgesia in postoperative pain. *Nature* 1979; 278:740–741.

Llewelyn MB, Azami J, Gibbs M, Roberts MH. A comparison of the sites at which pentazocine and morphine act to produce analgesia. *Pain* 1983; 16:313–331.

Malow RM. The effects of induced anxiety on pain perception: a signal detection analysis. *Pain* 1981; 11:397–405.

Manning BH. A lateralized deficit in morphine antinociception after unilateral inactivation of the central amygdala. *J Neurosci* 1998; 18:9453–9470.

Manning BH, Franklin KBJ. Morphine analgesia in the formalin test: reversal by microinjection of quaternary naloxone into the posterior hypothalamic area or periaqueductal gray. *Behav Brain Res* 1998; 92:97–102.

Manning BH, Mayer DJ. The central nucleus of the amygdala contributes to the production of morphine antinociception in the formalin test. *Pain* 1995a; 63:141–152.

Manning BH, Mayer DJ. The central nucleus of the amygdala contributes to the production of morphine antinociception in the rat tail-flick test. *J Neurosci* 1995b; 15:8199–8213.

Manning BH, Morgan MJ, Franklin K. Morphine analgesia in the formalin test: evidence for forebrain and midbrain sites of action. *Neuroscience* 1994; 63:289–294.

Manning BH, Merin NM, Meng ID, Amaral DG. Reduction in opioid- and cannabinoid-induced antinociception in rhesus monkeys after bilateral lesions of the amygdaloid complex. *J Neurosci* 2001; 21:8238–8246.

Manning BH, Martin WJ, Meng ID. The rodent amygdala contributes to the production of cannabinoid-induced antinociception. *Neuroscience* 2003; 120:1157–1170.

Mansour A, Fox CA, Burke S, et al. Mu, delta, and kappa opioid receptor mRNA expression in the rat CNS: an in situ hybridization study. *J Comp Neurol* 1994; 350:412–438.

Mason P. Contributions of the medullary raphe and ventromedial reticular region to pain modulation and other homeostatic functions. *Annu Rev Neurosci* 2001; 24:737–777.

Mayer DJ, Hayes RL. Stimulation-produced analgesia: development of tolerance and cross-tolerance to morphine. *Science* 1975; 188:941–943.

Mayer DJ, Liebeskind JC. Pain reduction by focal electrical stimulation of the brain: an anatomical and behavioral analysis. *Brain Res* 1974; 68:73–94.

Mayer DJ, Manning BH. The role of opioid peptides in environmentally-induced analgesia. In: Tseng LF (Ed). *The Pharmacology of Opioid Peptides.* Chur: Harwood Academic, 1995, pp 345–395.

Mayer DJ, Price DD. Central nervous system mechanisms of analgesia. *Pain* 1976; 2:379–404.

Mayer DJ, Wolfle TL, Akil H, Carder B, Liebeskind JC. Analgesia from electrical stimulation in the brainstem of the rat. *Science* 1971; 174:1351–1354.

McCleane G. Pharmacological management of neuropathic pain. *CNS Drugs* 2003; 17:1031–1043.

Meagher MW, Ferguson AR, Crown ED, et al. Shock-induced hyperalgesia: IV. Generality. *J Exp Psychol Anim Behav Process* 2001; 27:219–238.

Melzack R, Wall PD. Pain mechanisms: a new theory. *Science* 1965; 150:971–979.

Millan MJ. The induction of pain: an integrative review. *Prog Neurobiol* 1999; 57:1–164.

Millan MJ. Descending control of pain. *Prog Neurobiol* 2002; 66:355–474.

Mitchell JM, Lowe D, Fields HL. The contribution of the rostral ventromedial medulla to the antinociceptive effects of systemic morphine in restrained and unrestrained rats. *Neuroscience* 1998; 87:123–133.

Morgan MM, Whitney PK. Immobility accompanies the antinociception mediated by the rostral ventromedial medulla of the rat. *Brain Res* 2000; 872:276–281.

Nandigama P, Borszcz GS. Affective analgesia following the administration of morphine into the amygdala of rats. *Brain Res* 2003; 959:343–354.

Noordenbos W. *Pain.* Amsterdam: Elsevier, 1959.

Oley N, Cordova C, Kelly ML, Bronzino JD. Morphine administration to the region of the solitary tract nucleus produces analgesia in rats. *Brain Res* 1982; 236:511–515.

Ossipov MH, Kovelowski CJ, Nichols ML, Hruby VJ, Porreca F. Characterization of supraspinal antinociceptive actions of opioid delta agonists in the rat. *Pain* 1995; 62:287–293.

Ossipov MH, Hong ST, Malan P Jr, Lai J, Porreca F. Mediation of spinal nerve injury induced tactile allodynia by descending facilitatory pathways in the dorsolateral funiculus in rats. *Neurosci Lett* 2000; 290:129–132.

Pavlovic ZW, Bodnar RJ. Opioid supraspinal analgesic synergy between the amygdala and periaqueductal gray in rats. *Brain Res* 1998; 779:158–169.

Pert CB, Snyder SH. Opiate receptor: demonstration in nervous tissue. *Science* 1973; 179:1011–1014.

Pert A, Yaksh T. Sites of morphine induced analgesia in the primate brain: relation to pain pathways. *Brain Res* 1974; 80:135–140.

Pert CB, Snowman AM, Snyder SH. Localization of opiate receptor binding in synaptic membranes of rat brain. *Brain Res* 1974; 70:184–188.

Pert CB, Kuhar MJ, Snyder SH. Autoradiographic localization of the opiate receptor in rat brain. *Life Sci* 1975; 16:1849–1853.

Pertovaara A, Wei H. A dissociative change in the efficacy of supraspinal versus spinal morphine in the neuropathic rat. *Pain* 2003; 101:237–250.

Petrovic P, Kalso E, Petersson KM, Ingvar M. Placebo and opioid analgesia—imaging a shared neuronal network. *Science* 2002; 295:1737–1740.

Peyron R, Garcia-Larrea L, Deiber MP, et al. Electrical stimulation of precentral cortical area in the treatment of central pain: electrophysiological and PET study. *Pain* 1995; 62:275–286.

Pitman RK, van der Kolk BA, Orr SP, Greenberg MS. Naloxone-reversible analgesic response to combat-related stimuli in posttraumatic stress disorder: a pilot study. *Arch Gen Psychiatry* 1990; 47:541–544.

Porreca F, Burgess SE, Gardell LR, et al. Inhibition of neuropathic pain by selective ablation of brainstem medullary cells expressing the mu-opioid receptor. *J Neurosci* 2001; 21:5281–5288.

Przewlocki R, Przewlocka B. Opioids in chronic pain. *Eur J Pharmacol* 2001; 429:79–91.

Reynolds DV. Surgery in the rat during electrical analgesia induced by focal brain stimulation. *Science* 1969;164:444–445.

Rhudy JL, Meagher MW. Fear and anxiety: divergent effects on human pain thresholds. *Pain* 2000; 84:65–75.

Rhudy JL, Meagher MW. Individual differences in the emotional reaction to shock determine whether hypoalgesia is observed. *Pain Med* 2003; 4:244–256.

Richardson DE, Akil H. Pain reduction by electrical brain stimulation in man. Part 1: Acute administration in periaqueductal and periventricular sites. *J Neurosurg* 1977a; 47:178–183.

Richardson DE, Akil H. Pain reduction by electrical brain stimulation in man. Part 2: Chronic self-administration in the periventricular gray matter. *J Neurosurg* 1977b; 47:184–194.

Rodgers RJ. Elevation of aversive threshold in rats by intra-amygdaloid injection of morphine sulphate. *Pharmacol Biochem Behav* 1977; 6:385–390.

Rossi GC, Pasternak GW, Bodnar RJ. Mu and delta opioid synergy between the periaqueductal gray and the rostro-ventral medulla. *Brain Res* 1994; 665:85–93.

Saminin R, Valzelli L. Increase of morphine-induced analgesia by stimulation of the nucleus raphe dorsalis. *Eur J Pharmacol* 1971; 16:298–302.

Sato M, Takagi H. Effect of morphine on the pre- and postsynaptic inhibitions in the spinal cord. *Eur J Pharmacol* 1971; 14:150–154.

Schlaepfer TE, Strain EC, Greenberg BD, et al. Site of opioid action in the human brain: mu and kappa agonists' subjective and cerebral blood flow effects. *Am J Psychiatry* 1998; 155:470–473.

Schulz S, Schreff M, Koch T, et al. Immunolocalization of two mu-opioid receptor isoforms (MOR1 and MOR1B) in the rat central nervous system. *Neuroscience* 1998; 82:613–622.

Schumacher R, Velden M. Anxiety, pain experience, and pain report: a signal-detection study. *Percept Mot Skills* 1984; 58:339–349.

Seltzer Z, Dubner R, Shir Y. A novel behavioral model of neuropathic pain disorders produced in rats by partial sciatic nerve injury. *Pain* 1990; 43:205–218.

Shane R, Acosta J, Rossi GC, Bodnar RJ. Reciprocal interactions between the amygdala and ventrolateral periaqueductal gray in mediating Q/N(1-17)-induced analgesia in the rat. *Brain Res* 2003; 980:57–70.

Stacher G, Abatzi TA, Schulte F, et al. Naloxone does not alter the perception of pain induced by electrical and thermal stimulation of the skin in healthy humans. *Pain* 1988; 34:271–276.

Takagi H. The nucleus reticularis paragigantocellularis as a site of analgesic action of morphine and enkephalin. *Trends Pharmacol Sci* 1980; 1:182–184.

Takagi H, Satoh M, Akaike A, Shibata T, Kuraishi Y. The nucleus reticularis of the medulla oblongata is a highly sensitive site in the production of morphine analgesia in the rat. *Eur J Pharmacol* 1977; 45:91–92.

ter Riet G, de Craen AJ, de Boer A, Kessels AG. Is placebo analgesia mediated by endogenous opioids? A systematic review. *Pain* 1998; 76:273–275.

Terenius L. Stereospecific interaction between narcotic analgesics and a synaptic plasma membrane fraction of rat cerebral cortex. *Acta Pharmacol Toxicol* 1973; 32:317–320.

Thorat SN, Hammond DL. Modulation of nociception by microinjection of delta-1 and delta-2 opioid receptor ligands in the ventromedial medulla of the rat. *J Pharmacol Exp Ther* 1997; 283:1185–1192.

Tsou K. Antagonism of morphine analgesia by the intracerebral microinjection of nalorphine. *Acta Physiol Sin* 1963; 26:332–337.

Tsou K, Jang CS. Studies on the site of analgesic action of morphine by intracerebral micro-injection. *Sci Sin* 1964; 8:1099–1109.

Tsubokawa T, Katayama Y, Yamamoto T, Hirayama T, Koyama S. Chronic motor cortex stimulation for the treatment of central pain. *Acta Neurochir Suppl (Wien)* 1991a; 52:137–139.

Tsubokawa T, Katayama Y, Yamamoto T, Hirayama T, Koyama S. Treatment of thalamic pain by chronic motor cortex stimulation. *Pacing Clin Electrophysiol* 1991b; 14:131–134.

Vidal C, Jacob J. Hyperalgesia induced by non-noxious stress in the rat. *Neurosci Lett* 1982; 32:75–80.

Vidal C, Jacob J. Hyperalgesia induced by emotional stress in the rat: an experimental animal model of human anxiogenic hyperalgesia. *Ann NY Acad Sci* 1986; 467:73–81.

Watkins LR, Mayer DJ. Involvement of spinal opioid systems in footshock-induced analgesia: antagonism by naloxone is possible only before induction of analgesia. *Brain Res* 1982a; 242:309–316.

Watkins LR, Mayer DJ. Organization of endogenous opiate and nonopiate pain control systems. *Science* 1982b; 216:1185–1192.

Watkins LR, Cobelli DA, Mayer DJ. Classical conditioning of front paw and hind paw footshock induced analgesia (FSIA): naloxone reversibility and descending pathways. *Brain Res* 1982a; 243:119–132.

Watkins LR, Cobelli DA, Mayer DJ. Opiate vs non-opiate footshock induced analgesia (FSIA): descending and intraspinal components. *Brain Res* 1982b; 245:97–106.

Watkins LR, Kinscheck IB, Mayer DJ. The neural basis of footshock analgesia: the effect of periaqueductal gray lesions and decerebration. *Brain Res* 1983; 276:317–324.

Watkins LR, Kinscheck IB, Mayer DJ. Potentiation of opiate analgesia and apparent reversal of morphine tolerance by proglumide. *Science* 1984; 224:395–396.

Watson SJ, Khachaturian H, Akil H, Coy DH, Goldstein A. Comparison of the distribution of dynorphin systems and enkephalin systems in brain. *Science* 1982; 218:1134–1136.

Weisenberg M, Aviram O, Wolf Y, Raphaeli N. Relevant and irrelevant anxiety in the reaction to pain. *Pain* 1984; 20:371–383.

Wiertelak EP, Maier SF, Watkins LR. Cholecystokinin antianalgesia: safety cues abolish morphine analgesia. *Science* 1992; 256:830–833.

Willer JC, Dehen H, Chambier J. Stress-induced analgesia in humans: endogenous opioids and naltrexone-reversible depression of pain reflexes. *Science* 1981; 212:689–691.

Yaksh TL, Rudy TA. Analgesia mediated by a direct spinal action of narcotics. *Science* 1976; 192:1357–1358.

Yaksh TL, Rudy TA. Studies on the direct spinal action of narcotics in the production of analgesia in the rat. *J Pharmacol Exp Ther* 1977; 202:411–428.

Yaksh TL, Yeung JC, Rudy TA. Systematic examination in the rat of brain sites sensitive to the direct application of morphine: observation of differential effects within the periaqueductal gray. *Brain Res* 1976; 114:83–103.

Yang ZJ, Tang JS, Jia H. Morphine microinjections into the rat nucleus submedius depress nociceptive behavior in the formalin test. *Neurosci Lett* 2002; 328:141–144.

Yeung JC, Rudy TA. Multiplicative interaction between narcotic agonisms expressed at spinal and supraspinal sites of antinociceptive action as revealed by concurrent intrathecal and intracerebroventricular injections of morphine. *J Pharmacol Exp Ther* 1980a; 215:633–642.

Yeung JC, Rudy TA. Sites of antinociceptive action of systemically injected morphine: involvement of supraspinal loci as revealed by intracerebroventricular injection of naloxone. *J Pharmacol Exp Ther* 1980b; 215:626–632.

Young RF, Kroening R, Fulton W, Feldman RA, Chambi I. Electrical stimulation of the brain in treatment of chronic pain: experience over 5 years. *J Neurosurg* 1985; 62:389–396.

Zadina JE, Martin-Schild S, Gerall AA, et al. Endomorphins: novel endogenous mu-opiate receptor agonists in regions of high mu-opiate receptor density. *Ann NY Acad Sci* 1999; 897:136–144.

Zambotti F, Zonta N, Parenti M, et al. Periaqueductal gray matter involvement in the muscimol-induced decrease of morphine antinociception. *Naunyn Schmiedebergs Arch Pharmacol* 1982; 318:368–369.

Zimmermann M. Pathobiology of neuropathic pain. *Eur J Pharmacol* 2001; 429:23–37.

Zubieta JK, Smith YR, Bueller JA, et al. Regional mu opioid receptor regulation of sensory and affective dimensions of pain. *Science* 2001; 293:311–315.

Correspondence to: Barton H. Manning, PhD, Department of Neuroscience, Amgen Inc., One Amgen Center Drive, Mail Stop 29-2-B, Thousand Oaks, CA 91320-1799, USA. Tel: 805-447-7618; Fax: 805-480-1347; email: bmanning@ amgen.com.

Psychological Methods of Pain Control: Basic Science and Clinical Perspectives, Progress in Pain Research and Management, Vol. 29, edited by Donald D. Price and M. Catherine Bushnell, IASP Press, Seattle, © 2004.

4

Strategies to Decrease Pain and Minimize Disability

Patricia A. McGrath[a,b] and Lauren A. Dade[a]

[a]Chronic Pain Program, Departments of Anaesthesia and Psychology, The Hospital for Sick Children, and the Brain and Behavior Program, Research Institute at The Hospital for Sick Children, Toronto, Ontario, Canada; [b]Department of Anaesthesia, The University of Toronto, Toronto, Ontario, Canada

The impact of psychological factors on pain modulation has been recognized and discussed since antiquity. In the 10th century, in his *Canon of Medicine,* Avicenna recommended several behavioral and cognitive-behavioral interventions for relieving pain including massage, relaxing exercise, "walking about gently for a considerable time" to soften the tissues, listening to agreeable music, and "being occupied with something very engrossing" to reduce the severity of pain (Gruner 1930, p. 529). Avicenna's wording clearly reveals that he recognized a critical component of effective psychological pain modulation—the need to focus one's attention fully. Centuries later, we remain intrigued by the power of psychological factors to decrease pain, directing our research efforts toward identifying all the critical components and determining their mechanisms of action.

As described throughout this volume, data accrued from animal behavior studies and human psychophysical studies have confirmed that several psychological factors modify the experience of pain. Attention, perceived control, expectations, and the pain's meaning or relevance influence the ultimate perception of any pain. Moreover, because our beliefs guide what we do to relieve pain and shape our emotional responses to a pain problem, these psychological factors not only affect the immediate perception of pain but also influence pain-related disability and subsequent distress.

Our increasing recognition that pain is not simply and directly related to the nature and extent of tissue damage has had profound implications for pain assessment and management. The emphasis has shifted gradually from an almost exclusively disease-centered model focusing on detecting and treating the putative source of tissue damage to a more individual-centered perspective that includes assessing the individual with pain, identifying contributing psychological and contextual factors, and targeting interventions accordingly. In this chapter, we describe how to apply an individual-centered framework for assessing and treating pain within routine clinical practice. This practical clinical approach is based on our improved understanding of the psychological factors that modulate pain. Using case examples, we will illustrate simple and effective strategies for decreasing pain, minimizing pain-related disability, and alleviating emotional distress.

ACUTE PAIN

CONTEXTUAL AND PSYCHOLOGICAL FACTORS

The vast majority of pains that infants, children, and adults experience are acute pains caused by injuries. Acute pains usually have a rapid onset and a protective significance, warning us to avoid further physical harm. These pains are symptoms that diminish progressively as injuries heal. A wide array of over-the-counter analgesics can provide effective pain relief. We usually do not experience any prolonged emotional distress because acute pains are understandable and can be controlled easily. Thus, the psychological factors associated with most acute pains can be regarded as positive—an accurate understanding of the pain source, positive expectations for pain relief, and perceived control. The aversive significance is determined primarily by the pain intensity and by disruptions to normal activities.

However, consider the very different set of factors that can be associated with acute procedural pain. Invasive procedures such as blood sampling, injections, dressing changes, lumbar punctures, or endoscopic procedures are generally approached with some trepidation by adults and children alike. Patients often do not know what to expect with respect to the quality or intensity of the sensations that they will feel. Unsure whether the pain will be manageable, they may worry about how well they will cope. Perhaps believing that they have little control during the intervention, they may anxiously watch staff to assess how well it is proceeding. They also may be fearful about an underlying health problem.

Thus, the psychological factors associated with acute procedural pains are often negative—uncertainty, little perceived control, apprehension, fear, anxiety, and distress. The aversive significance is determined not only by the strength of the pain, but also by the impact of the underlying health condition on an individual's life. The adverse consequence of these negative factors on an individual's pain experience can be enormous. Nevertheless, health care providers can easily modify these factors to lessen pain and distress, even in very young children, as shown in the following case example.

CASE STUDY: INCREASED PAIN AND DISTRESS DURING CANCER TREATMENT

David, a 3-year-old boy with acute lymphoblastic leukemia, had become very anxious about many invasive medical procedures, especially lumbar punctures and bone marrow aspirations. He cried, stalled, refused treatment, and when finally sedated, fought the effects of the sedative so that staff needed to physically restrain him during painful procedures. David was receiving treatment at a time when little research had been conducted on childhood pain. Pain management was based on an acute injury model, wherein a child's pain was predictably and directly related only to the level of tissue injury. In general, the pains caused by repeated lumbar punctures were judged as almost equivalent, regardless of differences in contextual and psychological factors, although investigators had already demonstrated the power of these factors for modifying nociceptive activity in animals and altering pain experiences in adults (Johnson 1973; Barrell and Price 1975; von Graffenried et al. 1978; Dubner et al. 1981; McGrath et al. 1981; McGrath 1983).

Thus, our approach with David was to evaluate whether any of the factors that had been identified in the animal research and in studies conducted in adults were contributing to his procedural pain, and if so, to change those factors. Lumbar punctures were extremely difficult procedures for him. In these procedures, a needle is inserted into the cerebrospinal fluid between the lumbar vertebrae at the base of the spine, fluid is withdrawn, and chemotherapy is administered. In order to make the space between the vertebrae more accessible, children are bent into a tight "nose on your knees ball" and held tightly in this uncomfortable position. Children typically receive a sedative by oral or intramuscular injection before the procedure. Nurses help children to curl onto their sides with their backs close to the edge of the treatment table and hold them while the oncologist applies antiseptic and a topical anesthetic spray to their lower backs, holding them more tightly when the oncologist infiltrates the spinal region with a local anesthetic and inserts the needle into the cerebrospinal fluid. Staff frequently remind children to remain still, telling them that it will soon be over.

From David's perspective, everything about a lumbar puncture was awful. He was frightened when he started to feel drowsy after receiving a sedative and tried to stay alert. David was small, so he felt smothered when nurses immobilized his arms and legs to maintain the tight "nose on your knees" position. He hated losing a whole day for these appointments, for which he arrived in the morning and did not leave until late afternoon; when the procedure was completed, he was exhausted and slept deeply for several hours. Despite experiencing several lumbar punctures, David could not explain what happened behind his back (even in a very cursory manner). He said that he heard different noises and felt different sensations but they did not make sense to him. David vividly described the cold sensation from the topical anesthetic. He then knew that the other needles were coming and tried to fight to get away, even though he had promised his parents he would be good. Surprisingly (from our perspective as observers), David did not identify the spinal tap as the most painful aspect of the procedure. Instead, the whole sequence of events from the topical anesthetic until the final spinal needle was withdrawn blurred for him into one continuously painful event.

MODIFYING THE RESPONSIBLE COGNITIVE, BEHAVIORAL, AND EMOTIONAL FACTORS

From observing typical procedures and speaking with David, we noted many contextual and psychological factors that were probably intensifying his pain and distress, as listed in Fig. 1. David lacked an age-appropriate understanding of what was happening during a procedure, and he had few choices and no sense of control. He expected the entire procedure to be awful, as did his parents and most staff. He concentrated on every word, sound, and feeling—each aspect contributing to the overall aversive situation. The curled and restrained position made him feel vulnerable, particularly when he was under sedation.

Staff encouraged David to remain still, unintentionally emphasizing that he must behave himself and endure the ordeal. The more David flailed, the tighter the nursing staff held him (and the more his mother attempted to comfort and protect him). David became anxious a few days before lumbar punctures (as did his parents), as was evidenced by irritability, sleeping difficulties, and headache attacks. He expressed his frustration openly about the dreaded lumbar puncture days, particularly the fact that he was losing a whole day, and was very open about his anger toward the health care providers. Although David explained his cancer by saying that his blood was "sick," his behaviors suggested that he was also afraid about what cancer really meant.

We designed an educational program for David to modify the cognitive, behavioral, and emotional factors that contributed to his pain and distress. We used stuffed animals to explain what happened during a lumbar puncture,

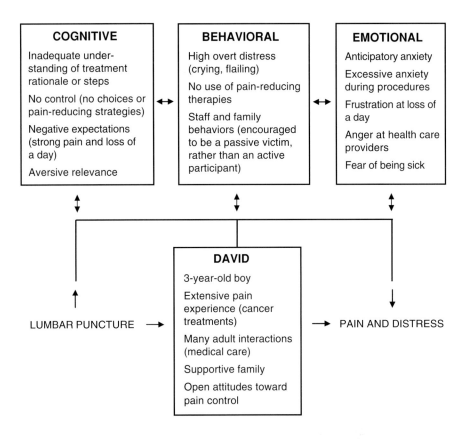

Fig. 1. Situational factors affecting David's pain experience.

demonstrating the equipment used and answering his questions. David was surprised to see the different bottles, swabs, and even the green cloth with a square cut-out for the back area that he had worn many times before. David quickly understood how much easier it was to see the back seam on the teddy bear when it was curled into the same position as his during a lumbar puncture, and then how difficult it was to inject the teddy bear's back when it moved around. David was initially frightened by the sight of the needles, but watched intently as we conducted a lumbar puncture on the bear. At a second practice, he prompted us about what to do next (so that we could gauge his understanding) and helped us to understand what the bear was feeling. Although at first, David did not want to touch any of the equipment, within a couple of sessions he confidently conducted the procedure on the bear.

Because David hated being restrained, we taught him to breathe deeply and relax while he remained in a curled position. He practiced this position during mock lumbar punctures in the clinic and at home with his parents. Soon David was able to maintain his relaxed curled-up position for a much longer time period than was required for the usual lumbar puncture. Because he still was startled by the topical anesthetic, we altered its aversive significance for him. We emphasized the sensations he described as "wet, cold, tingling, and stinging." David liked sledding in the snow, so we asked if the sensations from the anesthetic were similar to snow getting under his jacket when he was sledding. David was able to imagine the stinging of the anesthetic as a more familiar and comfortable sensation, and its application no longer startled him.

David learned two simple pain-reducing strategies to engage his mind and to provide him with a concrete activity. First, David learned that when he breathed deeply and slowly and matched the breathing rhythm of his therapist, he might become so relaxed that his back would become numb and the procedure would hurt less. We also taught David to imagine that any pain he felt in his lower back could be moved up his back and then down along his arm and into his hand, where he could squeeze the pain into his mother's hand and she would throw it onto the floor. We stressed that he could not just squeeze her hand hard; instead, he should squeeze it proportionately to how much pain he felt. Because David hated the effects of sedation, we agreed that he could forgo sedation for his next lumbar puncture and use only the psychological strategies he had learned.

The next lumbar puncture was a very positive experience for David, his parents, and all staff. He did not require restraint at any time. Throughout the procedure, the psychologist rubbed his shoulder to remind him to relax and praised him for maintaining his position. She described each phase of the procedure and asked David if he was ready (i.e., relaxed enough) before proceeding. She reminded him to use his breathing to numb his back or to squeeze his mother's hand, whichever he wanted. David reported only a little pain at the spinal needle insertion and was very happy about the whole experience. He was alert after the procedure and did not spend the rest of the day sleeping.

RECOMMENDATIONS FOR DECREASING ACUTE PAIN

In David's case, pain management consisted of identifying and modifying the cognitive, behavioral, and emotional factors listed in Fig. 1. These factors are regarded more globally as situational factors because they represent a unique interaction between the individual and the context in which the pain is experienced. Thus, they can vary dynamically, depending on the specific circumstances. Although the causal relationship between an injury and a consequent pain seems direct and obvious, what we understand, do, and feel affects our experience of pain. Differences in these situational factors may account for why the same tissue damage can evoke pains that vary in intensity, and may partially explain why proven analgesics can vary in effectiveness for different individuals and for the same individual at different times. As shown for David, health care providers can dramatically improve pain and lessen disability by modifying these factors.

The main cognitive factors that affect acute pain are individuals' understanding of the pain source and its significance, their ability to control what will happen, their expectations regarding the quality and strength of pain sensations that they will experience, their primary focus of attention (distracted away from or directed primarily toward the pain), and their knowledge of pain control strategies. Practical recommendations for lessening acute pain are listed in Table I. Generally, accurate information, realistic expectations, choices, control, and the use of some independent pain-reducing strategies will diminish pain. Strategies will vary according to individual preference and interest, and are most effective when patients can concentrate fully and actively engage in them. As an example, some adults prefer to visualize a relaxing setting and listen to music during an invasive procedure, while others prefer to attend to the different stages of the procedure and talk with health care providers.

While adults have developed a repertoire of different coping strategies, children require special attention because they depend on parents and health care staff for suggestions. Regrettably, health care providers often neglect a child's interest and preferences when suggesting a strategy. They may consider asking a child: "When your mom pulls out a sliver, do you watch or

Table I
Guidelines for minimizing acute pain and distress from invasive procedures

Explain what will happen clearly, in developmentally appropriate language.

Emphasize the qualitative sensations that patients may experience such as cold, tingling, and pressure so that they focus on what they are feeling, rather than only on the painful aspect.

If the procedure will cause some pain, describe the pain in familiar terms that the patient will understand, using examples of pains that they may have already experienced in situations that were not unduly stressful.

Help the patient to make the procedure less distressing and less painful, using attention and distraction, relaxation, and guided imagery or by attending to the various stages of the procedure (depending on their preference for being involved or distracted).

Remember that choice, control, and predictability are very important, particularly for children receiving invasive treatments. Allow children as much choice as possible, such as choosing which arm to use for injections, whether to watch or look away, and which pain-reducing tool to use.

look away?" "When you need to remove a Band-Aid, do you like to do it or do you like your mom to do it?" or "What makes you feel better when you have a stomach ache?" The answers will reveal whether the child prefers to attend to the situation or be distracted away from it, whether he or she prefers to be actively involved or passive, and whether he or she already has some comforting strategies that can be used in the clinical situation.

Our emotional reactions to acute pain depend on the nature of the pain and its meaning. Generally, the more threat the pain signifies, the stronger or more unpleasant the pain experience will be. Whether the pain sensations are caused by injury, disease, surgery, or invasive treatments, almost all individuals carefully appraise these sensations to assess how well they are recovering. They are alert for any changes in the expected pain (its quality, intensity, location, and frequency) that may signify that something might be wrong. Their appraisal of the pain determines what they feel emotionally— relatively neutral acceptance, annoyance, frustration, anxiety, fear, anger, or sadness. To minimize emotional distress, health care providers should educate patients about what sensations to expect and help them to accurately interpret the significance of any variation.

CHRONIC PAIN

CONTEXTUAL AND PSYCHOLOGICAL FACTORS

Although defined traditionally as any pain that persists beyond a 3-month period, chronic pain is not simply a prolongation of acute pain, nor is it always a symptom of active disease or injury. Chronic pain may have multiple sources, comprising nociceptive and neuropathic components, rather than a single nociceptive source. The pain often lacks a protective biological significance. Even when triggered by injury, the pain may not lessen progressively as the injury heals. Treatments that relieve acute pain may be wholly ineffective, with the result that individuals do not know whether they will ever be pain-free again. The continuing pain adversely affects all interpersonal relationships and all aspects of life—family, social activities, sports, work, and education. Individuals with chronic pain can experience prolonged psychological distress, impaired physical functioning, decreased independence, and often an uncertain prognosis. Effective treatment of chronic pain usually requires a multimodal approach comprising drug therapy, physical therapy, and psychological counseling, rather than a single therapy.

The common cognitive, behavioral, and emotional factors associated with chronic pain are listed in Table II. Complex and dynamic interactions occur among these factors. Patients' understanding of the cause of pain,

Table II
Key situational factors that can increase pain, distress, and disability

Cognitive:
    Inaccurate understanding from a "disease model" perspective
    Negative expectations about treatment efficacy
    Little perceived control
    Belief that certain environmental factors trigger attacks or exacerbations
    Belief that disability behaviors are wholly related to pain
    Failure to recognize or know how to resolve stress*

Behavioral:
    Inconsistent use of drug therapies
    Little use of flexible nondrug therapies
    Individual or family responses that reinforce disability
    Excessive withdrawal from activities
    Failure to fully resolve stressful situations (work, social, family, sports, and school)*

Emotional:
    Anxiety regarding true etiology
    Frustration at disruption to life activities
    Fear that the pain cannot be relieved
    Anger at health care providers for failing to treat pain effectively
    Depression about continuing pain and disability
    Anxiety about achieving at extremely high levels (work, social, family, sports, and school)*

* Particularly relevant for adolescents with chronic headache.

possible treatments, and long-term prognosis guides their behaviors and shapes their emotional responses to the pain problem. Individuals with chronic pain usually try to understand their condition from an acute disease perspective, where pain is due to a single cause and can be relieved by a single treatment. They do not understand that chronic pain, unlike most pains that they have already experienced, may have several interrelated causes. Thus, they continue medical investigations as they search for the clear-cut physical etiology and concentrate on finding one treatment that will immediately stop the pain. Patients may reject potentially effective treatments after only one attempt, even if the treatment addresses some of the causes and might lessen pain severity over time. Some individuals expect that they will remain disabled until the "right treatment" is found and believe that they have no control in changing the future course of continuing pain and disability.

    Irrespective of the etiology of chronic pain (whether it is known or unknown), several situational factors typically contribute to an individual's pain experience, emotional distress, and physical disability. To optimally control chronic pain, health care providers must target interventions to the relevant situational factors as well as to the primary pain source, as shown in the following case example.

CASE STUDY: CHRONIC PAIN AND DISABILITY AFTER INJURY

Kristina, a 13-year-old girl, developed pain in her right forearm shortly after her elbow was injured when "banged" by her younger sister. The pain persisted throughout the next day, so she was taken to the emergency department, where she had an X-ray that was normal. The pain continued, and Kristina returned to the hospital a few days later for another X-ray, which was normal. Two weeks later, Kristina was taken to another hospital for an additional X-ray, which was also normal. However, she received a splint cast that she wore for approximately 6 weeks. Eventually Kristina received physical therapy (two hour-long sessions per week), but the pain persisted. Kristina tried amitriptyline, acetaminophen, ibuprofen, acupuncture, physiotherapy, and transcutaneous electrical nerve stimulation, without any appreciable improvement in her pain level (usually 8–10 on a 0–10-point scale).

At the time of referral to our pain clinic, Kristina had experienced a constant "jabbing" pain in her right forearm for 6 months. The most painful region was on the proximal and lateral aspect. The pain increased with movement and also when her arm was touched. Kristina was no longer using her right arm and had learned to write with her left hand. On examination, her right arm was markedly different than her left arm—less muscle bulk in her right forearm (1 cm), increased hair growth in the most painful region of her forearm, and more shiny and brittle nails on her right hand. She had significant mechanical allodynia and hyperalgesia. Although her range of motion was excellent in the upper right extremity, Kristina kept her arm flexed at a 90º angle and held it close against her body.

Kristina was diagnosed with complex regional pain syndrome type I (CRPS-I). Her treatment recommendations included medication (continuing an amitriptyline prescription that she had just begun before her consultation at our clinic, with the possible addition of gabapentin within a few weeks), physical therapy, and a more comprehensive psychosocial assessment to identify any situational factors that were contributing to her pain and disability. The team emphasized that she should try to use her right arm as much as possible, beginning with desensitization techniques to acclimatize her skin to various sensations.

Kristina's psychosocial assessment was conducted a week later. A psychologist interviewed Kristina and her mother individually to evaluate the situational factors listed in Table II (see McGrath and Hillier [2001] for the structured interview for chronic pain). Kristina also completed standardized questionnaires to assess anxiety, depression, self-perception, and relationships within the family. Kristina presented as a happy and personable child. She was very well groomed and dressed conservatively. Her grades were high;

she had many friends and enjoyed competitive dance and gymnastics. While Kristina readily discussed her life, she denied all the daily problems that children typically encounter in their activities and relationships. She had difficulty expressing how she felt about her pain, particularly its impact on her life.

Kristina was very willing and eager to please, observing the therapist closely as if trying to figure out what might be the appropriate response to each inquiry. In fact, Kristina indicated that she always tried very hard in school and athletics, and that it was important to her to do the right things and not upset people. Kristina's responses on the psychological tests were within the normal range, except for elevated scores on the perfectionism and anxious coping subscales of the anxiety measure.

Her mother described Kristina as the "good and easy-going" child within the family, the daughter who always did the right thing. She reported that Kristina was comfortable in all situations and was well liked by her peers, teachers, and coaches. Although Kristina continued to achieve high marks in school despite her pain, teachers allowed her extra time to complete school assignments. Her mother was proud that Kristina coped with her pain in the same way that she did everything, rising to the challenge without complaining. She was very reluctant to push Kristina to use her right arm because any activity increased her pain, so she continued to help her daughter dress, bathe, and brush her hair.

Although some contributing factors were revealed during the interviews, we typically review all the information before providing specific feedback to families. The family was unable to schedule a feedback appointment until 6 weeks later, so the psychologist reminded them to follow the recommendations they had already received from the pain clinic (physical therapy, desensitization, and encouraging Kristina to use her right arm and hand as much as possible).

MODIFYING THE RESPONSIBLE COGNITIVE, BEHAVIORAL, AND EMOTIONAL FACTORS

At the feedback session, 6 weeks after the psychosocial assessment, Kristina continued to hold her arm protectively against her body. She had not followed any of the team's recommendations for desensitizing her skin or using her arm. Kristina's mother had requested that the school provide a computer to assist Kristina in completing her assignments. She was still worried that anything causing her arm to hurt would cause further damage. After reviewing what Kristina and her parents had done to relieve her pain since the assessment, the psychologist reviewed some of the common factors that affect individuals with chronic pain. She then presented a model to illustrate the specific cognitive, behavioral, and emotional factors that were relevant to Kristina's pain problem (shown in Fig. 2). The psychologist emphasized that Kristina was developing a severe disability problem as well as a pain problem.

Kristina and her family still understood her pain problem from an acute disease model. They expected that her pain would be fully relieved once the right medication was prescribed and that she would then be able to use her arm normally. Thus, they had continued to investigate alternative medications, as well as complementary therapies. The family remained uncertain because they had received differing medical opinions throughout the previous 6 months and because the pain continued despite supposedly appropriate therapies.

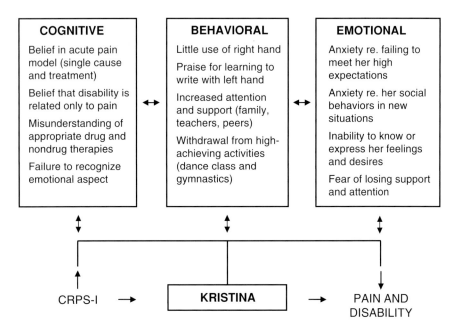

TREATMENT RECOMMENDATIONS

1. Learn and reinforce appropriate use of prescribed medication and physical therapy

2. Receive a cognitive-behavioral program (multifactorial etiology of CRPS-I, treatment rationale, prognosis)

3. Learn practical nondrug pain-reducing strategies (e.g., attention and distraction, relaxation, or self-hypnosis)

4. Modify the behavioral factors that inadvertently maintain disability

5. Consider counseling to address anxiety issues

Fig. 2. Factors relevant to Kristina's pain problem, and treatment recommendations.

The psychologist reviewed the key features differentiating chronic from acute pain, explaining the rationale for each treatment recommendation that Kristina had already received. She addressed the family's concerns about rehabilitating Kristina's arm, even though her skin remained sensitive to touch and activity increased her pain. The psychologist described how the same protective behaviors appropriate for an acute injury could eventually increase or prolong disability for certain chronic pains problems such as CRPS-I. While Kristina's guarding behaviors were appropriate immediately after her injury, they were very inappropriate 6 months later given the diagnosis of her pain condition. Unintentionally, Kristina's parents had encouraged her disability because they feared further damage. Moreover, their praise for her extraordinary efforts to cope by learning to do so much with her left hand (including writing legibly) further reinforced her disabling behaviors. Thus, they needed to switch their praise from disability to ability, encouraging her to resume her usual activities.

Despite Kristina's image as an easy-going child, she was extremely conscientious about fulfilling every responsibility—familial, social, academic, and athletic. She was anxious in many situations because she tried so hard to judge what was expected of her and behave accordingly. The constant pain relieved Kristina from her normal workload (at home and in school) and forced her to withdraw from competitive athletics, thus relieving the anxiety associated with these situations. The painful injury, clearly evident by the way she held her right arm, protected Kristina because she no longer had to compete at her previous level. Her teachers and family provided increased attention and support, and importantly, lowered their expectations for her achievement. Given Kristina's anxiety about doing the right thing in all situations, the pain had an extremely positive emotional significance. Kristina needed assistance to learn how to set realistic expectations for her performance. Because she had adopted a pattern of simply doing what she believed was expected as the "good child" within the family, Kristina also needed assistance to identify what she felt, and to understand that she was valued for herself—not just for complying in particular situations. The psychologist emphasized that we needed to address both Kristina's pain problem and her disability problem and outlined a treatment program to modify the contributing emotional factors (summarized at the bottom of Fig. 2).

Kristina agreed to participate in our recommended cognitive-behavioral program. At her next appointment 2 weeks after the feedback session, she held her arm in a less flexed position and had already started eating and writing with her right hand despite some continuing pain. Kristina showed considerable improvement over the 2-week period following the feedback appointment. While our recommendations for desensitization and using her arm were not different from those that she had received (and not followed) from the pain clinic 6 weeks earlier, the emphasis was very different. In addition to a diagnosis, we provided a more detailed framework for understanding and treating Kristina's chronic pain problem, especially the specific cognitive, behavioral, and emotional factors that contributed to her pain and disability. With this approach, we were able to quickly modify Kristina's beliefs and expectations and those of her family, and subsequently, they modified their behaviors. Kristina is only in the first phase of her cognitive-behavioral program. The longer patients have held unrealistically high expectations for their performance, the more time will be required for them to truly change how they evaluate themselves. Please see McGrath and Hillier (2001) for a more detailed description of this program.

RECOMMENDATIONS FOR DECREASING CHRONIC PAIN AND MINIMIZING DISABILITY

Irrespective of etiology, chronic pain has profound and prolonged physical, behavioral, and psychological consequences. Concurrently, what patients know, do, and feel exerts a profound impact on their subsequent pain and disability. Thus, to adequately treat chronic pain, we must evaluate the primary pain sources and ascertain which situational factors are relevant for which patients and families. Treatment emphasis accordingly shifts from an exclusively disease-centered framework to a more patient-centered focus. Clinicians can then select specific therapies to target the responsible central and peripheral mechanisms *and* to mitigate the pain-exacerbating impact of situational factors, recognizing that the multiple causes and contributing factors will vary over time.

Drug therapies (analgesics, analgesic adjuvants, and anesthetics) are essential for pain control, but nondrug therapies (cognitive, physical, and behavioral) are also essential. As we monitor the patient's improvement in response to the therapies initiated, we refine our pain diagnosis and treatment plan accordingly. Pain control is achieved practically by adjusting both drug and nondrug therapies in a rational, patient-centered manner based on the assessment process, as outlined by the treatment algorithm in Fig. 3. Controlling chronic pain requires an integrated approach because many factors are responsible, no matter how seemingly clear-cut the etiology. Adequate analgesic prescriptions, administered at regular dosing intervals, must be complemented by a practical cognitive-behavioral approach to ensure optimal pain relief.

---

1. Assess the Individual with Pain

Assess the sensory characteristics of pain

Conduct a medical examination and appropriate diagnostic tests

Evaluate the probable involvement of nociceptive and neuropathic mechanisms

Appraise situational factors contributing to pain, distress, and disability

2. Diagnose the Primary and Secondary Causes

Current nociceptive and neuropathic components

Attenuating physical symptoms

Relevance of key cognitive, behavioral, and emotional factors

3. Select Appropriate Therapies

Drug Therapies	*Nondrug Therapies*
Analgesics	Cognitive
Adjunct analgesics	Physical
Anesthetics	Behavioral

4. Implement Pain Management Plan

Provide feedback on causes and contributing factors

Provide rationale for integrated treatment plan

Measure pain regularly

Evaluate effectiveness of treatment plan

Revise plan as needed

Fig. 3. Treatment algorithm for chronic pain.

DIAGNOSING CHRONIC PAIN: "STOP, LOOK, AND LISTEN"

Every health care provider uses a particular cognitive-behavioral approach when treating patients. However, very few realize that they are already psychologically modulating a patient's pain experience through their personal approach. Pain modulation begins at the first consultation, where providers first shape what patients understand, what they will do, and how they will feel. To mitigate the factors that can intensify chronic pain, providers can "stop, look, and listen": *stop* an exclusive disease focus, *look* at the big picture in assessing the individual with pain, and *listen* to the individual's pain history, appreciating the potential impact of situational factors.

Typically, patients undergo a series of medical examinations and diagnostic tests to determine whether their pain is caused by disease, an underlying health condition, a neural dysfunction, or a psychological disorder. The diagnostic process may last several days, weeks, or even months as different specialists rule out various diagnoses. Patients and their families become increasingly anxious throughout this period. By the time the etiology (or probable etiology) is known, most patients have become extremely focused on their physical signs and symptoms in their search for clues as to what is wrong. If their pain is controlled during this period, they may have been able to continue many of their usual activities. If their pain is uncontrolled, patients may be unable to work, enjoy sports, or socialize, and their fears, frustration, and anxiety about the future may escalate.

In essence, the situational factors shown in Table II become progressively relevant as contributing factors for chronic pain, especially for patients with complex problems due to multiple etiologies or for those whose pain may have a primary psychological component. When medical consultations focus exclusively on pain features—location, frequency, quality, severity, duration, and accompanying physical symptoms—and fail to consider the relevant situational factors, health care providers inadvertently reinforce the disease model of pain. As such, they strengthen patients' beliefs that the pain is caused only by a particular physical abnormality and confirm their expectations that disability will persist until the right treatment is found.

Specialists may emphasize negative test findings, "a failure to find something," rather than a positive confirmation of an understandable, and therefore treatable, pain condition. Lacking a confirmatory and concise diagnosis, patients continue to be anxious and worried about why they have pain, fearing that the pain signifies an undiagnosed disease or medical condition. Primary care providers should be able to guide patients though the diagnostic phase of a chronic pain problem, helping them to understand the test results and reports from different specialists, alleviating their unfounded fears, and explaining why their assessment will focus on several aspects of the individual and not just on the pain symptom. Building on their knowledge of the patient and family history, primary care providers are also uniquely poised to evaluate the extent to which certain situational factors might contribute to pain and disability.

The communication of a diagnosis is a critical component of pain management. Even when some aspects of the pain condition are puzzling, health care providers should honestly describe what they know and explain what they need to explore further in a straightforward and reassuring manner. Accurate information about the pain source can mitigate the increased distress caused by patients' misinterpretations and anxieties. Moreover, given that expectancies can profoundly affect treatment effectiveness, health care providers may wish to directly address their patients' expectations within the diagnostic appointment.

CONTROLLING CHRONIC PAIN: MATCHING TREATMENTS TO THE PATIENT WITH PAIN

An accurate diagnosis is the foundation for pain management. For patients with chronic pain, the diagnosis should include information about both the primary causes and the secondary contributing factors so that treatments can be targeted at each relevant factor. Because these factors may vary over time, pain assessment remains a critical component of any treatment regimen. The focus of continuing assessment is the individual with pain—not only the pain features but also the situational factors that modulate pain. Even when pain is due to actively progressing disease, such as for patients with advanced cancer, many other factors can affect pain and suffering. Health care providers need to assess these factors and target their treatments accordingly.

For example, we have been consulted by clinicians treating children receiving palliative care, whose pain had been well controlled with large (and presumably appropriate) opioid doses, but who were now experiencing increasingly frequent episodes of breakthrough pain. For some children, the increased pain signified advancing disease, requiring increased medication. But for other children, it signified increasing emotional distress related to their fears about death. These children needed counseling to relieve their distress and concomitantly lessen their pain.

Ongoing patient-centered assessments need not be onerous. In our clinic, we use the pain model (shown in Figs. 1 and 2) to provide a general framework for assessing the relevant factors that can increase pain, intensify distress, and exacerbate disability. We have shaped this model in stages over the past 20 years as we have applied the principles of pain modulation, accruing from laboratory studies in humans and primates, to the clinical management of different pain problems in adults and children (McGrath 1983, 1990; McGrath and Hillier 2003). This model enables us to communicate easily with patients about the need for a patient-centered assessment, explain the results of the diagnostic pain consultation, and present the rationale for a particular treatment regimen.

The effective treatment of chronic pain usually requires a multimodal approach comprising physical, pharmacological, and psychological therapies. Psychological interventions are an essential component of most treatment programs because of the many cognitive, behavioral, and emotional factors that can affect pain and disability. Individualized programs are potentially the optimal and most practical interventions because they match treatments to the particular needs of each patient. Specific therapies based on the assessment results can target the responsible central and peripheral mechanisms and mitigate the pain-exacerbating impact of situational factors.

Thus, the emphasis is on the multifactorial etiology of pain and the need for a multimodal treatment approach. This treatment rationale is in direct contrast to the "single cause and single treatment" approach that is normally adequate for relieving acute pain.

PRACTICAL PSYCHOLOGICAL STRATEGIES IN CLINICAL PRACTICE

The renewed interest in the use of psychological interventions to reduce pain is a natural consequence of our increased knowledge of nociceptive processing, particularly the nature of endogenous pain-modulating systems, and the varied psychological factors that affect pain, as revealed by advanced imaging techniques. Prior to recent positron emission tomography and functional magnetic resonance imaging studies (see Chapters 5, 11), the choice of psychological intervention was frequently assumed as indicative of the psychological or functional nature of a pain complaint. However, today psychological methods are used routinely to treat acute and chronic pain problems for both adults and children.

The psychological interventions used to treat pain include stress management, attention and distraction techniques, art therapies, play therapies, guided imagery, hypnosis, counseling, psychotherapy, relaxation training, biofeedback, modeling, desensitization, and behavioral management. Many such therapies share a common individual-centered focus, addressing the unique factors contributing to each person's pain, distress, and disability.

COGNITIVE-BEHAVIORAL THERAPIES: SPECIALIZED PROGRAMS

Cognitive therapies focus on modifying an individual's beliefs, expectations, and coping abilities. They are a major component of specialized pain management programs for children (McGrath 1990; McGrath and Finley 1999; McGrath and Hillier 2001; Berde and Solodiuk 2003) and for adults (Gil et al. 1988; Turk and Monarch 2002; Turk and Gatchel 2002). Health care providers educate patients and families about the circumstances that exacerbate pain, often counseling them about how they can alter those circumstances (e.g., through lifestyle management, diet, sleep, and exercise). Therapists can teach patients how to use specific cognitive pain control methods such as attention and distraction, guided imagery, and self-hypnosis to complement their pharmacological pain management.

Behavioral interventions, often used in combination with cognitive therapy, are used to modify any behaviors that may increase pain or prolong disability. These interventions are targeted either for patients or for the family members (or health care staff) who respond to them when they experience pain. At the initial consultation, health care providers assess whether a patient's behaviors or those of significant others are influencing the pain. They recommend changes that will improve pain control and lessen disability. Alternatively, psychologists and therapists counsel families about the impact of their behaviors and help families to make changes using different reinforcement and conditioning strategies to positively alter behavior. In addition, they may teach patients specific behavioral pain control techniques, such as relaxation and biofeedback.

Often cognitive and behavioral methods are used in combination, as in our case examples, rather than independently. In fact, the term "cognitive-behavioral therapy" (CBT) has gradually emerged as the most appropriate description of comprehensive treatment programs for chronic pain. While the specific cognitive, behavioral, and physical components vary, these programs generally combine several treatment strategies and techniques to target the patient, family, and environmental factors contributing to pain and pain-related disability.

CBT programs have proven effective for lessening many types of acute and chronic pain, including postoperative pain (Good et al. 2002; LaMontagne et al. 2003), low back pain (Linton and Andersson 2000; Storheim et al. 2003), burn pain (Haythornthwaite et al. 2001), rheumatoid arthritis pain (Freeman et al. 2002), fibromyalgia (Walco and Ilowite 1992; Turk and Sherman 2002), complex regional pain syndrome (Lee et al. 2002; Nelson 2002), cancer pain (Liossi and Hatira 2003; Dalton et al. 2004), sciatica pain (Hasenbring et al. 1999), temporomandibular pain (Mishra et al. 2000), headache (McGrath et al. 1992; Kröner-Herwig et al. 1998; Sartory et al. 1998; McGrath and Hillier 2001), sickle cell disease (Gil et al. 2001), and procedural pain (Pederson 1996; Dahlquist et al. 2002). All CBT programs are based on a biopsychosocial perspective of pain wherein a dynamic interaction of biomedical, psychological, social, and environmental factors contributes to the experience of pain and to behavioral and emotional responses. Almost all randomized trials of CBT include pain severity or disability as the main outcome measures to evaluate its effectiveness. In contrast, relatively few controlled trials of CBT are designed to enable us to study the impact on the targeted psychosocial factors as well as pain outcomes.

Nevertheless, studies on patient beliefs specific to the clinical context of pain and its treatment support the importance of cognitive factors in pain management (DeGood and Shutty 1992; DeGood and Tait 2001; Pruitt and Von Korff 2002; Turk and Gatchel 2002). Beliefs, attitudes, and expectancies affect patients' reports of pain, the impact of pain on their lives, and their response to treatment (Flor and Turk 1988; Turk and Okifuji 1996;

Jensen et al. 1999, 2001; Burns et al. 2003). Chronic pain patients who believe that their pain is inexplicable show higher levels of psychological distress and have poor treatment compliance in comparison with patients who believe that health care providers understand their pain (Williams and Thorn 1989). Patients' feelings of helplessness and uncontrollability are associated with stronger pain and greater disability (Flor and Turk 1988; Keefe et al. 1989), while perceived control and appropriate information about active coping strategies are associated with less pain (Manning and Wright 1983; Mizener et al. 1988; Lawson et al. 1990; Burton et al. 1999). As demonstrated by such studies and illustrated in our previous case examples, cognitive factors shape our behaviors and emotions and affect our pain experience.

COGNITIVE-BEHAVIORAL THERAPIES: ROUTINE CLINICAL PRACTICE

Fortunately, many CBT principles can be applied regularly within clinical practice and not only in specialized pain clinics. These are high-impact and low-technology interventions. From a clinical perspective, our major challenge is to integrate what we already know about psychological pain modulation into our daily practice. Clinicians might find it helpful to "stop, look, and listen" when patients describe their pain problems. Irrespective of etiology, pain is plastic and complex. We cannot completely control pain by gearing our treatment solely to the putative source of tissue damage. Instead, we must also identify the contributing situational factors and target our interventions accordingly.

Patients may have similar pain features, but their pain problems may have very different causal and contributing factors. Certain cognitive, behavioral, and emotional factors are present for many patients with a similar pain condition, but their relevance as a primary cause or a secondary contributing factor varies. The diagnosis of a pain condition is more accurate when it includes an assessment of the relevant factors that can trigger pain attacks, intensify pain and distress, and prolong pain-related disability for particular individuals. An objective appraisal of these factors enables us to select the most appropriate drug or nondrug therapy for each patient with pain.

In the first consultation appointment, primary care providers have an opportunity to educate patients about the common factors that can exacerbate pain and make explicit recommendations for managing pain and preventing disability. For patients with complex pain problems, providers may wish to highlight the multifactorial etiology of the pain and the need for a multimodal treatment approach. Educating patients in this way may help them to become more attuned to the cognitive, behavioral, and emotional factors that could be contributing to their pain. In addition, this dialogue could facilitate the discussion of sensitive psychosocial factors that would otherwise remain hidden.

FUTURE CHALLENGES

Our major challenges are twofold—research and clinical practice. Although investigators are focusing renewed attention on conducting randomized clinical trials to evaluate the efficacy of many of the physical, pharmacological, and psychological interventions used extensively in clinical practice, we need to build from what we have learned and design studies to achieve research objectives broader than a simple determination of "Which treatment works better?" In particular, we need data on the efficacy of patient-centered treatment, in which psychological interventions are selected for the individual with pain, based on an assessment of the specific cognitive, behavioral, and emotional factors contributing to his or her pain and disability (McGrath and Holohan 2003).

Researchers should consider identifying the pain characteristics, individual factors, or social factors that might differentially affect treatment response. Although a biopsychosocial perspective is the cornerstone for chronic pain management, inadvertently many studies have focused almost exclusively on the intervention itself rather than on the intervention in relation to the person with pain. Clinically, psychological interventions are chosen to modify certain factors contributing to an individual's pain, emotional distress, and impaired functioning, and the impact of these problems on the family. However, researchers often fail to evaluate interventions within the context of these modulating factors and do not select outcomes appropriate to clinical goals. A broader focus would include more refined questions about treatment efficacy, aimed at matching treatments to the individual with pain.

We must recognize that we may compromise the efficacy of psychological interventions for chronic pain when we structure them into artificial formats (i.e., ones that we would not rigidly follow as clinicians) for the purpose of evaluating them in controlled trials. In most such trials, all patients receive certain "doses" of each component (e.g., imagery, biofeedback) over a prescribed number of sessions. In contrast, experienced therapists in clinical practice not only select psychological interventions for patients based on the initial assessment results, but also "titrate doses" (or add components) in accordance with how each patient progresses through the clinical sessions. To truly understand the efficacy of CBT for chronic pain, future study designs should demonstrate our knowledge of the dynamic interactions among the multiple factors that affect pain and disability.

Finally, we also need to address the longer-term efficacy of psychological interventions, the cost-effectiveness of treatments, and issues of treatment compliance and acceptance. In clinical practice, therapists shape CBT programs and treatment demands according to the needs of patients and their families. The emphasis is on selecting the best tools to address the specific factors responsible for pain and disability, rather than indiscriminately applying a particular set of tools. Typically, pain improvement is achieved after patients overcome a series of smaller milestones so that they (and their families) remain motivated to continue. Progress is evaluated over the long term rather than only at one discrete point. We need to creatively build these components into future studies.

In addition to these significant research challenges, we face a major clinical challenge in applying what we have learned to clinical practice. We already have a repertoire of effective therapies, individual-centered multimodal programs, and innovative ideas for implementing treatment guidelines in clinical practice. Optimal treatment for all patients begins with a differential diagnosis of pain that includes the relevant causative and contributing factors. A creative clinical approach enables health care providers to select the most appropriate therapies to modify the different factors that trigger pain attacks, intensify pain, and prolong disability for each patient with pain. We need to build from the research of the past two decades and incorporate our knowledge of the plasticity and complexity of pain into an effective biopsychosocial model for understanding and treating pain.

REFERENCES

Barrell JJ, Price DD. The perception of first and second pain as a function of psychological set. *Percept Psychophys* 1975; 17:163–166.
Berde CB, Solodiuk J. Multidisciplinary programs for management of acute and chronic pain in children. In: Schechter NL, Berde CB, Yaster M (Eds). *Pain in Infants, Children, and Adolescents.* Baltimore: Lippincott Williams & Wilkins, 2003, pp 471–486.
Burns JW, Kubilus A, Bruehl S, Harden RN, Lofland K. Do changes in cognitive factors influence outcome following multidisciplinary treatment for chronic pain? A cross-lagged panel analysis. *J Consult Clin Psychol* 2003; 71:81–91.
Burton AK, Waddell G, Tillotson KM, Summerton N. Information and advice to patients with back pain can have a positive effect: a randomized controlled trial of a novel educational booklet in primary care. *Spine* 1999; 24:2484–2491.
Dahlquist LM, Busby SM, Slifer KJ, et al. Distraction for children of different ages who undergo repeated needle sticks. *J Pediatr Oncol Nurs* 2002; 19:22–34.
Dalton JA, Keefe FJ, Carlson J, Youngblood R. Tailoring cognitive-behavioral treatment for cancer pain. *Pain Manag Nurs* 2004; 5:3–18.
DeGood DE, Shutty MS. Assessment of pain beliefs, coping, and self-efficacy. In: Turk DC, Melzack R (Eds). *Handbook of Pain Assessment.* New York: Guilford Press, 1992, pp 214–234.

DeGood DE, Tait RC. Assessment of pain beliefs and coping. In: Turk DC, Melzack R (Eds). *Handbook of Pain Assessment*. New York: Guilford Press, 2001, pp 320–345.

Dubner R, Hoffman DS, Hayes RL. Neuronal activity in medullary dorsal horn of awake monkeys trained in a thermal discrimination task. III. Task-related responses and their functional role. *J Neurophysiol* 1981; 46:444–464.

Flor H, Turk DC. Chronic back pain and rheumatoid arthritis: predicting pain and disability from cognitive variables. *J Behav Med* 1988; 11:251–265.

Freeman K, Hammond A, Lincoln NB. Use of cognitive-behavioural arthritis education programmes in newly diagnosed rheumatoid arthritis. *Clin Rehabil* 2002; 16:828–836.

Gil KM, Ross SL, Keefe FJ. Behavioral treatment of chronic pain: four pain management protocols. In: France RD, Krishnan KR (Eds). *Chronic Pain*. New York: American Psychiatric Association, 1988, pp 376–414.

Gil KM, Anthony KK, Carson JW, et al. Daily coping practice predicts treatment effects in children with sickle cell disease. *J Pediatr Psychol* 2001; 26:163–173.

Good M, Anderson GC, Stanton-Hicks M, Grass JA, Makii M. Relaxation and music reduce pain after gynecologic surgery. *Pain Manage Nurs* 2002; 3:61–70.

Gruner OC. *Treatise on the Canon of Medicine of Avicenna*. London: Luzac, 1930.

Hasenbring M, Ulrich HW, Hartmann M, Soyka D. The efficacy of a risk factor-based cognitive behavioral intervention and electromyographic biofeedback in patients with acute sciatic pain: an attempt to prevent chronicity. *Spine* 1999; 24:2525–2535.

Haythornthwaite JA, Lawrence JW, Fauerbach JA. Brief cognitive interventions for burn pain. *Ann Behav Med* 2001; 23:42–49.

Jensen MP, Romano JM, Turner JA, Good AB, Wald LH. Patient beliefs predict patient functioning: further support for a cognitive-behavioural model of chronic pain. *Pain* 1999; 81:95–104.

Jensen MP, Turner JA, Romano JM. Changes in beliefs, catastrophizing, and coping are associated with improvement in multidisciplinary pain treatment. *J Consult Clin Psychol* 2001; 69:655–662.

Johnson JE. Effects of accurate expectations about the sensations on the sensory and distress components of pain. *J Pers Soc Psychol* 1973; 27:261–275.

Keefe FJ, Brown GK, Wallston KA, Caldwell DS. Coping with rheumatoid arthritis pain: catastrophizing as a maladaptive strategy. *Pain* 1989; 37:51–56.

Kröner-Herwig B, Mohn U, Pothmann R. Comparison of biofeedback and relaxation in the treatment of pediatric headache and the influence of parent involvement on outcome. *Appl Psychophysiol Biofeedback* 1998; 23:143–157.

LaMontagne LL, Hepworth JT, Cohen F, Salisbury MH. Cognitive-behavioral intervention effects on adolescents' anxiety and pain following spinal fusion surgery. *Nurs Res* 2003; 52:183–190.

Lawson K, Reesor KA, Keefe FJ, Turner JA. Dimensions of pain-related cognitive coping: cross-validation of the factor structure of the Coping Strategy Questionnaire. *Pain* 1990; 43:195–204.

Lee BH, Scharff L, Sethna NF, et al. Physical therapy and cognitive-behavioral treatment for complex regional pain syndromes. *J Pediatr* 2002; 141:135–140.

Linton SJ, Andersson T. Can chronic disability be prevented? A randomized trial of a cognitive-behavior intervention and two forms of information for patients with spinal pain. *Spine* 2000; 25:2825–2831.

Liossi C, Hatira P. Clinical hypnosis in the alleviation of procedure-related pain in pediatric oncology patients. *Int J Clin Exp Hypn* 2003; 51:4–28.

Manning MM, Wright TL. Self-efficacy expectancies, outcome expectancies, and the persistence of pain control in childbirth. *J Pers Soc Psychol* 1983; 45:421–431.

McGrath PA. Biologic basis of pain and analgesia: the role of situational variables in pain control. *Anesth Prog* 1983; 30:137–146.

McGrath PA. *Pain in Children: Nature, Assessment and Treatment*. New York: Guilford Press, 1990.

McGrath PA, Hillier LM (Eds). *The Child with Headache: Diagnosis and Treatment,* Progress in Pain Research and Management, Vol. 19. Seattle: IASP Press, 2001.

McGrath PA, Hillier LM. Modifying the psychological factors that intensify children's pain and prolong disability. In: Schechter NL, Berde C, Yaster M (Eds). *Pain in Infants, Children, and Adolescents.* Baltimore: Lippincott, Williams & Wilkins, 2003, pp 85–104.

McGrath PA, Holahan A-L. Psychological interventions with children and adolescents: evidence for their effectiveness in treating chronic pain. *Semin Pain Med* 2003; 1:99–109.

McGrath PA, Brooke R, Varkey M. Analgesic efficacy and subject expectation for clinical and experimental pain. *Pain* 1981; (Suppl 1):S13.

McGrath PJ, Finley GA (Eds). *Chronic and Recurrent Pain in Children and Adolescents,* Progress in Pain Research and Management, Vol. 13. Seattle: IASP Press, 1999.

McGrath PJ, Humphreys P, Keene D, et al. The efficacy and efficiency of a self-administered treatment for adolescent migraine. *Pain* 1992; 49:321–324.

Mishra KD, Gatchel RJ, Gardea MA. The relative efficacy of three cognitive-behavioral treatment approaches to temporomandibular disorders. *J Behav Med* 2000; 23:293–309.

Mizener D, Thomas M, Billings R. Cognitive changes of migraineurs receiving biofeedback training. *Headache* 1988; 28:339–343.

Nelson DV. Treating patients with complex regional pain syndrome. In: Turk DC, Gatchel RJ (Eds). *Psychological Approaches to Pain Management: A Practitioner's Handbook.* New York: Guilford Press, 2002, pp 470–488.

Pederson C. Promoting parental use of nonpharmacologic techniques with children during lumbar punctures. *J Pediatr Oncol Nurs* 1996; 13:21–30.

Pruitt SD, Von Korff M. Improving the management of low back pain: a paradigm shift. In: Turk DC, Gatchel RJ (Eds). *Psychological Approaches to Pain Management: A Practitioner's Handbook.* New York: Guilford Press, 2002, pp 301–316.

Sartory G, Muller B, Metsch J, Pothmann R. A comparison of psychological and pharmacological treatment of pediatric migraine. *Behav Res Ther* 1998; 36:1155–1170.

Storheim K, Brox JI, Holm I, Koller AK, Bo K. Intensive group training versus cognitive intervention in sub-acute low back pain: short-term results of a single-blind randomized controlled trial. *J Rehabil Med* 2003; 35:132–140.

Turk DC, Gatchel RJ. *Psychological Approaches to Pain Management: A Practitioner's Handbook.* New York: Guilford Press, 2002.

Turk DC, Monarch ES. Biopsychosocial perspective on chronic pain. In: Turk DC, Gatchel RJ (Eds). *Psychological Approaches to Pain Management: A Practitioner's Handbook.* New York: Guilford Press, 2002, pp 3–29.

Turk DC, Okifuji A. Perception of traumatic onset, compensation status, and physical findings: impact on pain severity, emotional distress, and disability in chronic pain patients. *J Behav Med* 1996; 19:435–453.

Turk DC, Sherman JF. Treatment of patients with fibromyalgia. In: Turk DC, Gatchel RJ (Eds). *Psychological Approaches to Pain Management: A Practitioner's Handbook.* New York: Guilford Press, 2002, pp 390–416.

von Graffenried B, Adler R, Abt K, Nuesch E, Spiegel R. The influence of anxiety and pain sensitivity on experimental pain in man. *Pain* 1978; 4:253–263.

Walco GA, Ilowite NT. Cognitive-behavioral intervention for juvenile primary fibromyalgia syndrome. *J Rheumatol* 1992; 19:1617–1619.

Williams DA, Thorn BE. An empirical assessment of pain beliefs. *Pain* 1989; 36:351–358.

Correspondence to: Patricia A. McGrath, PhD, Chronic Pain Program, Department of Anaesthesiology, The Hospital for Sick Children, 555 University Avenue, Toronto, ON, Canada M5G 1X8. Tel: 416-813-6467; Fax: 416-813-7543; email: patricia.mcgrath@sickkids.ca.

Part II

Modulation of Pain by Attention, Cognitive Factors, and Emotions

Psychological Methods of Pain Control: Basic Science and Clinical Perspectives, Progress in Pain Research and Management, Vol. 29, edited by Donald D. Price and M. Catherine Bushnell, IASP Press, Seattle, © 2004.

5

Psychophysical and Neurophysiological Studies of Pain Modulation by Attention

M. Catherine Bushnell,[a,b] Chantal Villemure,[a] and Gary H. Duncan[c]

[a]Centre for Research on Pain and [b]Departments of Anesthesia and Dentistry, McGill University, Montreal, Quebec, Canada; [c]Faculty of Dental Medicine, University of Montreal, Montreal, Quebec, Canada

A child bumps her knee and runs crying to her mother. What does the parent do? She gives the child a hug, which helps improve mood and reduce anxiety, and then finds something to distract the child—an ice cream cone, a game, the child's favorite video. We all instinctively know that changes in psychological state somehow help to reduce pain. Nevertheless, until recently little was known about how psychological modulation of pain is achieved, nor whether it changes the pain experience itself or only pain-related behavior. This chapter will describe studies of attentional modulation of pain in the clinical setting, controlled psychophysical studies that objectively assess the effects of attention on pain, and human and animal neurophysiological studies that address the mechanisms of attentional modulation of pain.

CLINICAL STUDIES OF ATTENTION AND DISTRACTION

The use of distraction and directed attention to reduce pain and distress in patients has a long history in health care. The clinical application of distraction has been described in many settings, including injections in children, dental procedures, wound cleaning in burn patients, and procedures such as tissue biopsies and lumbar punctures in cancer patients (Hoffman et al. 2000; Frere et al. 2001; Haythornthwaite et al. 2001; Aitken et al. 2002; Cohen 2002; Landolt et al. 2002; Sander et al. 2002; Bentsen et al. 2003;

Kwekkeboom 2003). Different types of distractors have been used, including music (Kwekkeboom 2003), cartoon movies (Landolt et al. 2002), and most recently 3D (three-dimensional) video glasses (Bentsen et al. 1999, 2003; Hoffman et al. 2000, 2001; Frere et al. 2001; Sander et al. 2002). The results of clinical distraction studies are variable, with some reports of excellent pain relief and others finding no relief at all. Such variability can be attributed both to a lack of control of the patient's attentional state in some studies and to pain conditions that are too severe to be adequately controlled by psychological state. Nevertheless, as we will describe below, strong psychophysical and neurophysiological evidence shows that changes in attention alter activity in pain-related pathways and consequently modify the painful experience.

PSYCHOPHYSICAL STUDIES OF ATTENTION

Attention can be manipulated in several ways. The most general attentional manipulation used to modify pain is to distract the individual either by presenting an interesting stimulus, such as music or a video, or by having the person perform some attention-demanding task, such as mental arithmetic. Such manipulations are fairly simple to employ, but usually attention is not the only variable that changes. When a person is performing mental arithmetic, his anxiety may well increase, his mood may be altered, and he may become more alert and vigilant. The presentation of music or a video also is likely to alter mood, anxiety, arousal, and vigilance. Each of these variables could contribute to changes in the pain experience. An additional problem with interpreting data from simple distraction tasks is that there is no measure of the subject's attentional state. Some people may pay attention to music in the face of pain, whereas others may continue to focus on the pain. Although the performance of mental arithmetic requires attention to that task, for those who are mathematically gifted, the amount of attention required is much less than for other, less mathematically inclined individuals.

A more controlled manner in which to change attention utilizes a psychophysical paradigm involving two balanced conditions. For example, in the cross-modality attention paradigm, stimuli from two sensory modalities (such as lights and tones) are presented simultaneously, and subjects are asked to perform tasks that require attention to one or the other modality in order to maximize their psychophysical performance. The tasks can be equated for difficulty, and task performance can be used as a parametric measure of attentional status. Such paradigms have the advantage of controlling for level of arousal and vigilance because the same stimuli are presented in all trials, task difficulty is equated between the two modalities, and only the direction of attention changes.

A variant of the balanced-condition psychophysical approach is the intra-modal spatial attention paradigm. Tasks can be utilized in which identical stimuli are presented simultaneously to different receptive fields (different body regions for somatosensory stimuli), and subjects are directed to perform tasks that require their attention to one or the other location. Intramodal spatial attention has been studied extensively in the visual and auditory systems (Andersen 1995; Hikosaka et al. 1996; Corbetta and Shulman 2002). Nevertheless, when this paradigm is applied to the pain system, a complication arises that is not present for other sensory modalities, because the simultaneous presentation of two noxious stimuli may engage another modulatory system, diffuse noxious inhibitory controls (DNICs), which could evoke changes in pain perception (Le Bars et al. 1979a,b; Talbot et al. 1987; Bouhassira et al. 1988; Price and McHaffie 1988) independent of those occasioned by shifts of spatial attention.

Finally, a balanced-condition psychophysical approach can involve shifts of attention to different dimensions of the same stimulus, within a single stimulus modality. When looking at a visual stimulus, for example, one can attend to different features, such as color, shape, motion, or texture. Attentional shifts from one feature to another alter neural activity in different parts of the visual system that process specific features of visual stimuli (Barrett et al. 2001; Vandenberghe et al. 2001; Giesbrecht et al. 2003; Liu et al. 2003). Similarly, when a painful stimulus is presented, subjects can be asked to attend to the quality of the sensation, such as the burning, stinging, or aching associated with the pain. Conversely, they can be asked to attend to the unpleasantness associated with the sensation. As described below, such manipulations can alter both the pain experience and pain-evoked neural activity.

EXPERIMENTAL STUDIES OF DISTRACTION

A number of studies have compared ratings of experimental pain stimuli with and without a distracter present. The cold pressor paradigm, in which subjects immerse their hand into a cold-water bath, has been used in various studies (e.g., Leventhal et al. 1979; McCaul and Haugtvedt 1982; Hodes et al. 1990; Johnson and Petrie 1997; Bentsen et al. 1999; Keogh et al. 2000). In some studies, subjects were simply asked to distract themselves, to focus their attention toward or away from the pain, or to imagine something else

(Leventhal et al. 1979; McCaul and Haugtvedt 1982; Arntz et al. 1991; Janssen and Arntz 1996; Johnson and Petrie 1997). In others, they performed some attention-demanding task such as mental arithmetic or word shadowing (Hodes et al. 1990; Johnson and Petrie 1997). Finally, some studies have used sensory distracters such as 3D video glasses (Bentsen et al. 1999). Although these studies differ somewhat in their findings, overwhelmingly they show that subjects report less pain when they are distracted. Nevertheless, as indicated above, the specificity of this modulation to mechanisms of directed attention is difficult to infer because other factors, such as vigilance, mood, or anxiety, are not controlled in these paradigms and thus could contribute to the overall modulatory effect.

CROSS-MODAL ATTENTION STUDIES

Several studies have more specifically examined the modulatory effects of directed attention within the context of cross-modality psychophysical paradigms where subjects must switch their attention between pain and another sensory modality, such as vision, audition, or olfaction. Miron et al. (1989) presented painful heat pulses simultaneously with a visual stimulus (white light) and asked subjects to detect small changes in the intensity of one stimulus or the other. The detection task was made difficult enough that subjects could not perform with 100% accuracy, and stimulus changes were chosen so that level of performance was similar when subjects were detecting changes in the painful heat or the visual stimulus. Both speed and accuracy of detecting the stimulus changes decreased when the subject attended to another stimulus modality. Further, direction of attention affected the perceived intensity and unpleasantness of the painful stimulus. When subjects were asked to try to divide their attention between the two modalities, both their reaction times and pain ratings indicated that they attended more to the painful stimulus than to the visual stimulus. These results suggest that although we are able to divert our attention away from pain, if we do not actively do so, pain will tend to automatically attract our attention. Spence et al. (2002) extended the findings of Miron et al.'s study to a situation in which a visual stimulus and a pain stimulus were presented on the same skin site, using a painful laser heat stimulus and a spot illuminated by a light-emitting diode. These investigators observed cross-modality attentional changes in speed of detecting a stimulus change, even when the spatial location of the stimuli was the same.

Bushnell et al. (1999) found similar attentional effects when subjects alternated their attention between painful heat stimuli and auditory stimuli.

Further, this study observed greater changes in perceived pain intensity than in pain unpleasantness, suggesting a more robust effect within circuitry underlying the sensory dimension of pain. Similarly, Villemure et al. (2003), using a cross-modality attention paradigm involving olfactory stimuli and painful heat pulses, found that direction of attention significantly altered perceived pain intensity, with a lesser nonsignificant effect on pain unpleasantness, thus further supporting the idea that cross-modality attention may alter the sensory dimension of pain more than the unpleasantness dimension (Fig. 1a). Nevertheless, all of the above studies required that subjects attend to a sensory feature of the stimulus (i.e., stimulus intensity); attending to emotional aspects of a stimulus might well alter the affective aspect of pain perception more than the sensory (see Chapter 6).

SPATIAL ATTENTION STUDIES

Bushnell et al. (1985) used a spatial attention task in which two contact thermodes were placed above the upper lip, one on each side of the face. Both thermodes were heated simultaneously to a painful temperature, and after an unpredictable time, the temperature of one increased again. Subjects were instructed to release a lever in response to the second stimulus change, regardless of the perceived location. The desired direction of spatial attention was signaled to the subject by indicator lights representing either one or the other of the two thermode locations; attention to the desired location was reinforced by an 80% probability that the stimulus change would occur at that position, thus bestowing a behavioral advantage for subjects trying to maximize their speed in detecting the changes in pain intensity. Results of this study confirmed that subjects followed instructions to switch their attention between two stimulus locations, in that stimulus changes were detected more rapidly when they occurred on the signaled thermode. In addition, these results indicated that spatial attention modulates the perception of the perceived intensity of pain stimuli, because subjects were less accurate in detecting the stimulus change if it occurred outside their attentional focus. This study also suggests that mechanisms of directed attention in the spatial domain most likely involve areas of the nervous system that exhibit a fine somatotopic organization (and separation) of nociceptive information. Such perceptual effects of spatial attention are not unique to pain, but instead are shared with other sensory modalities such as vision and audition and are essential for orienting to important features of our environment (Posner 1980).

a. Main effect of attention

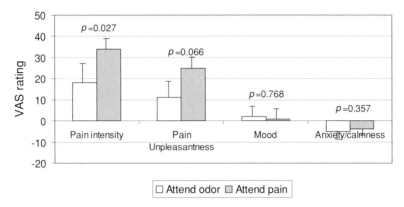

b. Main effect of odor valence

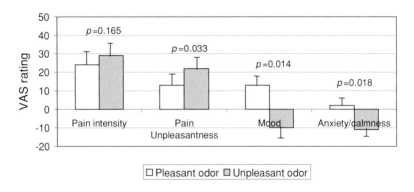

Fig. 1. Main effects of attention and odor valence on visual analogue scale (VAS) ratings of pain intensity, pain unpleasantness, mood, and anxiety/calmness. Because as a group subjects rated the thermal stimuli as painful and unpleasant, the original scales of pain intensity and hedonics were transformed for more clarity so that 0 represents pain threshold/neutral and 100 represents the most intense pain tolerable/extremely unpleasant. For mood, 0 is neutral, 100 is extremely good, and −100 is extremely bad. For anxiety/calmness, 0 is neutral, 100 is extremely calm, and −100 is extremely anxious. (a) Direction of attention had no effect on mood and anxiety, but altered both perceived pain intensity and unpleasantness. (b) Odor valence altered mood, anxiety, and pain unpleasantness ratings but did not significantly affect perceived pain intensity. (Reprinted from Villemure et al. 2003, with permission.)

INTRA-MODAL ATTENTION STUDIES

In addition to focusing attention on another stimulus modality or another spatial location, it is possible to move attention from one feature or dimension of a stimulus to another. Several studies indicate that the unpleasantness or overall painfulness of the pain can be decreased by attending to its sensory features, such as the burning, pricking, or aching sensation. Haythornthwaite et al. (2001) found that sensory focusing in burn patients having their dressings changed led to greater pain relief than did music distraction. Similarly, Hadjistavropoulos et al. (2000) observed that chronic pain patients who were particularly anxious about their health reported less anxiety and discomfort when they restricted their attentional focus to the physical sensations associated with their chronic pain. In the experimental situation, Keogh et al. (2000) observed that men reported less cold-pressor pain when they attended to the sensation of the pain than when they tried to avoid it altogether; this effect did not occur in female subjects. One possible explanation for the paradoxical findings that men felt less pain by attending to it could be that they were focusing on the cold sensation, and this sensory focusing reduced the painfulness of the situation.

EFFECTS OF PERSONALITY VARIABLES ON ATTENTIONAL MODULATION OF PAIN

There has been little direct experimental investigation of the effects of personality variables on pain processing. James and Hardardottir (2002) observed that subjects with low trait anxiety had a greater effect of distraction on cold-pressor pain tolerance than did subjects with high trait anxiety. Unpublished data from our laboratory indicate that personality variables such as neuroticism, extraversion, openness, agreeableness, and conscientiousness, as measured by the NEO Five-Factor Inventory (McCrae 1991), do not alter the degree of attentional modulation of pain, although there was a tendency for subjects low in neuroticism to have a greater effect of distraction on pain unpleasantness. However, when an embedded figures test was used to assess cognitive style (Witkin et al. 1971), subjects with high field independence (those who could more easily pick out the embedded figure) showed more robust attentional effects on perceived pain intensity than did those with low field independence (C. Villemure, M.C. Bushnell, T. Peixe, and L. Mozessohn, unpublished data).

SEPARATING ATTENTION FROM EMOTIONS

Clinical studies indicate that a patient's attitude and emotional state can affect his or her perception of pain associated with chronic disease (Haythornthwaite and Benrud-Larson 2000; Schanberg et al. 2000). Laboratory studies confirm these observations, demonstrating that pleasant stimuli, such as music and humorous films, improve mood and generally reduce pain perception (Cogan et al. 1987; Zelman et al. 1991; Good 1996; Weisenberg et al. 1998; De Wied and Verbaten 2001; Meagher et al. 2001; Marchand and Arsenault 2002). However, such stimuli will usually alter attentional state as well as mood, so the effects of the two variables are confounded. Villemure et al. (2003) used a cross-modality attention task similar to those of Miron et al. (1989) and Bushnell et al. (1999), except that attention was alternated between painful heat and olfactory stimuli. In this study, instead of using hedonically neutral stimuli, such as white lights and pure tones, the investigators used odors that the subjects perceived as clearly pleasant or unpleasant. They then independently manipulated direction of attention and emotional state, using tasks involving heat pain and pleasant and unpleasant odors. Shifts in attention between the thermal and olfactory modalities altered pain perception, but not mood or anxiety. However, when subjects focused attention on the pain, they perceived it as clearly more intense and somewhat more unpleasant than when they attended to the odor (Fig. 1a). In contrast, odor valence altered mood, anxiety level, and pain unpleasantness, but did not change the perception of pain intensity (Fig. 1b). Although odor valence modulated both mood and pain unpleasantness, the changes in pain unpleasantness correlated only with mood, and not with odor valence, suggesting that emotional changes, triggered by differences in odor valence, underlie the selective modulation of pain affect. The results of this study show that the effects of emotion and attention can be separated and that these variables differentially alter pain perception.

EFFECT OF ATTENTION AND DISTRACTION ON PAIN-EVOKED ACTIVITY IN THE BRAIN

A few studies have been performed in nonhuman primates in which attentional state was manipulated and action potentials were recorded from isolated nociceptive neurons in the spinal cord and brain (Bushnell et al. 1984; Bushnell and Duncan 1989). These studies revealed that for some neurons in the dorsal horn and the thalamus, the activity evoked by a noxious stimulus was enhanced when the monkey performed a task that required attention to the noxious stimulus, compared to that observed when the monkey received the same noxious stimulus, but performed a task that required attention to be diverted to a visual stimulus (Fig. 2). These studies were the first to demonstrate that the modulatory effect of attention on nociceptive processing involves descending pathways from the brain to the first synapse in the dorsal horn. This type of modulation had been anticipated by

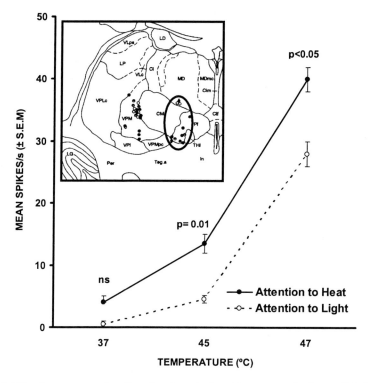

Fig. 2. Stimulus-response function showing single-cell responses in the medial thalamus (location shown in inset) during thermal stimuli of 35°C, 45°C, and 49°C presented with a 1-cm² thermode on the maxillary face of a monkey. The solid line shows the responses when the monkey was required to attend to the thermal stimuli, and the dashed line shows responses to the same temperatures when the monkey was required to attend to a visual stimulus. (Adapted from Bushnell and Duncan 1989, with permission.)

existing theories of pain (e.g., the gate control theory), but had never before been demonstrated in a behavioral context.

Human studies, using non-invasive imaging techniques to examine the effects of attention and distraction, show modulation of pain-evoked activity in the thalamus and in several cortical regions, including the primary soma-tosensory cortex (S1), anterior cingulate cortex (ACC), and insular cortex (IC) (Bushnell et al. 1999; Longe et al. 2001; Bantick et al. 2002; Brooks et al. 2002). Peyron et al. (1999) compared a pain-attention condition, in which subjects counted the number of painful heat pulses that they received, to a condition in which they were asked to perform a repetitive iteration from 1 to 10. Fig. 3 shows that several brain regions were more activated when the subjects focused on the painful stimulus than when they did not. Using a cross-modality attention task involving painful heat and auditory stimuli, as described above, Bushnell et al. (1999) showed the greatest attentional modulation of pain-evoked activity in the S1 cortex, perhaps because the subjects were attending to a sensory feature of the stimulus (Fig. 4, top panel). A reciprocal modulation was observed in the primary auditory cortex, in that this region was activated more when the subjects attended to the auditory stimulus than to the painful heat stimulus (Fig. 4, bottom panel), thus showing the generality of attentional modulation across sensory modalities. As shown in Fig. 5, other regions, including the periaqueductal gray matter (PAG), parts of the ACC, and the orbitofrontal cortex show activation when subjects are distracted from pain, suggesting that these regions may be involved in the modulatory circuitry related to attention (Petrovic et al. 2000; Frankenstein et al. 2001; Tracey et al. 2002).

Electroencephalogram (EEG) and magnetoencephalograph (MEG) studies show that modulation of pain by attention probably involves both early sensory processing in the S2 and IC (Nakamura et al. 2002; Legrain et al. 2002) and later processing in the ACC (Beydoun et al. 1993a; Kanda et al. 1996; Siedenberg and Treede 1996; Garcia-Larrea et al. 1997). Involvement of early processing would be expected on the basis of the dorsal horn studies described above. Perceptual changes in pain related to attentional state appear to reflect in part a change in cortical processing and in part a decrease in ascending afferent input from the spinal cord due to activation of descending inhibitory controls. EEG signals can document this type of inhibitory control in humans (Plaghki et al. 1994; Reinert et al. 2000; Hoshiyama and Kakigi 2000).

Recent single-unit studies in nonhuman primates (Roy et al. 2000; Steinmetz et al. 2000) have suggested a local process within the somatosensory cortices that may underlie attention-related modulation of stimulus-evoked activity. In monkeys participating in a cross-modal attention task, similar to those described above, Steinmetz et al. (2000) reported that most neuron pairs responsive to the tactile stimuli fired in synchrony. Approximately 30% of those neuron pairs showing synchronous activity demonstrated a modulation in the degree of synchrony related to the monkey's

---

Fig. 4. Top row shows regions of increased pain-evoked activity when subjects were required to attend to the noxious heat stimulus presented with a 9-cm^2 thermode on the arm, compared to that observed when they were required to attend to a simultaneously presented auditory stimulus. The primary somatosensory cortex (S1) showed the largest attention-related modulation, but lesser effects were observed in the anterior cingulate cortex (ACC) and insular cortex (Insula). The bottom row shows regions in which there was more auditory-evoked activation when subjects attended to the auditory stimulus than to the painful stimulus. The only significant attention-related enhancement was observed in the primary auditory cortex, in the temporal lobe. (Adapted from Bushnell et al. 1999, with permission.) →

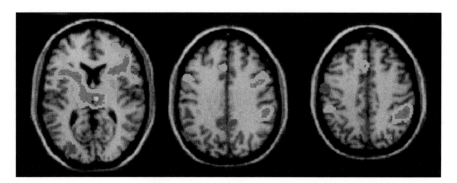

Fig. 3. Comparison of attentional versus non-attentional conditions, irrespective of stimulus intensity, showed a large network of attention-related rCBF increases involving the anterior cingulate cortex, thalami, and prefrontal and posterior parietal cortices bilaterally (shown as green, red, and white, respectively). Significantly decreases in rCBF were observed in the primary motor cortex contralateral to the stimulated hand, in the parieto-occipital cortex, and in the posterior cingulate cortex (shown as blue). (Adapted from Peyron et al. 1999, with permission.)

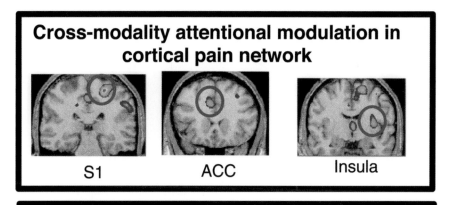

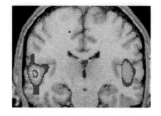

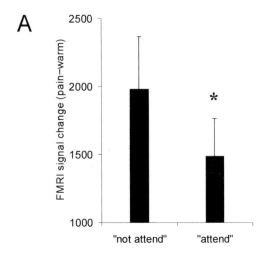

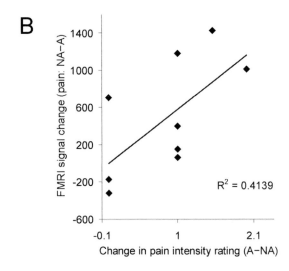

Fig. 5. (A) Total signal intensity (arbitrary units) within the periaqueductal gray (PAG) for the two attentional conditions (mean ± SE; *$P < 0.05$). (B) Correlation of total signal intensity change (arbitrary units) within the PAG and total change in pain intensity (visual analogue score) between the two conditions ($P < 0.025$). (From Tracey et al. 2002, with permission.)

attentional state—attending either to the tactile or to the visual stimuli during discrimination tasks. Although these results were obtained using innocuous tactile stimuli, a similar process is likely to underlie the modulation of pain-related activity by attentional processes.

EFFECT OF ANTICIPATION ON PAIN-EVOKED ACTIVITY

Anticipation or expectation of pain relief is a powerful means for producing placebo analgesia (see Chapters 8, 9, and 10). Conversely, the anticipation or expectation that something is going to be painful can activate pain-related areas, even in the absence of a physical pain stimulus. For example, regions such as S1, ACC, PAG, IC, prefrontal cortex, and cerebellum show activation during a period of expectation before the pain itself is presented (Beydoun et al. 1993b; Hsieh et al. 1999; Ploghaus et al. 1999; Sawamoto et al. 2000; Porro et al. 2002; Villemure and Bushnell 2002). Similarly, anticipation of painful stimuli, or priming with pain-related adjectives, significantly enhances EEG signals (Miyazaki et al. 1994; Dillmann et al. 2000). An example of enhancement of ACC activation when subjects anticipate a painful stimulus is shown in Fig. 6. When subjects received painful laser stimulation, there was significant activation in the ACC. Nonpainful stimulation showed only a small trend toward activation in the same region. However, when the nonpainful stimulus was presented, but the subjects expected a painful stimulus, ACC activity was enhanced and resembled that evoked by the "real" pain stimulus. A previous positron emission tomography (PET) imaging study (Drevets et al. 1995) suggested an attention-related focusing mechanism that might underlie enhanced responses to noxious stimuli that are anticipated or expected. In this study, expectation of an impending noxious stimulus did not, by itself, increase regional cerebral blood flow (rCBF) within the somatosensory cortices, but it did result in a general suppression of rCBF in both contralateral and ipsilateral regions of S1 outside the projected somatotopic target of the anticipated stimulus.

Anticipation-related changes in cerebral activity, reported above, may underlie numerous behavioral responses associated with changes in emotional state, preparation for dealing with the pending stimulus, and even activation of endogenous analgesic processes. However, few data support the notion that anticipation of pain, without the actual noxious stimulus, results in the perception of pain itself. Therefore, one must interpret with caution the direct relationship between pain perception and anticipation-related changes in activity within regions of the cortex that have been associated with pain-related activity (S1, ACC, and IC).

SUMMARY

In clinical situations, if a patient's pain changes with his or her psychological state, it is often believed that the pain is "inorganic," and the patient

Painful Stimulation   **Non-Painful Stimulation**   **Non-painful Stimulation**
                                 with Expectation of Pain   **Alone**

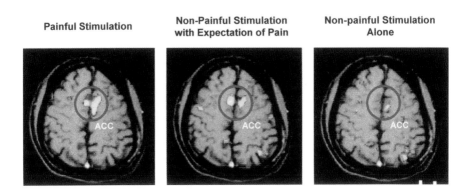

Fig. 6. Activation in the anterior cingulate cortex (ACC) for painful stimulation (left), nonpainful stimulation when expecting pain (center), and nonpainful stimulation when expecting warmth (right). Activated areas, which showed significant transient signal increase time-locked to the stimulus, are superimposed on the subject's own structural MRI. (Adapted from Sawamoto et al. 2000, with permission.)

is dismissed as being neurotic, unstable, attention-seeking, or worse. However, as shown above, overwhelming evidence indicates that psychological modulation of pain has genuine physiological underpinnings. Our ability to focus attention is essential to our well-being and allows us to extract relevant information from the environment. Because pain is normally an alerting signal that leads us to escape or avoid tissue damage, it has a strong attentional demand. When pain becomes chronic, the need for it to attract our attention is diminished, so it is in our best interest to direct our attention elsewhere. As shown above, directing attention away from pain reduces its perceived intensity, as well as inhibiting underlying neural activity that is responsible for our pain perception. Thus, we may be able to better serve chronic pain patients by helping them to understand the importance of attentional state on their pain and, when appropriate, teaching them techniques of self-distraction.

REFERENCES

Aitken JC, Wilson S, Coury D, Moursi AM. The effect of music distraction on pain, anxiety and behavior in pediatric dental patients. *Pediatr Dent* 2002; 24:114–118.

Andersen RA. Encoding of intention and spatial location in the posterior parietal cortex. *Cereb Cortex* 1995; 5:457–469.

Arntz A, Dreessen L, Merckelbach H. Attention, not anxiety, influences pain. *Behav Res Ther* 1991; 29:41–50.

Bantick SJ, Wise RG, Ploghaus A, et al. Imaging how attention modulates pain in humans using functional MRI. *Brain* 2002; 125:310–319.

Barrett NA, Large MM, Smith GL, et al. Human cortical processing of colour and pattern. *Hum Brain Mapp* 2001; 13:213–225.

Bentsen B, Svensson P, Wenzel A. The effect of a new type of video glasses on the perceived intensity of pain and unpleasantness evoked by a cold pressor test. *Anesth Prog* 1999; 46:113–117.

Bentsen B, Wenzel A, Svensson P. Comparison of the effect of video glasses and nitrous oxide analgesia on the perceived intensity of pain and unpleasantness evoked by dental scaling. *Eur J Pain* 2003; 7:49–53.

Beydoun A, Morrow TJ, Shen JF, Casey KL. Variability of laser-evoked potentials: attention, arousal and lateralized differences. *Electroencephalogr Clin Neurophysiol* 1993a; 88:173–181.

Beydoun A, Morrow TJ, Shen JF, Casey KL. Variability of laser-evoked potentials: attention, arousal and lateralized differences. *Electroencephalogr Clin Neurophysiol* 1993b; 88:173–181.

Bouhassira D, Villanueva L, Le Bars D. Intracerebroventricular morphine decreases descending inhibitions acting on lumbar dorsal horn neuronal activities related to pain in the rat. *J Pharmacol Exp Ther* 1988; 247:332–342.

Brooks JC, Nurmikko TJ, Bimson WE, Singh KD, Roberts N. fMRI of thermal pain: effects of stimulus laterality and attention. *Neuroimage* 2002; 15:293–301.

Bushnell MC, Duncan GH. Sensory and affective aspects of pain perception: is medial thalamus restricted to emotional issues? *Exp Brain Res* 1989; 78:415–418.

Bushnell MC, Duncan GH, Dubner R, He LF. Activity of trigeminothalamic neurons in medullary dorsal horn of awake monkeys trained in a thermal discrimination task. *J Neurophysiol* 1984; 52:170–187.

Bushnell MC, Duncan GH, Dubner R, Jones RL, Maixner W. Attentional influences on noxious and innocuous cutaneous heat detection in humans and monkeys. *J Neurosci* 1985; 5:1103–1110.

Bushnell MC, Duncan GH, Hofbauer RK, et al. Pain perception: is there a role for primary somatosensory cortex? *Proc Natl Acad Sci USA* 1999; 96:7705–7709.

Cogan R, Cogan D, Waltz W, McCue M. Effects of laughter and relaxation on discomfort thresholds. *J Behav Med* 1987; 10:139–144.

Cohen LL. Reducing infant immunization distress through distraction. *Health Psychol* 2002; 21:207–211.

Corbetta M, Shulman GL. Control of goal-directed and stimulus-driven attention in the brain. *Nat Rev Neurosci* 2002; 3:201–215.

De Wied M, Verbaten MN. Affective pictures processing, attention, and pain tolerance. *Pain* 2001; 90:163–172.

Dillmann J, Miltner WH, Weiss T. The influence of semantic priming on event-related potentials to painful laser-heat stimuli in humans. *Neurosci Lett* 2000; 284:53–56.

Drevets WC, Burton H, Videen TO, et al. Blood flow changes in human somatosensory cortex during anticipated stimulation. *Nature* 1995; 373:249–252.

Frankenstein UN, Richter W, McIntyre MC, Remy F. Distraction modulates anterior cingulate gyrus activations during the cold pressor test. *Neuroimage* 2001; 14:827–836.

Frere CL, Crout R, Yorty J, McNeil DW. Effects of audiovisual distraction during dental prophylaxis. *J Am Dent Assoc* 2001; 132:1031–1038.

Garcia-Larrea L, Peyron R, Laurent B, Mauguiere F. Association and dissociation between laser-evoked potentials and pain perception. *Neuroreport* 1997; 8:3785–3789.

Giesbrecht B, Woldorff MG, Song AW, Mangun GR. Neural mechanisms of top-down control during spatial and feature attention. *Neuroimage* 2003; 19:496–512.

Good M. Effects of relaxation and music on postoperative pain: a review. *J Adv Nurs* 1996; 24:905–914.

Hadjistavropoulos HD, Hadjistavropoulos T, Quine A. Health anxiety moderates the effects of distraction versus attention to pain. *Behav Res Ther* 2000; 38:425–438.

Haythornthwaite JA, Benrud-Larson LM. Psychological aspects of neuropathic pain. *Clin J Pain* 2000; 16:S101–S105.

Haythornthwaite JA, Lawrence JW, Fauerbach JA. Brief cognitive interventions for burn pain. *Ann Behav Med* 2001; 23:42–49.

Hikosaka O, Miyauchi S, Shimojo S. Orienting a spatial attention—its reflexive, compensatory, and voluntary mechanisms. *Brain Res Cogn Brain Res* 1996; 5:1–9.

Hodes RL, Howland EW, Lightfoot N, Cleeland CS. The effects of distraction on responses to cold pressor pain. *Pain* 1990; 41:109–114.

Hoffman HG, Doctor JN, Patterson DR, Carrougher GJ, Furness TA III. Virtual reality as an adjunctive pain control during burn wound care in adolescent patients. *Pain* 2000; 85:305–309.

Hoffman HG, Garcia-Palacios A, Patterson DR, et al. The effectiveness of virtual reality for dental pain control: a case study. *Cyberpsychol Behav* 2001; 4:527–535.

Hoshiyama M, Kakigi R. After-effect of transcutaneous electrical nerve stimulation (TENS) on pain-related evoked potentials and magnetic fields in normal subjects. *Clin Neurophysiol* 2000; 111:717–724.

Hsieh JC, Stone-Elander S, Ingvar M. Anticipatory coping of pain expressed in the human anterior cingulate cortex: a positron emission tomography study. *Neurosci Lett* 1999; 262:61–64.

James JE, Hardardottir D. Influence of attention focus and trait anxiety on tolerance of acute pain. *Br J Health Psychol* 2002; 7:149–162.

Janssen SA, Arntz A. Anxiety and pain: attentional and endorphinergic influences. *Pain* 1996; 66:145–150.

Johnson MH, Petrie SM. The effects of distraction on exercise and cold pressor tolerance for chronic low back pain sufferers. *Pain* 1997; 69:43–48.

Kanda M, Fujiwara N, Xu X, et al. Pain-related and cognitive components of somatosensory evoked potentials following CO_2 laser stimulation in man. *Electroencephalogr Clin Neurophysiol* 1996; 100:105–114.

Keogh E, Hatton K, Ellery D. Avoidance versus focused attention and the perception of pain: differential effects for men and women. *Pain* 2000; 85:225–230.

Kwekkeboom KL. Music versus distraction for procedural pain and anxiety in patients with cancer. *Oncol Nurs Forum* 2003; 30:433–440.

Landolt MA, Marti D, Widmer J, Meuli M. Does cartoon movie distraction decrease burned children's pain behavior? *J Burn Care Rehabil* 2002; 23:61–65.

Le Bars D, Dickenson AH, Besson J-M. Diffuse noxious inhibitory controls (DNIC). I. Effects on dorsal horn convergent neurones in the rat. *Pain* 1979a; 6:283–304.

Le Bars D, Dickenson AH, Besson J-M. Diffuse noxious inhibitory controls (DNIC). II. Lack of effect on non-convergent neurones, supraspinal involvement and theoretical implications. *Pain* 1979b; 6:305–327.

Legrain V, Guerit JM, Bruyer R, Plaghki L. Attentional modulation of the nociceptive processing into the human brain: selective spatial attention, probability of stimulus occurrence, and target detection effects on laser evoked potentials. *Pain* 2002; 99:21–39.

Leventhal H, Brown D, Shacham S, Engquist G. Effects of preparatory information about sensations, threat of pain, and attention on cold pressor distress. *J Pers Soc Psychol* 1979; 37:688–714.

Liu T, Slotnick SD, Serences JT, Yantis S. Cortical mechanisms of feature-based attentional control. *Cereb Cortex* 2003; 13:1334–1343.

Longe SE, Wise R, Bantick S, et al. Counter-stimulatory effects on pain perception and processing are significantly altered by attention: an fMRI study. *Neuroreport* 2001; 12:2021–2025.

Marchand S, Arsenault P. Odors modulate pain perception: a gender-specific effect. *Physiol Behav* 2002; 76:251–256.

McCaul KD, Haugtvedt C. Attention, distraction, and cold-pressor pain. *J Pers Soc Psychol* 1982; 43:154–162.

McCrae RR. The five-factor model and its assessment in clinical settings. *J Pers Assess* 1991; 57:399–414.

Meagher MW, Arnau RC, Rhudy JL. Pain and emotion: effects of affective picture modulation. *Psychosom Med* 2001; 63:79–90.

Miron D, Duncan GH, Bushnell MC. Effects of attention on the intensity and unpleasantness of thermal pain. *Pain* 1989; 39:345–352.

Miyazaki M, Shibasaki H, Kanda M, et al. Generator mechanism of pain-related evoked potentials following CO_2 laser stimulation of the hand: scalp topography and effect of predictive warning signal. *J Clin Neurophysiol* 1994; 11:242–254.

Nakamura Y, Paur R, Zimmermann R, Bromm B. Attentional modulation of human pain processing in the secondary somatosensory cortex: a magnetoencephalographic study. *Neurosci Lett* 2002; 328:29–32.

Petrovic P, Petersson KM, Ghatan PH, Stone-Elander S, Ingvar M. Pain-related cerebral activation is altered by a distracting cognitive task. *Pain* 2000; 85:19–30.

Peyron R, Larrea L, Gregoire MC, et al. Haemodynamic brain responses to acute pain in humans: sensory and attentional networks. *Brain* 1999; 122:1765–1780.

Plaghki L, Delisle D, Godfraind JM. Heterotopic nociceptive conditioning stimuli and mental task modulate differently the perception and physiological correlates of short CO_2 laser stimuli. *Pain* 1994; 57:181–192.

Ploghaus A, Tracey I, Gati JS, et al. Dissociating pain from its anticipation in the human brain. *Science* 1999; 284:1979–1981.

Porro CA, Baraldi P, Pagnoni G, et al. Does anticipation of pain affect cortical nociceptive systems? *J Neurosci* 2002; 22:3206–3214.

Posner ME. Orienting of attention. *Q J Exp Psychol* 1980; 32:3–25.

Price DD, McHaffie JG. Effects of heterotopic conditioning stimuli on first and second pain: a psychophysical evaluation in humans. *Pain* 1988; 34:245–252.

Reinert A, Treede R, Bromm B. The pain inhibiting pain effect: an electrophysiological study in humans. *Brain Res* 2000; 862:103–110.

Roy A, Steinmetz PN, Niebur E. Rate limitations of unitary event analysis. *Neural Comput* 2000; 12:2063–2082.

Sander WS, Eshelman D, Steele J, Guzzetta CE. Effects of distraction using virtual reality glasses during lumbar punctures in adolescents with cancer. *Oncol Nurs Forum* 2002; 29:E8–E15.

Sawamoto N, Honda M, Okada T, et al. Expectation of pain enhances responses to nonpainful somatosensory stimulation in the anterior cingulate cortex and parietal operculum/posterior insula: an event-related functional magnetic resonance imaging study. *J Neurosci* 2000; 20:7438–7445.

Schanberg LE, Sandstrom MJ, Starr K, et al. The relationship of daily mood and stressful events to symptoms in juvenile rheumatic disease. *Arthritis Care Res* 2000; 13:33–41.

Siedenberg R, Treede RD. Laser-evoked potentials: exogenous and endogenous components. *Electroencephalogr Clin Neurophysiol* 1996; 100:240–249.

Spence C, Bentley DE, Phillips N, McGlone FP, Jones AK. Selective attention to pain: a psychophysical investigation. *Exp Brain Res* 2002; 145:395–402.

Steinmetz PN, Roy A, Fitzgerald PJ, et al. Attention modulates synchronized neuronal firing in primate somatosensory cortex. *Nature* 2000; 404:187–190.

Talbot JD, Duncan GH, Bushnell MC, Boyer M. Diffuse noxious inhibitory controls (DNICs): psychophysical evidence in man for intersegmental suppression of noxious heat perception by cold pressor pain. *Pain* 1987; 30:221–232.

Tracey I, Ploghaus A, Gati JS, et al. Imaging attentional modulation of pain in the periaqueductal gray in humans. *J Neurosci* 2002; 22:2748–2752.

Vandenberghe R, Gitelman DR, Parrish TB, Mesulam MM. Location- or feature-based targeting of peripheral attention. *Neuroimage* 2001; 14:37–47.

Villemure C, Bushnell MC. Cognitive modulation of pain: how do attention and emotion influence pain processing? *Pain* 2002; 95:195–199.

Villemure C, Slotnick BM, Bushnell MC. Effects of odors on pain perception: deciphering the roles of emotion and attention. *Pain* 2003; 106:101–108.

Weisenberg M, Raz T, Hener T. The influence of film-induced mood on pain perception. *Pain* 1998; 76:365–375.

Witkin HA, Oltman PK, Raskin E, Karp SA. *A Manual for the Embedded Figures Tests.* Palo Alto, CA: Consulting Psychologists Press, 1971.

Zelman DC, Howland EW, Nichols SN, Cleeland CS. The effects of induced mood on laboratory pain. *Pain* 1991; 46:105–111.

Correspondence to: M. Catherine Bushnell, PhD, McGill Centre for Research on Pain, 3640 University Street, Room M19, Montreal, Quebec, Canada H3A 2B2. Email: catherine.bushnell@mcgill.ca.

Psychological Methods of Pain Control: Basic Science and Clinical Perspectives, Progress in Pain Research and Management, Vol. 29, edited by Donald D. Price and M. Catherine Bushnell, IASP Press, Seattle, © 2004.

6

Pain and Emotions

Pierre Rainville

Department of Stomatology, Faculty of Dental Medicine, University of Montreal, Montreal, Quebec, Canada

The importance of emotions for the well-being of patients is generally acknowledged, but the specific psychological and physiological mechanisms by which emotions affect health are far from being fully understood. Emotions are intimately related to pain in many ways. The notion of suffering from pain corresponds to the strong negative emotion associated with the pain experience. Emotions also share a number of features with pain, including visceromotor responses and several experiential dimensions. Growing evidence shows that emotions do not simply occur in parallel with pain but rather play a critical role in its modulation, perhaps reflecting the important overlap between pain and emotion-related neurophysiological processes. This chapter introduces several perspectives on emotions and provides several examples taken from the experimental literature, demonstrating how each perspective may contribute to our understanding of the effects of emotion on pain. Clinical studies are briefly considered, and possible brain mechanisms are outlined.

NEGATIVE EMOTIONS AS A CONSTITUENT OF PAIN

The International Association for the Study of Pain defines pain as a "an unpleasant sensory and emotional experience associated with actual or potential tissue damage, or described in terms of such damage" (Merskey and Bogduk 1994). Price (1999) has proposed a slightly different definition in which pain is "a somatic perception containing (1) a bodily sensation with qualities like those reported during tissue-damaging stimulation, (2) an experienced threat associated with this sensation, and (3) a feeling of unpleasantness or other negative emotion based on this experienced threat" (pp. 1–2). In both definitions, negative emotions, at least in their most basic expression, are a constituent of the pain experience.

Price (1999) has further described stages of pain processing that distinguish between primary pain affect and secondary emotions (see Chapter 1). The primary affective stage refers to the immediate unpleasantness that is integral to the pain experience and intimately related to the sense of threat. The second stage is characterized by emotions related to the broader meaning of pain and by the evaluation of the consequences of pain. While the sensory experience and the first stage of pain affect are necessary and sufficient for an experience to be characterized as painful, the emotions associated with the secondary stage of pain affect complement the experience in relation to its broader significance and future implications.

WHAT IS AN EMOTION?

Several features are common to most theories of emotions. Emotions are triggered or induced by objects or events that are immediately present or evoked mentally and are evaluated, consciously or unconsciously, in order to appraise their relevance. Emotions include behavioral and expressive components along with a variety of responses that affect the physiological state of the body, which are considered to be adaptive and are at least partly inherited through evolutionary processes (e.g., Plutchik 1980). A subjective experience generally accompanies the perception of the emotion inducer and the associated responses. Although most theories of emotions will usually include each of those aspects, they disagree on several points regarding the general organization of emotion systems and the relative importance and causal role of each component.

DIMENSIONS OF EMOTIONS OR DISCRETE EMOTIONS

Emotions have been described along the dimension of valence based on opposite experiences (pleasure versus displeasure), action tendencies (approach versus avoidance), and arousal levels (calm versus excited). Although this view has provided an adequate model to begin investigating basic aspects and neural determinants of positive and negative emotions (e.g., Davidson 1999), it may be insufficient to account for the richness of emotional experiences. In contrast, the popular notion of emotion generally refers to the existence of discrete emotions such as fear, disgust, sadness, happiness, and surprise. Darwin (1872) had recognized some essential features of emotion expression across species and identified stereotypical

patterns of expressive behaviors (also see Ekman 1999). This original description has motivated several investigations of the distinctive features of
basic emotions (reviewed in Ortony and Turner 1990). This line of work has
been extended more recently to include the study of brain systems involved
in the recognition and experience of discrete basic emotions (e.g., Lane et al.
1997b; Damasio et al. 2000; Adolphs 2002).

VISCEROSOMATIC ACTIVITY DURING EMOTIONS

One aspect of emotion theories that has been quite controversial is the
nature and role of peripheral activity during emotions. In contrast to the
convincing evidence provided by Ekman (1999) about the universal stereotypical facial expression of basic emotions, the demonstration of distinctive
patterns of autonomic activity associated with separate emotions has been
more difficult to achieve. Unfortunately, peripheral activity has traditionally
been reduced to a single dimension of arousal to describe emotional states.
This reduction is an unacceptable oversimplification and does not account
for the complexity of somatic regulatory systems.

Over the last 20 years or so, specific patterns of autonomic activity have
been observed during the voluntary production of emotional facial expression and reliving of past emotional experiences (Ekman et al. 1983; also see
Levenson et al. 1990), and in response to visual (Collet et al. 1997) and
olfactory stimuli (Vernet-Maury et al. 1999). Similarly, we have observed
that the recall and reliving of emotional events produces patterns of cardio-
respiratory activity that distinguish fear, sadness, anger, and happiness
(Rainville et al. 2000; P. Rainville, unpublished manuscript). As physiological measurements are refined and expanded to include the visceral,
skeletomotor, hormonal, and immune systems, this line of research promises
to provide additional support to James's century-old theory that the felt
afferent signals from the viscera may contribute to the unique feelings associated with emotions (reprinted in James 1994).

COGNITIVE PROCESSES

The role of cognitive factors has been emphasized in some theories in
which peripheral activity contribute only to the felt level of arousal and not
to the quality of the emotion experienced. Evaluative processes (or appraisal)
are known to affect the emotion felt, as suggested by the seminal study
of Schacter and Singer (1962). Several versions of cognitive theories have
been proposed in which initial evaluative processes of an inducer and a
situation may occur unconsciously and trigger automatic emotional responses,

followed by secondary, more elaborate deliberations and elaboration of meanings (e.g., Lazarus 1991). Interestingly, these positions are consistent with the existence of at least two processing pathways in the brain involved in the analysis of, and response to, emotional inducers (Izard 1993; LeDoux 1996; Morris et al. 1998). These neurophysiological studies contribute to a reconciliation of the peripheral and cognitive views, in that a rudimentary appraisal and the activation of the corresponding neural mechanisms are sufficient to trigger autonomic responses and produce the corresponding "gut feelings" that characterize emotions and emotion-guided behaviors (e.g., Bechara et al. 1997, 1999; Bechara and Naqvi 2004). However, the complexity of autonomic responses associated with this basic appraisal remains to be determined, and we do not know whether higher-order evaluation processes are necessary to produce full-blown emotional states.

EXPERIENTIAL DIMENSIONS OF EMOTION

The last aspect of emotions that most theories acknowledge is the subjective experience, including the thoughts and feelings that accompany emotions. However, there are at least three distinct and partly complementary approaches to the phenomenology of emotions that are closely related to the theoretical perspective on emotion described above.

Self-report measures inspired by theories of discrete emotions typically require subjects to indicate, and rate the intensity of, each emotion felt. These measures are sometimes used in pain assessment questionnaires (e.g., see Wade et al. 1990). In contrast, self-reports of emotions, inspired by dimensional theories of emotions, are often limited to ratings of valence (positive versus negative) and arousal (calm versus excited) (Lang et al. 1998; Bradley 2000; Bradley and Lang 2000).

Price and Barrell (1980) have promoted another line of investigation of emotion-related experiences. In these studies, emotions experienced in a variety of real and imagined situations have been described according to the positive (approach) or negative (avoidance) goal experienced by the subject and by the felt intensity of the desire and expectation regarding the attainment of that goal (also see Chapter 10; Price and Barrell 1984; Price et al. 1985). This approach clearly relates conceptually to the basic approach/avoidance theory of emotion; it is consistent with cognitive approaches because it includes the subject's goal as a primary determinant of the experienced emotion. However, it also contributes to the refinement of those models in several ways. First, the experiential approach emphasizes the importance of the *subject's experience* of an approach or avoidance goal rather than relying solely on the observation of overt behavioral responses. Second, the model identifies the felt desire and expectation toward that goal as a critical determinant of the emotion. Third, the model specifies the interrelations between those experiential dimensions in the determination of the emotion (see Fig. 2 in Chapter 10).

The experiential model further provides some link to the theories of discrete emotions by specifying the combination of positive and negative goals, desires, and expectations that lead to some specific emotions (satisfaction, excitement, anxiety, frustration, and depression). For example, study participants have frequently described feelings of anxiety in response to an avoidance goal that they had an uncertain expectation of achieving. In contrast, frustration is associated with avoidance goals (e.g., removing an obstacle) when the expectation that these goals can be achieved is low. Depression is associated with an avoidance goal (e.g., avoiding a loss) when there is little or no expectation that the goal can be achieved. Positive emotions are generally associated with high expectations of achieving positive goals (satisfaction and excitement) or negative goals (e.g., the satisfaction of successfully avoiding a negative consequence). Stronger desires to achieve the specified goal generally produce stronger emotional feelings.

The experiments conducted by Price and Barrell (1985) also demonstrate that subjective somatic sensations are part of the emotional experience and vary considerably among emotions. Satisfaction is associated with relaxation, warmth, and calmness, while excitement involves urges to move. In contrast, anxiety is associated with inner tension felt in the viscera, frustration is often described as somatic tension, and depression usually involves generalized weakness, numbness, heaviness, and lack of desire to move. We suspect that each of those bodily experiences reflects specific patterns of somatic activity, consistent with the hypothesis that distinct emotions are associated with distinct body states.

IS PAIN AN EMOTION?

The multiple aspects covered by emotion theories clearly relate to pain processes in many ways. The main difference between pain and emotion may be that pain requires the presence of "a bodily sensation with qualities like those reported during tissue-damaging stimulation" (Price 1999; p. 1). In this respect, pain sensations may be considered a specific inducer of a primitive emotional response, consistent with the view that emotion systems are intimately related to adaptive biological processes (e.g., Plutchik 1980; Izard 1993). Prototypical facial expressions of pain have been documented that can be differentiated from the basic emotions of fear, anger, and sadness

(Craig and Patrick 1985; LeResche and Dworkin 1988; reviewed in Williams 2002). Patterns of autonomic responses to nociceptive stimuli are well documented, mainly in animals (Sato et al. 1997), and may contribute to pain-related emotional responses as well as subjective feelings of unpleasantness (e.g., Fillingim et al. 1998; Rainville et al. 1999). It is also noteworthy that the model of pain discussed above includes primary and secondary affective stages (Price 1999), where the first corresponds to the basic experience of a threat, or the fear of tissue damage, and may include self-perception of autonomic and motor responses triggered automatically. The second stage reflects secondary evaluative processes consistent with modern views on the role of cognitive evaluative processes in emotions. This model is also consistent with the experiential model in which emotional experiences are related to goals, desires, and expectations. This experiential model of emotions has been shown to predict variations in pain unpleasantness, but not pain intensity (Price et al. 1980), consistent with the view that pain-related affective processes may be considered emotional responses to pain sensations.

EFFECTS OF EMOTION ON PAIN: EXPERIMENTAL STUDIES

The effects of emotions on pain may take various forms. First, one must distinguish emotions associated with the meaning of pain from those that may occur during pain but have a different cause, independent of pain. When emotions are related to the pain felt, they constitute secondary affective responses to pain. In this case, the interpretation of the meaning of pain may give rise to secondary emotions associated with pain-related goals that could enhance or reduce pain. When emotions are not related to pain, they may be considered distracters and may produce physiological responses that increase or decrease pain.

THE EXPERIENCE OF PAIN-RELATED EMOTIONS

In a series of studies conducted in normal volunteers, an experimental paradigm has been developed in our laboratory to test the effect of pain-related emotions on pain using hypnosis. Hypnotic suggestions were given to normal subjects to produce specific emotional feelings during the immersion of the hand in painfully hot water. In the first experiment, feelings of sadness-depression, fear-anxiety, and frustration-anger were induced in the negative emotion conditions, and expectations of imminent relief or experiences of satisfaction associated with the ability to tolerate the pain were induced in the positive emotion conditions. Compared to a prehypnotic baseline and to hypnotic relaxation, ratings of pain intensity and unpleasantness generally increased in the negative emotion conditions and decreased in the positive emotion conditions. However, consistent with the mediating effects of emotions on observed pain modulation, selective examination of trials in which the target emotion was specifically elicited led to stronger and highly significant increases, mainly in pain unpleasantness, most consistently during negative emotion conditions (see Fig. 1). Stronger negative emotions also predicted greater increases in pain unpleasantness, independent of changes reported in pain intensity (Table I). This study therefore confirmed that negative emotions related to pain mainly increase pain unpleasantness.

In a follow-up experiment, we examined the effects of anger and sadness in more detail because these were the two conditions that we could induce most reliably and that produced the strongest and most reliable effects on pain (Huynh Bao and Rainville 2003). In this experiment, subjects rated their felt desire and expectation to avoid or escape pain during the

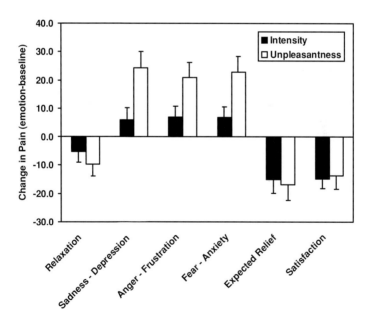

Fig. 1. Changes in pain intensity and pain unpleasantness produced by 1-minute immersions of the hand in hot water, from a baseline control condition and following the hypnotic induction of emotions. Significant increases in pain ($P < 0.05$) are found in response to negative emotions relative to the baseline ($y = 0$) and relaxation conditions, with larger effects observed in pain unpleasantness than in pain intensity. Decreases in pain during positive emotions did not reach significance relative to relaxation.

Table I
Correlation between changes in pain and changes in emotional valence, rated
on a scale ranging from –5 to +5 for negative to positive emotion

Pearson R	Pain Intensity	Pain Unpleasantness	Partial Intensity	Partial Unpleasantness
All conditions ($n = 120$)	–0.46***	–0.76***	–0.11	–0.68***
Relaxation ($n = 24$)	+0.08	–0.17	+0.13	–0.20
Sadness ($n = 22$)	–0.05	–0.69***	+0.02	–0.69**
Anger ($n = 23$)	–0.37	–0.79***	–0.10	–0.76***
Fear ($n = 18$)	–0.63**	–0.73***	–0.41	–0.59*
Relief ($n = 13$)	–0.44	–0.64*	–0.30	–0.58
Satisfaction ($n = 20$)	–0.09	–0.44	–0.31	–0.52*

Note: Increases in pain unpleasantness are associated to a decrease in positive emotions
and to increase in negative emotions (negative changes on the emotion scale). The
correlation between the magnitude of changes in emotions and in pain is more
pronounced for pain unpleasantness than pain intensity, and is significant mainly in the
negative emotion conditions. Similar effects were observed after accounting for
changes in pain intensity (see Partial Unpleasantness). In contrast, no correlations
between changes in emotion and changes in pain intensity reach significance after
accounting for changes in pain unpleasantness (see Partial Intensity). Values of n
correspond to the number of subjects who experienced the target emotional state in each
condition and entered the correlation analyses (out of a total sample of 26 subjects).
* Uncorrected, $P < 0.05$; ** uncorrected, $P < 0.01$; *** uncorrected, $P < 0.001$.

experimental pain test. Subjects also rated the valence of their emotion, their
felt arousal, and their feeling of being in control (dominance) (Lang 1980).
Hypnotic suggestions for sadness and anger were associated with significant
increases in desire and reductions in expectations of avoiding or escaping
pain, compared to both a prehypnotic and a hypnotic relaxation control (Fig.
2A). Consistently, ratings of negative valence and arousal increased significantly in the negative emotion conditions, and dominance decreased significantly in sadness but not in anger. Pain unpleasantness increased robustly
and pain intensity increased to a lesser extent in both sadness and anger
(Fig. 2B). Critically, changes in pain unpleasantness, and to a lesser extent
in pain intensity, were predicted by changes in emotions (Table II). Again,
correlations between emotion dimensions and pain ratings indicated a primary effect on pain unpleasantness, with the exception of expectation, which
contributed some unique variance in changes in pain intensity (see partial
correlation in Table II). We have recently confirmed that the specific manipulation of the desire to avoid or escape pain using hypnosis does lead to a
significant modulation of pain unpleasantness, independent of changes in
pain intensity or in expectation (P. Chrétien and P. Rainville, unpublished
manuscript).

In the experiment on sadness and anger, in which we also included
autonomic measures, we found a significant modulation of heart rate responses

to the experimental heat pain test. The interbeat interval decreased (i.e., heart rate increased) significantly more during negative emotions, compared to the prehypnotic baseline or to the hypnotic relaxation condition. Furthermore, this increase in cardiac response to pain was positively correlated with changes in pain and emotional experience (Table III). We calculated partial

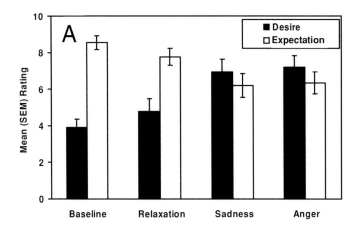

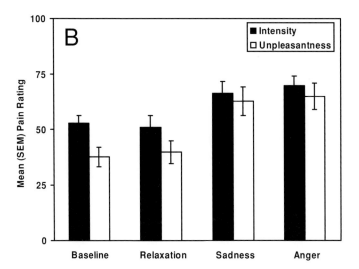

Fig. 2. Effects of hypnotic relaxation and hypnotic induction of anger and sadness on subjective desires and expectations to avoid/escape pain (A) and on the pain intensity and unpleasantness produced by 1-minute immersion of the hand in hot water (B). Desire increased and expectation decreased in the negative emotion conditions ($P < 0.05$). As a result, pain unpleasantness, and to a lesser extent, pain intensity, increased in both conditions ($P < 0.05$).

Table II
Correlation coefficients between changes in pain intensity and unpleasantness,
and changes in several emotional dimensions

Pearson R	Pain Intensity	Pain Unpleasantness	Partial Intensity	Partial Unpleasantness
Desire	+0.74***	+0.83***	+0.16	+0.56***
Expectation	−0.36**	−0.65***	+0.43*	−0.68***
Valence	+0.65***	+0.76***	+0.04	+0.52***
Felt arousal	+0.52***	+0.67***	−0.09	+0.50***
Dominance	−0.47***	−0.53***	−0.05	−0.29*

Note: Pain increases significantly with increases in desire to avoid or escape pain, negative affect (valence) and arousal, and with decreases in expectations to avoid or escape pain and in feelings of being in control (dominance). Similar effects are observed in pain unpleasantness after accounting for changes in pain intensity (see Partial Unpleasantness). In contrast, and with the exception of expectation, no correlations between changes in emotion and changes in pain intensity reached significance after accounting for changes in pain unpleasantness (Partial Intensity). * $P < 0.05$; ** $P < 0.01$; *** $P < 0.001$.

correlation analyses testing for the residual correlations after controlling for changes in pain intensity, pain unpleasantness, or felt arousal. Changes in pain unpleasantness were positively correlated with changes in cardiac responses after we accounted for changes in pain intensity or felt arousal. However, cardiac responses did not predict pain intensity after we accounted for pain unpleasantness and only marginally after we accounted for arousal. Changes in felt arousal were consistently positively correlated with cardiac responses, consistent with the idea that this dimension of experience reflects the perceived viscerosomatic activity. However, this effect was considerably reduced after we accounted for changes in pain unpleasantness, which suggests that feelings of arousal and pain unpleasantness may be closely related but not completely overlapping phenomena.

Findings of experiential studies examining the effect of pain-related emotions on pain are summarized in Fig. 3. In this model, the nociceptive stimulus contributes to pain sensation intensity, which in turn contributes to pain unpleasantness (Price 1999, 2000; Rainville et al. 1999). The nociceptive input also triggers autonomic responses and somatic feedback that contribute to felt arousal and pain unpleasantness. Pain-related goals and the associated desire and expectation contribute to the modulation of pain. Desire to avoid or escape pain appears mainly to affect pain unpleasantness, independent of pain sensation intensity (Table II, Partial Unpleasantness). In contrast, expectation may exert a modulatory influence on both pain intensity and pain unpleasantness (see partial correlations in Table II), consistent with studies on placebo showing robust modulation of pain intensity by

Table III
Correlation between changes in pain-evoked cardiac responses
and changes in pain- and emotion-related dimensions

Pearson R	Modulation of Cardiac Response	Residual (–INT)	Residual (–UNP)	Residual (–Arousal)
Pain intensity	+0.48***		–0.02	+0.27*
Pain unpleasantness	+0.59***	+0.38**		+0.35**
Desire to avoid or escape	+0.47***	+0.19	–0.03	+0.26
Expectation of avoiding or escaping	–0.44***	–0.33	–0.10	–0.16
Valence	+0.37**	+0.09	–0.14	+0.13
Felt arousal	+0.55***	+0.40**	+0.27*	
Dominance	–0.30*	–0.10	+0.01	–0.10

Note: Larger cardiac responses (larger heart rate increase or interbeat interval decrease) are associated with increases in pain intensity and unpleasantness, desire to avoid pain, negative valence, and arousal, and with decreases in expectation of avoiding pain and in felt control or dominance. Partial correlations are shown after controlling for changes in pain intensity (–INT), in pain unpleasantness (–UNP), and in arousal. * $P < 0.05$; ** $P < 0.01$; *** $P < 0.001$.

expectation of relief (see Chapter 10). In addition, autonomic activity associated with pain may be facilitated or attenuated by the action of descending neurophysiological mechanisms following the modulation of pain unpleasantness (see Fig. 9 in Chapter 11). Taken together, these results demonstrate the usefulness of experiential measures to describe emotions related to pain and to predict emotion-induced pain modulation. Results confirm that pain-related

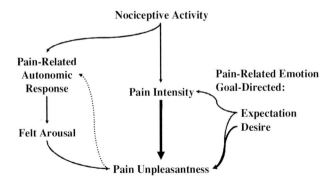

Fig. 3. Pain-related emotions are suggested to affect pain perception in several ways. Goal-directed desires appear to affect mainly pain unpleasantness, whereas goal-directed expectations influence both pain sensation intensity and pain unpleasantness. Emotion-related physiological activity may contribute to the felt arousal and to pain unpleasantness.

negative emotions contribute mainly to increases in pain unpleasantness and
to a lesser extent to increases in pain intensity.

PAIN ANTICIPATION AND PAIN-RELATED FEAR AND ANXIETY

Several additional experimental studies have examined the effects of
emotion on pain perception from a different perspective. One phenomenon
that has received considerable attention is pain anticipation and the associated negative emotions. The anticipation of pain may contribute to increased
vigilance and enhanced attention toward future painful stimulation, as discussed in Chapter 5, but may also produce fear-related responses and anxiety associated with the expectation of potential harm (see different interpretations of the effects of pain anticipation on pain in Vlaeyen and Linton
[2000]). Although the notions of pain-related anxiety, fear, and fear-avoidance have been elaborated most comprehensively in relation to pain in clinical contexts, these studies may relate to animal studies examining mechanisms of fear conditioning and stress-related responses.

Experimental studies conducted by Meagher, Grau, and colleagues have
attempted to bridge the gap between animal and human studies on pain-
related fear and anxiety. Experiments performed in rats showed that mild
electric shocks typically produce hyperalgesia, whereas exposing the animals to higher intensities generally results in stress-induced analgesia (e.g.,
Meagher et al. 2001). Rhudy and Meagher have tried to clarify the effects of
pain anticipation on pain perception and to relate the effects observed in
humans to those observed in animals. They first compared the effects on
heat pain threshold ("finger-withdrawal" latency) of a threat of electric shocks
(Rhudy and Meagher 2000) or a loud white noise (Rhudy and Meagher
2001), with or without prior exposure to the stressor. Compared to a control
condition, the threat alone (their "anxiety" condition) generally decreased
pain threshold while the threat with prior exposure to the stressor (their
"fear" condition) increased it. These authors have argued that these effects
are consistent with the animal literature suggesting anxiety-related hyperalgesia and fear- or stress-related analgesia. However, follow-up studies examining the effect of the threat of shocks on heat pain ratings produced
divergent results in which all conditions led to pain reductions (Rhudy and
Meagher 2003). Furthermore, closer examination of the results and follow-
up experiments also demonstrated that the specific emotion experienced and
the associated physiological response helped to predict pain modulation. For
example, in response to the loud noise, women reported experiences of fear
and showed increased sympathetic activity (skin conductance level and heart
rate) associated with decreased pain. In contrast, men reported experiences

of surprise rather than fear and showed no significant physiological arousal and no increase in pain. In another recent study, Rhudy and Meagher (2003) further reported that subjects responding with a sense of humor to the threat of, and exposure to, electric shocks experienced less analgesic effects. These mixed results pointed to important individual differences in the effect of the experimental manipulation and the critical effect of the emotion experienced on pain.

In a review of their early findings, Rhudy and Meagher (2001) had proposed that valence and arousal were the mediating mechanisms, with negative emotions leading to hyperalgesia at moderate levels of arousal and to analgesia at higher levels of arousal. However, in view of their divergent findings obtained with pain threshold and pain ratings, and following their more recent studies demonstrating that the specific emotion experienced may better predict the pain modulation observed, we suspect that a more comprehensive assessment of experiential dimensions associated with the experimental manipulation will further clarify their contradictory findings. Another aspect that may also contribute to the effects observed in those studies is the direction of attention. Indeed, although the emotion in those studies is evoked by the threat of pain or another aversive stimulus (the *stressor*), this stimulus is distinct from the pain stimulus used to assess pain perception. In those conditions it is therefore difficult to exclude the possibility that the impending potential stressor might have reduced the attentional resources available to process the less intense target pain stimulus.

In some experimental conditions, however, anticipation of pain is directly related to the pain assessment test. Pain sensitivity increases more clearly in response to pain-specific anxiety than non-specific anxiety (Dougher et al. 1987), consistent with the notion that pain-related and pain-unrelated emotions may affect pain differently. Sullivan et al. (2001a) have also suggested that pain expectancies mediate the effects of catastrophizing and depression on cold pressor pain in normal subjects. This interpretation suggests an influence of emotion on cognitive processes, which, in turn, affect pain perception. However, in that study, the expected mood rated by the subjects predicted the pain experienced better than did the expected pain. This intriguing result suggests that the anticipation of an emotional response may contribute to pain modulation.

EMOTIONS UNRELATED TO PAIN

We constantly encounter situations that may trigger emotions not directly related to pain. Several methods have been used to induce emotions or moods experimentally. Pictures displaying fear (e.g., angry face, animal rage) and disgust (e.g., mutilated body parts) presented before a cold pressor test reduced the onset latency (threshold) of pain intensity and unpleasantness (increased sensitivity), and those displaying fear significantly reduced pain tolerance (Meagher et al. 2001). In contrast, erotic pictures increased pain intensity and unpleasantness threshold in men. Cold-pressor pain tolerance also increased in proportion to the pleasantness of picture viewed during the pain test; negative pictures displaying pain-related contents decreased pain tolerance (De Wied et al. 2001). This effect is consistent with the proposed distinction between pain-related and pain-unrelated emotions, the former being generally associated with increased pain.

Other methods have been used to induce moods. Reading statements with positive or negative affective valence (Velten 1968) has been shown to increase or decrease cold pressor pain tolerance, respectively (Zelman et al. 1991). Decreases in cold pain tolerance were also suggested to relate to pain catastrophizing in a depressed mood induction condition using this method (Willoughby et al. 2002). Similarly, the induction of positive affect by films significantly reduced experimental pain perception, whereas negative affect produced nonsignificant increases in pain (Zillmann et al. 1996; Weisenberg et al. 1998). Soothing music increased experimental pain thresholds without changing innocuous tactile thresholds, while stimulating music increased both pain and tactile thresholds (Whipple and Glynn 1992). The analgesic effect of music on heat pain was also observed in our laboratory (Roy et al. 2003). In those studies, the effects of happy and pleasant music were specific to pain and did not alter nonpainful sensation. This absence of effect on nonpainful perception suggests that the effects of emotions and moods may be specific to pain processing and not simply due to nonspecific distracting effects.

Sweet taste (Lewkowski et al. 2003) and pleasant odors (Marchand and Arsenault 2002; Villemure et al. 2003) reduced experimental heat and cold pain, respectively. However, the effect occurred only in subjects with low arterial blood pressure in the study on taste and only in women in the study on odors by Marchand and Arsenault (2002). These findings generally confirm that the induction of positive moods decreases pain while that of negative moods generally increases pain, yet they also emphasize the importance of individual differences in the effects of mood induction on pain.

Finally, the stress induced by the administration of a difficult cognitive task may produce changes in pain mediated by emotions. However, these effects interact with the sex of subjects. In one study (Logan et al. 2001), subjects performed the Stroop color-word task and were urged several times to improve their performance. Immediately after the cognitive task, the pain produced by the intradermal injection of capsaicin was rated. Compared to the relaxation condition, the stress of the cognitive task increased pain significantly in women, while men showed a nonsignificant decrease in pain. Furthermore, increases in pain ratings were positively correlated with task-induced effects on plasma norepinephrine and cortisol, and with reduced self-ratings of relaxation. The interaction with the sex of the subject was particularly intriguing in view of the stronger correlation that men showed between pain increases and *physiological* indices of arousal (increases in blood pressure and norepinephrine) and the stronger correlation that women demonstrated between pain increases and *subjective* measures of arousal (reduction in self-ratings of relaxation). These findings suggest that the contribution of emotion-related physiological and subjective arousal to pain modulation may vary according to the sex of the subject. In the discussion of these results, the authors hypothesized that the specific emotion elicited during the cognitive task depends on the sex of the subject and mediates the effects of stress on pain. Another study using a similar cognitive-stress paradigm found that anger, produced by harassing instructions to improve performance, was associated with increases in cold pain tolerance (Janssen et al. 2001). At this point, we can only speculate that in the study by Logan et al. (2001), men might have experienced more anger and analgesia in the stress condition while women may have experienced different emotions. However, another aspect that may also prove to be relevant in those conditions is the possible distracting effect of anger on pain, the possible moderating effect of the object of anger (e.g., anger directed at oneself or others), and the tendency to express anger (see clinical studies below; Okifuji et al. 1999).

EMOTION OR ATTENTION?

Emotion stimuli naturally attract attention, and an emotional inducer unrelated to pain may therefore compete with pain for attentional resources. This possible confounding factor was identified in early studies investigating the analgesic effect of sound and music (e.g., Gardner and Licklider 1959; Gardner et al. 1960). Results from Villemure et al. (2003) show that pain may be modulated by mood, independent of the direction of attention (see Chapter 5). Furthermore, although distraction may explain the analgesic effect of positive emotions in some conditions, it does not provide an adequate explanation for increases in pain reported in response to negative emotions (e.g., Meagher et al. 2001). In addition, the effect of attention is generally observed on both intensity and unpleasantness (e.g., Miron et al. 1989), while the effects of emotions appear to be more robust on pain unpleasantness for both pain-unrelated emotions (e.g., Roy et al. 2003; Villemure 2003) and pain-related emotions (e.g., Huynh Bao and Rainville 2002, 2003).

Negative emotions and moods have been associated with increased self-focus characterized by increased attention to, and concern with, somatic signals (Mor and Winquist 2002; also see Salovey 1992). For example, anxiety has been argued to increase vigilance and attention to pain (e.g., Arntz et al. 1994; Eccleston et al. 1997; Crombez et al. 2002). The observation that negative pictures decrease cold pain tolerance, especially when they display pain-related contents, is consistent with this possibility (De Wied et al. 2001). Negative moods may facilitate pain processing and enhance the perception of somatic responses associated with pain. To the extent that viscerosomatic responses contribute to pain unpleasantness, as suggested in Fig. 3, it is possible that negative emotional states and moods increase pain unpleasantness by increasing the subjects' awareness of their viscerosomatic responses without affecting pain sensation intensity.

EFFECTS OF EMOTIONS ON PAIN: CLINICAL STUDIES

Clinical studies have generally examined the interaction between discrete emotions or emotion disorders and pain, rather than examining the effects of arousal, valence, or specific experiential dimensions of emotions. A large-scale study conducted by the World Health Organization has shown that patients with persistent pain have an elevated risk of having anxiety or depressive disorder (Gureje et al. 1998). Reciprocally, sustained negative emotional states increase pain; fear-anxiety and sadness-depression have been studied the most (see the review by Fernandez and Milburn 1994; Fernandez and Turk 1995; Huyser and Parker 1999; Keefe et al. 2001). A significant relationship has been demonstrated especially between pain unpleasantness and feelings of depression, anxiety, frustration, fear, and to a lesser degree anger, in large populations of chronic pain patients (Wade et al. 1990, 1996; see Chapter 2).

The emotions associated with pain are often dependent upon cognitive processes that attribute meaning to the pain (e.g., Price 1999). In a study performed in cancer pain patients participating in sessions of physical therapy, Smith et al. (1998) observed that patients who believed that their pain was due to the cancer experienced more pain than patients who did not have such beliefs. Such an effect might be mediated by pain-related emotions. Catastrophizing about pain and fear of pain (or injury) has been shown most consistently to contribute to pain severity and pain-related distress (Sullivan and D'Eon 1990; Sullivan and Neish 1998; Sullivan et al. 2001a,b; Crombez et al. 1999; Vlaeyen and Crombez 1999; Vlaeyen and Linton 2000; Eccleston et al. 2001). Similar to the effects of some emotional factors on experimental pain discussed above, these effects may be mediated by hypervigilance and increased attention to pain, as well as by changes in emotions and moods. Importantly, the effects of pain-related negative emotions, and particularly fear and catastrophizing, are generally strong predictors of pain-related disability.

Similarly, the effects of anger on pain seem to depend on several factors. Okifuji et al. (1999) observed that the anger experienced by chronic pain patients is most frequently directed at themselves or at their health care providers. Interestingly, pain severity was found to correlate specifically with anger directed at oneself, and with the overall anger experienced, and less so with anger directed at other targets including the health care provider or, when applicable, the person who caused the injury. Depression was also more strongly correlated with anger directed at oneself and with overall anger. These findings provide further support that the target of the emotion is critical in determining its effect on pain. Recently, additional factors have been identified that contribute to the effect of anger on pain (Greenwood et al. 2003). Those include gender, hostility (i.e., the tendency to perceive malicious intent or to anticipate aggression), and anger management style (i.e., the tendency to express ["anger-out"], suppress ["anger-in"], or control anger). Complex interactions between those factors have been reported. For example, anger exacerbates pain when it is associated with high hostility combined with high anger expression in women or low anger expression in men (Burns et al. 1996).

As a general rule, negative emotions generally increase clinical pain, particularly pain unpleasantness, and they are good predictors of pain-related behaviors and disability. Although the precise psychological mechanisms by which emotions affect clinical pain are not clearly established and are likely to vary with the specific emotion experienced, the relation between the emotions and pain again appears to be critical in the modulatory effect. Indeed, self-directed or pain-related negative emotions seem to be the most detrimental to the pain condition.

BRAIN SYSTEMS FOR PAIN AND EMOTION

There have been interesting developments in the study of physiological mechanisms of pain and emotion using functional brain-imaging methods. Studies of pain in humans have demonstrated activation in the classical ascending spinothalamocortical pathways up to the primary and secondary somatosensory cortices (S1 and S2), the insula, and the anterior cingulate cortex (ACC) (reviewed in Peyron et al. 2000). Additional subcortical activation

sites reported more sporadically include the cerebellum, brainstem, hypothalamus, amygdala, nucleus accumbens, and various divisions of the basal
ganglia. Fewer studies have been performed examining specifically the neural correlates of the subjective experience of emotions. Damasio and his
colleagues have examined brain activity when subjects indicated that they
experienced an emotional feeling triggered by the autobiographical recall of
experiences of happiness, sadness, fear, and anger (Damasio et al. 2000; see
also Lane et al. 1997b). Changes in regional cerebral blood flow (rCBF)
were observed in many pain-related areas, including the ACC, the insula,
and the parietal operculum, where the S2 cortex is located. Additional effects were reported in the orbitofrontal cortices and in several subcortical
areas involved in the regulation of body states, including many areas also
involved in nociception (e.g., brainstem nuclei, the amygdala, and the hypothalamus). This shared brain network for pain and emotion is consistent with
the involvement of common physiological processes and with the considerable interactions between pain and emotions.

Pain and emotion are associated with autonomic responses that may
relate to activity within the insula (Zhang et al. 1999; Craig et al. 2000;
Critchley et al. 2000a; Craig 2003). Similarly, pain and emotions may be
conceived as motivational states that involve reward-punishment and ap-
proach-avoidance systems, including the ventral striatum and the motor sec-
tor of the ACC. Interestingly, activity in different sectors of the ACC has
been related to changes in pain unpleasantness (Rainville et al. 1997), to
self-awareness of emotional responses (Lane et al. 1997a, 1998), and to the
higher-order regulation of motor activity (Picard and Strick 1996; Paus 2001)
and autonomic activity (Critchley et al. 2000a,b, 2003, 2004). In the study
by Damasio et al. (2000), ACC activity was found to increase in anger and
sadness and to decrease in happiness in portions of the ACC where pain-
related activity is usually observed (caudal to mid-ACC). Those areas may
be involved in the interaction between pain and emotion.

EMOTION, SELF-REGULATION, AND ENDOGENOUS
PAIN-MODULATORY SYSTEMS

The ACC constitutes an interface between motor, motivational, and cognitive processes (Paus 2001) and may play an important role in regulating
both pain and emotion (Rainville 2002). A model of attention further points
to the ACC as a regulator of both affective and cognitive processes (Bush et
al. 2000). This model is highly consistent with a potential role of the ACC in
pain-related fear, pain catastrophizing, and pain anticipation (Hsieh et al.

1999; Ploghaus et al. 1999). Indeed, the consequence of those cognitive-emotional states may be increased attention directed toward pain, and especially self-directed attention to the felt desires, expectations, and somatic sensations and responses associated with pain. However, the cerebral mechanisms associated with those dimensions of experience have not yet been examined specifically.

The ACC not only may be involved in the experience of pain affect, emotions, and attention, but also may trigger subcortical pain modulatory mechanisms affecting brainstem descending modulatory pathways. The effects of hypnotic analgesia on both ACC activity and spinal nociceptive reflexes (see Chapters 11 and 12) is consistent with the possibility that descending modulatory mechanisms may be triggered from the ACC, and with the possibility that these mechanisms may, in turn, affect both pain intensity and unpleasantness. A similar involvement of the ACC in self-regulation may occur during the voluntary inhibition of sexual arousal (Beauregard et al. 2001) and during relaxation biofeedback (Critchley et al. 2001). A reduction in rCBF in the subgenual portion of the ACC and the medial prefrontal cortex observed during anticipation of electric shocks has also been suggested to reflect the engagement of coping strategies to reduce anxiety (Simpson et al. 2001). This suggestion would be consistent with a role of the ACC in the self-regulation of emotional responses. Additional studies will be required to assess the specific mechanisms and the specific role of subsectors of the ACC in the regulation of pain and emotions by various strategies such as cognitive coping, relaxation, or hypnosis.

The pain/emotion network is also involved in endorphin-related analgesia. The μ-opioid receptor mRNA is expressed, and the μ-opioid receptor is found, in many areas of the brainstem, thalamus, amygdala, striatum, and the frontal cortices including the ACC (Arvidsson et al. 1995; Peckys and Landwehrmeyer 1999; Sim-Selley et al. 1999). Zubieta et al. (2001) observed that sustained pain is associated with activation of the endogenous opioid system in the ACC, the bilateral prefrontal cortices, the contralateral insula, thalamus, and hypothalamus, and the ipsilateral amygdala. Interestingly, stronger endogenous opioid activation in the ACC, the thalamus, and the ispilateral nucleus accumbens was also associated with lower pain affective ratings. Anger-related changes in pain may involve this system, as recently suggested by the observed reduction in endogenous opioid activity during anger (anger-related antianalgesia; Bruehl et al. 2002, 2003). Consistently, the experience of anger involves part of this network including nuclei of the brainstem, the amygdala, the nucleus accumbens, and the ACC (e.g., see the control condition in Damasio et al. 2000b; Kilts et al. 2001).

SUMMARY AND CONCLUSIONS

Pain and emotions are partly overlapping phenomena with reciprocal influences. One important conclusion that emerges from this chapter is that the specific experience felt by the subject or patient appears to predict the effect of emotions on pain better than the "objective" conditions of emotion induction. These experiential factors may eventually help to explain some differences between men and women, and between subjects with different tendencies to express emotions (e.g., anger-in versus anger-out). The effect of emotions on pain generally depends on the valence of the felt emotion and its object. Pain-related negative emotions increase pain, particularly pain unpleasantness. This effect is mediated by pain-related goals, by the associated desire and expectation of reaching these goals, and possibly by the felt arousal. In contrast, negative emotions unrelated to pain may decrease pain as a result of distraction, or they may increase pain as a result of negative mood induction. Pain-related and pain-unrelated negative emotions may also enhance self-directed attention and thereby contribute to increases in pain and somatic concerns.

The overlap among brain networks involved in pain and emotions reflects their common processes involving motivational, cognitive, expressive, skeletomotor, and visceromotor aspects. However, more research is required before we can further specify the brain areas and mechanisms underlying the multiple dimensions of pain and emotion experiences and the interaction between emotions and pain.

REFERENCES

Adolphs R. Neural systems for recognizing emotion. *Curr Opin Neurobiol* 2002; 12:169–177.

Arntz A, Dreessen L, De Jong P. The influence of anxiety on pain: attentional and attributional mediators. *Pain* 1994; 56:307–314.

Arvidsson U, Riedl M, Chakrabarti S, et al. Distribution and targeting of a mu-opioid receptor (MOR1) in brain and spinal cord. *J Neurosci* 1995; 15:3328–3341.

Beauregard M, Levesque J, Bourgouin P. Neural correlates of conscious self-regulation of emotion. *J Neurosci* 2001; 21:RC165.

Bechara A, Naqvi N. Listening to your heart: interoceptive awareness as a gateway to feeling. *Nat Neurosci* 2004; 7:102–103.

Bechara A, Damasio H, Tranel D, Damasio AR. Deciding advantageously before knowing the advantageous strategy. *Science* 1997; 275:1293–1295.

Bechara A, Damasio H, Damasio AR, Lee GP. Different contributions of the human amygdala and ventromedial prefrontal cortex to decision-making. *J Neurosci* 1999; 19:5473–5481.

Bradley MM. Emotion and motivation. In: Cacioppo JT, Tassinary LG, Berntson GG (Eds). *Handbook of Psychophysiology*. Cambridge, MA: Cambridge University Press, 2000.

Bradley MM, Lang PJ. Measuring emotion: behavior, feeling, and physiology. In: Lane RD, Nadel L (Eds). *Cognitive Neuroscience of Emotion*. New York: Oxford University Press, 2000.

Bruehl S, Burns JW, Chung OY, Ward P, Johnson B. Anger and pain sensitivity in chronic low back pain patients and pain-free controls: the role of endogenous opioids. *Pain* 2002; 99:223–233.

Bruehl S, Chung OY, Burns JW, Biridepalli S. The association between anger expression and chronic pain intensity: evidence for partial mediation by endogenous opioid dysfunction. *Pain* 2003; 106:317–324.

Burns JW, Johnson BJ, Mahoney N, Devine J, Pawl R. Anger management style, hostility and spouse responses: gender differences in predictors of adjustment among chronic pain patients. *Pain* 1996; 64:445–453.

Bush G, Luu P, Posner MI. Cognitive and emotional influences in anterior cingulate cortex. *Trends Cogn Sci* 2000; 4:215–222.

Collet C, Vernet-Maury E, Delhomme G, Dittmar A. Autonomic nervous system response patterns specificity to basic emotions. *J Auton Nerv Syst* 1; 62:45–57.

Craig AD. A new view of pain as a homeostatic emotion. *Trends Neurosci* 2003; 26:303–307.

Craig KD, Patrick CJ. Facial expression during induced pain. *J Pers Soc Psychol* 1985; 48:1080–1091.

Craig AD, Chen K, Bandy D, Reiman EM. Thermosensory activation of insular cortex. *Nat Neurosci* 2000; 3184–3190.

Critchley HD, Corfield DR, Chandler MP, Mathias CJ, Dolan RJ. Cerebral correlates of autonomic cardiovascular arousal: a functional neuroimaging investigation in humans. *J Physiol* 2000a; 523:259–270.

Critchley HD, Elliott R, Mathias CJ, Dolan RJ. Neural activity relating to generation and representation of galvanic skin conductance responses: a functional magnetic resonance imaging study. *J Neurosci* 2000b; 20:3033–3040.

Critchley HD, Melmed RN, Featherstone E, Mathias CJ, Dolan RJ. Brain activity during biofeedback relaxation: a functional neuroimaging investigation. *Brain* 2001; 124:1003–1012.

Critchley HD, Mathias CJ, Josephs O, et al. Human cingulate cortex and autonomic control: converging neuroimaging and clinical evidence. *Brain* 2003; 126:2139–2152.

Critchley HD, Wiens S, Rothstein P, Ohman A, Dolan RJ. Neural systems supporting intero-ceptive awareness. *Nat Neurosci* 2004; 7:189–195.

Crombez G, Vlaeyen JW, Heuts PH, Lysens R. Pain-related fear is more disabling than pain itself: evidence on the role of pain-related fear in chronic back pain disability. *Pain* 1999; 80:329–339.

Crombez G, Eccleston C, van den BA, van Houdenhove B, Goubert L. The effect of cata-strophic thinking about pain on attentional interference by pain: no mediation of negative affectivity in healthy volunteers and in patients with low back pain. *Pain Res Manage* 2002; 7:31–39.

Damasio AR, Grabowski TJ, Bechara A, et al. Subcortical and cortical brain activity during the feeling of self-generated emotions. *Nat Neurosci* 2000a; 3:1049–1056.

Darwin C. The expression of emotions in man and animals. New York: Appleton, 1872.

Davidson RJ, Irwin W. The functional neuroanatomy of emotion and affective style. *Trends Cogn Sci* 1993; 3:11–21.

De Wied M, Verbaten MN. Affective pictures processing, attention, and pain tolerance. *Pain* 2001; 90:163–172.

Dougher MJ, Goldstein D, Leight KA. Induced anxiety and pain. *J Anxiety Dis* 1987; 1:259–264.

Eccleston C, Crombez G, Aldrich S, Stannard C. Attention and somatic awareness in chronic pain. *Pain* 1997; 72:209–215.

Eccleston C, Crombez G, Aldrich S, Stannard C. Worry and chronic pain patients: a description and analysis of individual differences. *Eur J Pain* 2001; 5:309–318.

Ekman P. Facial expressions. In: Dalgleish T, Power M (Eds). *Handbook of Cognition and Emotion.* New York: John Wiley & Sons, 1999, pp 301–320.

Ekman P, Levenson RW, Friesen WV. Autonomic nervous system activity distinguishes among emotions. *Science* 1983; 221:1208–1210.

Fernandez E, Milburn TW. Sensory and affective predictors of overall pain and emotions associated with affective pain. *Clin J Pain* 1994; 10:3–9.

Fernandez E, Turk DC. The scope and significance of anger in the experience of chronic pain. *Pain* 1995; 61:165–175.

Fillingim RB, Maixner W, Bunting S, Silva S. Resting blood pressure and thermal pain responses among females: effects on pain unpleasantness but not pain intensity. *Int J Psychophysiol* 1998; 30:313–318.

Gardner WL, Licklider JC. Auditory analgesia in dental operations. *J Am Dent Assoc* 1959; 59:1144–1149.

Gardner WL, Licklider JC, Weisz AZ. Suppression of pain by sound. *Science* 1960; 132:32–33.

Gureje O, Von Korff M, Simon G, Gater R. Persistent pain and well-being: a World Health Organization study in primary care. *JAMA* 1998; 280:147–151.

Hsieh JC, Stone-Elander S, Ingvar M. Anticipatory coping of pain expressed in the human anterior cingulate cortex: a positron emission tomography study. *Neurosci Lett* 1999; 262:61–64.

Huynh Bao QV, Rainville P. Modulation of experimental pain by emotion induced using hypnosis. *Pain Res Manage* 2003; (Suppl 8):35B.

Huyser BA, Parker JC. Negative affect and pain in arthritis. *Rheum Dis Clin North Am* 1999; 25:105–121.

Izard CE. Four systems for emotion activation: cognitive and noncognitive processes. *Psychol Rev* 1993; 100:68–90.

James W. The physical bases of emotion. *Psychol Rev* 1994; 101:205–210.

Janssen SA, Spinhoven P, Brosschot JF. Experimentally induced anger, cardiovascular reactivity, and pain sensitivity. *J Psychosom Res* 2001; 51:479–485.

Keefe FJ, Lumley M, Anderson T, Lynch T, Carson KL. Pain and emotion: new research directions. *J Clin Psychol* 2001; 57:587–607.

Kilts CD, Schweitzer JB, Quinn CK, et al. Neural activity related to drug craving in cocaine addiction. *Arch Gen Psychiatry* 2001; 58:334–341.

Lane RD, Fink GR, Chau PM, Dolan RJ. Neural activation during selective attention to subjective emotional responses. *Neuroreport* 1997a; 8:3969–3972.

Lane RD, Reiman EM, Ahern GL, Schwartz GE, Davidson RJ. Neuroanatomical correlates of happiness, sadness, and disgust. *Am J Psychiatry* 1997b; 154:926–933.

Lane RD, Reiman EM, Axelrod B, et al. Neural correlates of levels of emotional awareness: evidence of an interaction between emotion and attention in the anterior cingulate cortex. *J Cogn Neurosci* 1998; 10:525–535.

Lang PJ. Behavioral treatment and bio-behavioral assessment: computer applications. In: Sidowski JB, Johnson JH, Williams EA (Eds). *Technology in Mental Health Care Delivery System*. Norwood, NJ: Ablex, 1980, pp 119–137.

Lang PJ, Bradley MM, Cuthbert BN. *International Affective Picture System (IAPS) Technical Manual and Affective Ratings*. Gainesville, FL, 1998.

Lazarus RS. Cognition and motivation in emotion. *Am Psychol* 1991; 46:352–367.

LeDoux JE. *The Emotional Brain: The Mysterious Underpinnings of Emotional Life.* New York: Simon & Shuster, 1996.

LeResche L, Dworkin SF. Facial expressions of pain and emotions in chronic TMD patients. *Pain* 1988; 35:71–78.

Levenson RW, Ekman P, Friesen WV. Voluntary facial action generates emotion-specific autonomic nervous system activity. *Psychophysiology* 1990; 27:363–384.

Lewkowski MD, Ditto B, Roussos M, Young SN. Sweet taste and blood pressure-related analgesia. *Pain* 2003; 106:181–186.

Logan H, Lutgendorf S, Rainville P, et al. Effects of stress and relaxation on capsaicin-induced pain. *Pain* 2001; 2:160–170.

Marchand S, Arsenault P. Odors modulate pain perception: a gender-specific effect. *Physiol Behav* 2002; 76:251–256.

Meagher MW, Ferguson AR, Crown ED, et al. Shock-induced hyperalgesia: IV. Generality. *J Exp Psychol Anim Behav Process* 2001; 27:219–238.

Merskey H, Bogduk N. *Classification of Chronic Pain: Descriptions of Chronic Pain Syndromes and Definition of Pain Terms,* 2nd ed. Seattle: IASP Press, 1994.

Miron D, Duncan GH, Bushnell MC. Effects of attention on the intensity and unpleasantness of thermal pain. *Pain* 1989; 39:345–352.

Mor N, Winquist J. Self-focused attention and negative affect: a meta-analysis. *Psychol Bull* 2002; 128:638–662.

Morris JS, Ohman A, Dolan RJ. Conscious and unconscious emotional learning in the human amygdala. *Nature* 1998; 393:467–470.

Okifuji A, Turk DC, Curran SL. Anger in chronic pain: investigations of anger targets and intensity. *J Psychosom Res* 1999; 47:1–12.

Ortony AF, Turner TJ. What's basic about basic emotions? *Psychol Rev* 1990; 97:315–331.

Paus T. Primate anterior cingulate cortex: where motor control, drive and cognition interface. *Nat Rev Neurosci* 2001; 2:417–424.

Peckys D, Landwehrmeyer GB. Expression of mu, kappa, and delta opioid receptor messenger RNA in the human CNS: a 33P in situ hybridization study. *Neuroscience* 1999; 88:1093–1135.

Peyron R, Laurent B, Garcia-Larrea L. Functional imaging of brain responses to pain: a review and meta-analysis. *Neurophysiol Clin* 2000; 30:263–288.

Picard N, Strick PL. Motor areas of the medial wall: a review of their location and functional activation. *Cereb Cortex* 1996; 6:342–353.

Ploghaus A, Tracey I, Gati JS, et al. Dissociating pain from its anticipation in the human brain. *Science* 1999; 284:1979–1981.

Plutchik R. A general psychoevolutionary theory of emotion. In: Plutchik R, Kellerman H (Eds). *Emotion: Theory, Research, and Experience,* Theories of Emotion, Vol. 1. New York: Academic Press, 1980, pp 3–33.

Price DD. *Psychological Mechanisms of Pain and Analgesia,* Progress in Pain Research and Management, Vol. 15. Seattle: IASP Press, 1999.

Price DD. Psychological and neural mechanisms of the affective dimension of pain. *Science* 2000; 288:1769–1772.

Price DD, Barrell JJ, Gracely RH. A psychophysical analysis of experiential factors that selectively influence the affective dimension of pain. *Pain* 1980; 8:137–149.

Price DD, Barrell JE, Barrell JJ. A quantitative-experiential analysis of human emotions. *Motivation Emotion* 1985; 9:19–38.

Price DD, Barrell JJ. Some general laws of human emotion: interrelationships between intensities of desire, expectation, and emotional feeling. *J Pers* 1984; 52:389–409.

Rainville P. Brain mechanisms of pain affect and pain modulation. *Curr Opin Neurobiol* 2002; 12:195–204.

Rainville P, Duncan GH, Price DD, Carrier B, Bushnell MC. Pain affect encoded in human anterior cingulate but not somatosensory cortex. *Science* 1997; 277:968–971.

Rainville P, Carrier B, Hofbauer RK, Bushnell MC, Duncan GH. Dissociation of pain sensory and affective dimensions using hypnotic modulation. *Pain* 1999; 82:159–171.

Rainville P, Naqvi N, Long J, Bechara A. Distinct body states associated with self-evoked basic emotions. *Soc Neurosci Abstracts* 2000; 756.13.

Rhudy JL, Meagher MW. Fear and anxiety: divergent effects on human pain thresholds. *Pain* 2000; 84:65–75.

Rhudy JL, Meagher MW. Noise stress and human pain thresholds: divergent effects in men and women. *J Pain* 2001; 2:57–64.

Rhudy JL, Meagher MW. Negative affect: effects on an evaluative measure of human pain. *Pain* 2003; 104:617–626.

Roy M, Peretz I, Rainville P. Effects of emotion induced by music on experimental pain. *Pain Res Manage* 2003; (Suppl 8):33B.

Salovey P. Mood-induced self-focused attention. *J Pers Soc Psychol* 1992; 62:699–707.

Sato A, Sato Y, Schmidt RF. The impact of somatosensory input on autonomic functions. In: Blaustein MP, Grunicke H, Konstanz DP, Schultz G, Schweiger M (Eds). *Rev Physiol Biochem Pharmacol* 1997; 130:1–310.

Schacter S, Singer JE. Cognitive, social, and physiological determinants of emotional state. *Psychol Rev* 1962; 69:379–399.

Sim-Selley LJ, Daunais JB, Porrino LJ, Childers SR. Mu and kappa-1 opioid-stimulated [^{35}S]guanylyl-5'-O-(gamma-thio)- triphosphate binding in cynomolgus monkey brain. *Neuroscience* 1999; 94:651–662.

Simpson JR Jr, Drevets WC, Snyder AZ, Gusnard DA, Raichle ME. Emotion-induced changes in human medial prefrontal cortex: II. During anticipatory anxiety. *Proc Natl Acad Sci USA* 2001; 98:688–693.

Smith WB, Gracely RH, Safer MA. The meaning of pain: cancer patients' rating and recall of pain intensity and affect. *Pain* 1998; 78:123–129.

Sullivan MJ, D'Eon JL. Relation between catastrophizing and depression in chronic pain patients. *J Abnorm Psychol* 1990; 99:260–263.

Sullivan MJ, Neish NR. Catastrophizing, anxiety and pain during dental hygiene treatment. *Community Dent Oral Epidemiol* 1998; 26:344–349.

Sullivan MJ, Rodgers WM, Kirsch I. Catastrophizing, depression and expectancies for pain and emotional distress. *Pain* 2001a; 91:147–154.

Sullivan MJ, Thorn B, Haythornthwaite JA, et al. Theoretical perspectives on the relation between catastrophizing and pain. *Clin J Pain* 2001b; 17:52–64.

Velten E. A laboratory task for induction of mood states. *Behav Res Ther* 1968; 6:473–482.

Vernet-Maury E, Alaoui-Ismaili O, Dittmar A, Delhomme G, Chanel J. Basic emotions induced by odorants: a new approach based on autonomic pattern results. *J Auton Nerv Syst* 1999; 75:176–183.

Villemure C, Slotnick BM, Bushnell MC. Effects of odors on pain perception: deciphering the roles of emotion and attention. *Pain* 2003; 106:101–108.

Vlaeyen JW, Crombez G. Fear of movement/(re)injury, avoidance and pain disability in chronic low back pain patients. *Man Ther* 1999; 4:187–195.

Vlaeyen JW, Linton SJ. Fear-avoidance and its consequences in chronic musculoskeletal pain: a state of the art. *Pain* 2000; 85:317–332.

Wade JB, Price DD, Hamer RM, Schwartz SM, Hart RP. An emotional component analysis of chronic pain. *Pain* 1990; 40:303–310.

Wade JB, Dougherty LM, Archer CR, Price DD. Assessing the multiple stages of pain processing: a multivariate analytical approach. *Pain* 1996; 68:157–167.

Weisenberg M, Raz T, Hener T. The influence of film-induced mood on pain perception. *Pain* 1998; 76:365–375.

Whipple B, Glynn NJ. Quantification of the effects of listening to music as a noninvasive method of pain control. *Sch Inq Nurs Pract* 1992; 6:43–58.

Williams AC. Facial expression of pain: an evolutionary account. *Behav Brain Sci* 2002; 25:439–455.

Willoughby SG, Hailey BJ, Mulkana S, Rowe J. The effect of laboratory-induced depressed mood state on responses to pain. *Behav Med* 2002; 28:23–31.

Zelman DC, Howland EW, Nichols SN, Cleeland CS. The effects of induced mood on laboratory pain. *Pain* 1991; 46:105–111.

Zhang ZH, Dougherty PM, Oppenheimer SM. Monkey insular cortex neurons respond to baroreceptive and somatosensory convergent inputs. *Neuroscience* 1999; 94:351–360.

Zillmann D, De Wied M, King-Jablonski C, Jenzowsky S. Drama-induced affect and pain sensitivity. *Psychosom Med* 1996; 58:333–341.

Zubieta JK, Smith YR, Bueller JA, et al. Regional mu opioid receptor regulation of sensory and affective dimensions of pain. *Science* 2001; 293:311–315.

Correspondence to: Pierre Rainville, PhD, Department of Stomatology, Faculty of Dental Medicine, University of Montreal, CP 6128, Montreal, PQ, Canada H3C 3J7. Tel: 514-343-6111; Fax: 514-343-2111; email: pierre.rainville@umontreal.ca.

Psychological Methods of Pain Control: Basic Science and Clinical Perspectives, Progress in Pain Research and Management, Vol. 29, edited by Donald D. Price and M. Catherine Bushnell, IASP Press, Seattle, © 2004.

7

Environmental and Learning Factors in the Development of Chronic Pain and Disability

Steven J. Linton

Department of Occupational and Environmental Medicine, Örebro University Hospital; and Department of Behavioral, Social, and Legal Sciences-Psychology, Örebro University, Örebro, Sweden

Persistent pain problems do not simply or suddenly occur, but rather they develop in an interaction with the environment. Although we often focus on the internal, biological causes of the painful stimuli, chronic pain also involves a host of behavioral, emotional, and cognitive aspects that change over time. These changes are shaped by the interplay among biological factors, the environment, and our behavior, emotions, and cognitions. Indeed, learning is the foremost mechanism by which the environment impinges upon the development of persistent pain.

There is good reason to be concerned about this process because medical problems involving pain develop into a chronic state surprisingly often. Undeniably, this outcome may represent the "treatment failures" that clinicians strive to avoid. In a wide range of painful illnesses, there is a real risk that the condition will develop into a chronic problem. Estimates of the prevalence of chronic pain range from 7% to 40% (Crombie and Davies 1999). For example, one study showed that 10% of the population may suffer from widespread chronic pain (McBeth and Macfarlane 2002). Moreover, long-term pain problems are not uncommon after a variety of illnesses including headache, stroke, surgery, stomach disorders, and most forms of musculoskeletal disorders (Crombie et al. 1999). In fact, back and neck pain are by far the most common sources of persistent pain (McBeth and Macfarlane 2002). This chapter puts spinal pain in the spotlight as an example of how chronic pain may develop. However, the processes described here are relevant to the development of long-term pain problems in general.

Although the term "chronic pain" is frequently employed to denote pain that persists beyond the normal time of healing, other terms such as "persistent pain" may be more appropriate. The word "chronic" holds the connotation that the problem is irreversible. However, one important message in this chapter is that understanding the influence of learning factors on pain opens new doors to treatment and prevention. In other words, if certain aspects of a persistent problem are learned, then it is possible to change these through learning as well. Thus, I prefer the term "persistent" or "long-term" rather than "chronic" because they simply refer to the length of the problem.

This chapter will explore the developmental process of how a pain problem develops into a chronic one. While pain intensity is the center of attention in the clinic, I will also concentrate on function and disability because persistent pain is characterized not only by the experience of pain, but above all by the devastating consequences it has on one's ability to function in daily life. I conclude the chapter by examining the consequences of our current knowledge for clinical practice. Better understanding of the process of the development of persistent pain should facilitate early identification and intervention.

THE TIME FACTOR: ACUTE, CHRONIC, OR RECURRENT

Time is a crucial factor because it provides a framework and plays a role in the chronification process itself. The development of persistent pain may be described in a series of stages (Vällfors 1985; Skevington 1995; Gatchel 1996). However, the road from acute injury to chronic dysfunction may be quite different for various individuals. Rather than being a stable phenomenon, this progression appears to be influenced by critical factors and incidents that determine its exact course for a given person. *Acute pain*, which is generally defined as pain lasting up to about 3 weeks, is characterized by temporary decreases in activity, reliance on medication, and help-seeking. It is accompanied by psychological distress such as fear, anxiety, and worry in addition to beliefs that pain is controllable through medication and active coping. The patient may have organic findings and muscle spasms. In the next stage, *subacute pain*, considered to last between 3 and 12 weeks, patients may exhibit altering patterns of increasing and decreasing activity and may withdraw or become reliant on medication. They often attempt to maintain their work, and they use various coping styles. Pain of varying intensity is experienced, and depressive symptoms may begin to develop. Patients tend to focus on the physical symptoms, which are affected by stress. Anxiety may persist, and anger and frustration are common. As time passes, the likelihood of finding organic pathology decreases. In *persistent* or *chronic pain*, often defined as pain lasting more than 3 months, activities may have decreased sharply, and patients may "doctor shop" and overuse medications. Acceptance of these lifestyle changes accompanies the sick role. The pain becomes more constant, although patients may experience "good" and "bad" periods. Depression and passive coping strategies become predominant. Similarly, a preoccupation with symptoms is common, as are beliefs that the patient has little control over the pain. Typically there are few organic findings that can be treated, but the patient may suffer from spasms, inflammation, and decreased muscle strength and endurance.

Although the above stages of pain development serve as a heuristic aid, it is vital to understand that musculoskeletal pain is almost always *recurrent*. While most episodes of back pain remit rather quickly, and most people return to work within 6 weeks (Reid et al. 1997), the majority of sufferers will experience several episodes of pain during the course of a year (Frymoyer 1992; Nachemson 1992; Von Korff 1994). In addition, it is rare indeed for someone with no history of such pain to be off work for 6 weeks or more during the first episode. Rather, persistent problems tend to develop over extended periods of time in which recurrent bouts become more frequent and last longer (Philips and Grant 1991; Rossignol et al. 1992; Von Korff 1994). More than 50% of patients with acute back pain will experience another bout within a year (Nachemson 1992), and prospective studies indicate that almost half will still have significant problems 6–12 months later (Philips and Grant 1991; Von Korff 1994; Linton and Halldén 1997).

To understand persistent musculoskeletal pain, it is helpful to view it as a developmental process, given that psychological factors work over time to produce the cognitive, emotional, and behavioral changes defining the syndrome. Interestingly, the psychological reactions associated with acute pain typically result in adequate adjustment to the pain until healing occurs and the pain subsides. A surprising number of people, moreover, cope with persistent pain so well that they require little sick leave or health care (Linton 1999). For a minority of people, however, the cognitive, emotional, and behavioral reactions are not sufficient and may even contribute to the development of persistent pain problems.

PSYCHOLOGICAL RISK FACTORS IN THE TRANSITION FROM ACUTE TO PERSISTENT PAIN

One way of approaching the development of persistent pain is to examine the risk factors associated with it. In this way, one might isolate variables that seem to promote chronicity. Psychological factors are known to play a significant role in chronic pain (Skevington 1995; Main and Spanswick 2000), and they appear to play a fundamental role in the *transition* from acute to chronic problems (Turk 1997; Burton et al. 1999; Linton 2000b).

To identify which psychological factors might be involved in the development of persistent pain, I conducted a systematic review of the literature, focusing on prospective studies. These studies are characterized by the fact that they first measure a psychological variable and then follow participants to determine outcome. In this way, the effects of a particular psychological variable in the *development* of the problem may be better ascertained. The literature search isolated 37 such studies that were deemed to be of relatively high quality (Linton 2000a,b). In fact, 26 of the studies first measured psychological factors either in healthy individuals or acute back pain patients and subsequently followed participants over several months to determine how the pain problem developed. These 26 studies are therefore particularly interesting for models concerning the development of persistent pain. A summary of the studies clearly demonstrated that psychological factors were consistently related to the onset and development of back pain problems.

The significant psychological risk factors isolated represented cognitive, emotional, and behavioral variables. For example, cognitive variables such as fear-avoidance beliefs and catastrophizing were stable features having a particularly significant relationship with the development of dysfunction. Further, anxiety, distress, and stress were related to back pain in every study that investigated them. Similarly, mood and depression were unfailingly reported to be significant risk factors. Behavioral aspects such as coping strategies and higher levels of pain behavior and dysfunction were also related to poor outcome. Similar findings have been reported in other reviews of the literature (Turk 1997; Pincus et al. 2002). Thus, psychological variables affecting the individual seem to be pivotal in the transition from acute to chronic pain.

While individual psychological factors have been highlighted above, one may also need to consider psychosocial factors at the workplace in the development of a persistent problem because work disability is a common feature. I conducted a review of the literature that featured prospective studies where psychological work factors were measured first and participants were then followed to determine outcome (Linton 2001). My review was consistent with others in underscoring several links between psychological factors at work and back pain (Bongers et al. 1993; Hoogendoorn et al. 2000; Linton 2001; National Research Council 2001). These included such risk factors as stress, perceived control, work pace, job content, and job satisfaction. Consequently, psychological factors at work appear to play a significant role in the development of persistent pain and disability.

To summarize, considerable evidence links psychological factors to the development of persistent pain problems including suffering, health care usage, and work disability. One possible explanation is that such variables create *barriers* for a return to work (Main and Spanswick 2000). Several obstacles for return to work in fact appear to be related to the interaction between individual patients and their psychological work environment (Marhold et al. 2002; Shaw et al. 2002).

Although my review of psychological risk factors underscores the importance of these variables, it does not provide a proper picture of how persistent pain develops over time. In order to understand the process one must examine the mechanisms that determine development. Unfortunately, our knowledge about mechanisms is fractional, and considerable work remains to be done. In part, this difficulty arises because developmental processes are by nature fluid and therefore difficult to capture in traditional scientific methodology aimed at looking at static relationships. However, some emerging ideas deserve our attention. Therefore, let us explore some concepts that may help us better understand the mechanisms involved in the development of persistent pain (Linton 2002).

DEVELOPMENTAL MECHANISMS

In this section I consider some of the mechanisms that appear to be involved when spinal pain extends to a persistent problem. No such appraisal could possibly cover every conception of operative mechanisms, of which a seemingly infinite number have been proposed. I have summarized some examples that I find particularly interesting for exploring the development of the problem over time.

ENVIRONMENTAL INFLUENCES (LEARNING)

Most of the things we do, say, and think when we experience a painful stimulus are learned behaviors. Whether we take an aspirin, go for a walk, or attempt to think about something else, these activities are all learned rather than innate behaviors. In essence, learning theory postulates that our behavior, including when we are in pain, is steered by its consequences and by the situation in which it occurs. Early on, Fordyce and others (Fordyce 1976; Keefe et al. 1978; Linton et al. 1984) described how learning factors influence behavior, referring to "pain" behavior as opposed to "well" behavior. Since then, learning paradigms have been developed and tested. Clearly, pain behaviors are controlled in part by their consequences. Interestingly, various sorts of pain-related behaviors are specific to the situation in which they occur (the setting or discriminative stimulus), but they may generalize to other situations. When reinforcement is provided according to certain schedules, the pain behavior may be maintained even though the nociceptive stimulus is no longer present. Simply stated, behaviors that successfully reduce or eliminate pain will tend to increase in frequency in similar situations, while behaviors that result in increases in pain will tend to decrease in frequency. This is a basic and powerful mechanism.

As a specific example, in one experiment we provided positive feedback to normal subjects who received painful stimuli in the form of pressure. At the same time as we systematically reduced the pressure, we provided reinforcement for high pain ratings, and subjects continued to rate the stimulus as clearly "painful" even though the pressure was reduced dramatically (Linton and Götestam 1985). Thus, we concluded that the consequences of the behavior (verbal reinforcement of higher pain ratings) influenced the pain ratings.

Although the learning model can nicely explain the increase in the frequency of pain behaviors and has resulted in a revolution in the way we view pain, it does have certain limitations. First, the theory in its most adamant forms from the 1970s suggests that learning might be the same for all people. That is, it suggests that learning occurs in "an empty box" and that all people might react in the same way given the proper stimuli and consequences. However, learning appears to be more complex, involving numerous individual differences. Further, the simple learning model does not seem to adequately explain why a few people increase their pain behavior while most people decrease it as healing occurs. Why is this the case when the contingencies seem to be quite similar?

COGNITIVE AND EMOTIONAL FACTORS

Psychologists attempted to expand the learning model by adding cognitive processes (Turk et al. 1983; Keefe et al. 1992; Turk 1996). In essence they maintained that learning does not take place in an empty box, but instead is influenced by cognitive and emotional processes that include beliefs, attitudes, and emotional states. As an example, the interpretations that a patient makes concerning a perceived painful stimulus may significantly influence coping behavior (i.e., how the pain is dealt with) as well as how environmental consequences are experienced. Interpretations of the cause of the pain are central. If a patient interprets the cause of a stomachache as being cancer, the emotional reaction is different than if the cause is interpreted as being benign (the garlic eaten last night). Indeed, our belief system seems to be associated with a host of factors that influence expectations about what constitutes a proper assessment, treatment, response from friends and family, and prognosis.

The literature on back pain demonstrates that the belief that activity increases pain is linked to several behaviors (Vlaeyen and Linton 2000). Back pain patients, for example, expect more pain when performing activities (even though the pain that is experienced is less than expected), and higher levels of the belief are associated with lower activity levels. In other words, people who hold this belief tend to avoid movements and activities that they believe will increase the pain or result in injury. Thus, the belief seems integrally related to what is learned and how the pain problem develops.

People may have conceptions of how the spine works that enhance and reflect negative beliefs. As an illustration, a person may believe that the spine has a limited number of movements before it wears out, much like the miles on a car. Given this belief, a good strategy would be to conserve movements so as to not waste the precious few remaining. This strategy results in avoidance of activity. Consequently, examining beliefs about back pain seems to provide insights into how patients behave.

Further, examining beliefs helps to explain how a given consequence may be experienced. That is, the same consequence, such as a stretching sensation in a muscle, may be experienced as positive or negative depending on one's cognitive system. A person who believes there is a risk that the back may break would experience this sensation negatively, which might strengthen the idea that movement is indeed harmful. Such beliefs in turn set the stage for avoidance behavior. On the other hand, a person who believes it is important to use stretching so as to prevent injury while being active may interpret the same sensation as positive. Thus, cognitive factors such as beliefs provide a link between the environment and behavior.

Emotional factors are also tied to the development of persistent problems. Experiences, thoughts, and cognitions trigger emotional responses. For example, the expectation that a movement will result in severe pain triggers fear and worry. Worry in turn serves the purpose of creating vigilance so that danger may be avoided. While this process is ordinarily helpful, we know that in the case of pain, vigilance seems to increase suffering. That is, focusing attention on a painful sensation tends to magnify the pain. As a result, emotions that are linked to cognitions might be said to set the stage for a particular behavior and learning process.

The fear-avoidance model is one concrete mechanism that illustrates the relationship between cognitions, emotions, and behavior (Vlaeyen and Linton 2000). The model features cognitions such as catastrophizing, emotions such as fear, worry, and associated vigilance, and behaviors such as avoidance. In brief, the model purports that if pain is interpreted as threatening, then catastrophizing occurs and fear evolves. Such fear leads to avoidance behaviors, followed by disability, disuse, and depression. This outcome in turn influences pain perception and increases the pain. As a result, a vicious circle evolves where increases in fear and avoidance increase pain, which in turn increases fear. Although this scenario certainly may not apply to all patients with persistent back pain, it represents an important, specific model that may help us to understand how a persistent pain problem develops.

Our view of learning has changed substantially from its first applications to pain. Rather than being a simple, mechanistic influence on an "empty" person, we now see that pain-related learning involves an integration of biological, cognitive, and emotional aspects. Moreover, it appears to be a powerful method for the environment to "select" behaviors. Taken together, the different aspects of learning represent an important means by which the environment asserts control over pain and can contribute to the development of a persistent problem. Below I will expand upon how the environment, through learning, influences the development of persistent pain.

THE PROCESS OF CHRONIFICATION

Most of us tend to view the development of chronic pain as a linear process that occurs relatively rapidly and that is directly related to a specific injury. Yet, as we saw above, musculoskeletal pain is recurrent. This feature sets the stage for the gradual development of persistent pain and disability. In turn, this gradual change seems to be related to cognitive and learning factors. Let us examine a variety of aspects of the chronification process.

INDIVIDUAL PROCESS

Although this chapter describes the general processes involved in the development of a persistent problem, it is important to emphasize that the process is unique to each individual. In fact, the differences among individuals may be quite large. While anxiety and fear avoidance may be important for one person, monotonous work and a poor relationship with a supervisor may be critical for another. Likewise, the pertinent risk factors may change over time. For example, anxiety and fear may be crucial in the acute stage, while depression and catastrophizing may become more important as the problem becomes nonrelenting.

RECURRENT NATURE OF BACK PAIN: REPEATED LEARNING

A key concept is an understanding of the natural history of back pain, where recurrent problems are the rule. First, a bout of back pain normally takes about 8 weeks to subside (van den Hoogen et al. 1998), even though patients may expect it to go away within a few days. Second, back pain is normally recurrent (von Korff 1994; van den Hoogen et al. 1997, 1998). Thus, once someone has experienced a back pain problem it is almost inevitable that he or she will suffer further bouts, usually within a year (van den Hoogen et al. 1998). In the development of a chronic problem, the interval between bouts may gradually become shorter and the length of the bouts longer. During the bouts, people will attempt a variety of ways of coping with the pain and the resultant disability. This experience provides an endless number of learning opportunities. In short, the environment shapes the coping strategies employed and thereby has a direct impact on pain behavior, thoughts, and emotions.

GRADUAL LIFESTYLE CHANGES

The recurrent nature of back pain allows ample opportunities for learning. Considering the large number of people who deal with their back pain effectively, this learning ordinarily seems to be helpful in coping with the problem. However, for some people, coping strategies that seem to work on the short term may enhance the development of a persistent problem in the long term. The process is gradual. Rather than the "straight line" often depicted in the literature, the road to persistent pain is crooked. It is not unusual to experience periods with little or no pain. With small alterations taking place during bouts of pain, a change in lifestyle may occur. However, because of the gradual nature of the change, the person may not be aware of the process until a major development has already taken place.

Gradual changes in lifestyle are particularly difficult to perceive. Therefore, on a cognitive-perceptual level, individuals may not become aware of the type and extent of the change until it is quite advanced. Contributing to these insidious lifestyle changes are expectations that the pain will resolve quickly and that "normality" will be restored. Patients may thereby incorporate coping strategies such as resting, taking medications, and reducing social activities because they believe they will only be temporary. As an illustration, a father who normally plays with his small children each day upon returning home from work may stop doing so when faced with back pain. He may believe that the pain will soon resolve and then the play may be resumed in its usual form. While this is one small lifestyle change involving a few minutes, it is quite likely that other small changes will be made in other sectors of this man's life. When these small changes are pieced together they involve a major change. The gradual character of the change may then circumvent feedback so that the problem continues to develop.

THE ROLE OF INJURY AND THE RESULTANT PAIN

Psychological models might be criticized because they always seem to assume that an injury has occurred, but often ignore this injury once nociception has been initiated. Indeed, many psychological models seem to omit the role of nociception. Nevertheless, we know that the intensity, duration, and quality of the pain can influence our psychological reaction. Thus, an intense "jolt" of pain is experienced very differently than a mild "ache."

These nuances have direct relevance for our understanding of the development of long-term pain problems. First, pain sensations generate reactions including central emotional processes. Intense pain that is quite unlike earlier pain experiences is linked to fear and worry, which may elicit certain beliefs such as "It must be dangerous or it wouldn't hurt so much." In addition, worry enhances vigilance, which influences whether pain signals will be detected. Vigilance and worry, if sufficiently strong, may result in misinterpretations, such that nonpainful signals such as pressure of movement are interpreted as painful.

Second, the pain signals from an injury are related to how the problem might best be dealt with. Coping is postulated to be directly related to the idiosyncrasies of the pain sensations. Distraction may work wonderfully to cope with low-intensity pain, but might be relatively useless for very intense pain, either because intense pain physiologically is programmed to elicit our attention or because it is difficult to maintain distraction techniques as intensity increases.

CRITICAL EVENTS

Certain critical events are hypothesized to account for the apparent "jumps" in the development of long-term pain problems. These critical events are decisive experiences that result in a new belief or behavior for the individual. In this section I will concentrate on negative thoughts and behaviors, but "positive" critical events also apply to the recovery process. An example of a negative critical event is when a patient attempts to return to work and the supervisor states: "Your back is too weak for this work." This event might be critical in changing the patient's beliefs about his or her ability to work ("If my supervisor doesn't believe I can do the job, I must be in really bad shape").

Another example might involve a visit to a health care practitioner. Let us assume that the person with back pain expects to get something to relieve the pain and that the pain will go away within a few days. The provider, however, states that there is probably degeneration in the spine and that the patient must rest to protect the back. This advice might trigger a dramatic change in beliefs and behavior in which the patient begins to entertain the thought that the pain may not resolve, that permanent functional problems will develop, and that it is necessary to restrict movement in order to "save" on wear and tear.

Critical events emphasize that development occurs in "leaps and bounds" rather than in an even, linear fashion. The increments may be relatively small, but in some cases they can be large. Here again, we see the individual nature of the development, as the exact events that trigger the critical events appear to be peculiar to the individual.

DYNAMIC PROCESS

Because they are easier to understand and test, static processes have been the focus of models to date, but a developmental process is by its very nature vibrant. Consequently, if we are to understand how and why chronic pain develops we need to consider longitudinal aspects. Static models are good at isolating important variables and demonstrating links between them. This information is vital for understanding which factors are involved and for developing an overview of the problem. However, static models are poor at elucidating the process involved. Indeed, if we consider the number of variables that may be important in the development of chronic pain and then multiply them by a time unit such as hours or days, a tremendous number of events can occur. To understand development, we need to know more about how these processes start and progress. A good model will incorporate dynamic aspects, although we certainly could not expect a detailed description of every possible road to a chronic problem.

Learning is an important concept because it incorporates a dynamic view. A learning approach includes the person's interaction with pain as well as with the environment. Modern theories of learning include cognitive and emotional aspects. Their advantage is that they serve as an aid in understanding the dynamics of the process because different stimuli, thoughts, emotions, behaviors, and consequences may be placed into the scheme. In this way an individual's situation may be entered into the scheme and analyzed to determine a reasonable explanation for the development of chronic pain. At present, however, it is more difficult to generate scenarios of common paths for the development of persistent pain disability. Such information is vital to identifying people at risk of developing persistent pain, as well as for developing effective preventive interventions. As a result, more work needs to be done to clarify how a persistent problem develops.

SUMMARY OF DEVELOPMENT

The development of long-term pain problems is a complex, multidimensional process whereby psychological factors, in interaction with the environment, play an important catalytic role. The evidence suggests that once a painful injury occurs, the environment shapes our behavior, emotions, and cognitions through psychological factors. These, in turn, influence the course of development. Usually this learning process is advantageous, and quite often the person copes adequately and recovers. However, sometimes the process results in further development of the problem. Thus, psychological factors interplay with other types of variables. Rather than being static, the development of a disabling chronic pain problem involves a dynamic process in which critical events trigger changes in beliefs and behavior. Small resultant changes in lifestyle may then gradually proceed without alarming the individual, who does not perceive the changes. The recurrent nature of musculoskeletal pain is an important feature because it presents numerous opportunities for learning. Thus, psychological factors are comparatively powerful in predicting disability, and they may offer important insights as to how persistent pain problems might be prevented.

IMPLICATIONS FOR CLINICAL PRACTICE

Considerable information about the development of persistent pain problems has been assembled. Such work has several implications for clinical practice. Scientific knowledge as well as the model of development described above give us important insights into how and why persistent pain problems may develop. As a result, we are in a better position to deal with these problems, and I assert that we are even in a position to begin with preventive interventions. Such interventions would admittedly be secondary prevention measures, aimed at those with pain who might develop persistent problems. Nevertheless, this possibility offers a new road for dealing with the problem of persistent pain and disability and could potentially reduce the indescribable amounts of suffering and high costs associated with these disorders.

These implications are directly linked to an early identification of patients risking the development of persistent pain and depend on methods of intervening to prevent this course of events. Let us examine these methods more closely with an eye on what might be done clinically.

EARLY IDENTIFICATION

Screening to identify the few patients who are at considerable risk of developing a persistent problem may be essential for the elaboration of a successful prevention program. This task is not an easy one. Most people will suffer from spinal pain at some point and will have recurrences (Crombie et al. 1999). Yet only a relatively small percentage of these people—an estimated 3–10%—will develop a long-term work absence after an acute bout of back pain (Reid et al. 1997). Given the large number of people who have back pain, the recurrent nature of the problem, and the relatively small number who develop persistent problems, it is a real challenge to identify "at-risk" patients early on. Nevertheless, it is an important challenge because these patients suffer greatly and consume the majority of the resources (Waddell 1996, 1998; Nachemson and Jonsson 2000). Moreover, given their large numbers, it would be difficult to provide all individuals with back pain with a special preventive intervention.

Screening offers several potentially valuable aspects to a clinical assessment. Primarily it provides an opportunity to concentrate limited resources on those patients most in need of help. In addition, early screening might elucidate and direct attention to those psychosocial factors that are most pertinent. Given that psychological factors are not normally included in clinical assessments of patients with acute or subacute pain, for example at a primary care facility, it is valuable to develop relevant targets for intervention. Finally, screening might complement primary care facilities that often simply lack the time and resources for assessing psychosocial factors. Assessing the large number of identified psychosocial risk factors through an interview would, for instance, be time-consuming, especially considering the large number of individuals seeking care for musculoskeletal pain. Some health care professionals may find it difficult to address delicate psychosocial issues such as depression or anxiety and lack skills in how these issues should be handled.

Given that psychological factors have been associated with the development of persistent pain problems, it is logical to explore the utility of such factors in screening. As described above, research has established a firm link between psychological factors and the development of a long-term pain problem (Turk 1996, 1997; Waddell 1998; Turk and Flor 1999; Linton 2000b; Main and Spanswick 2000; Vlaeyen and Linton 2000). Psychosocial factors then might represent key factors that could be utilized in screening (Gatchel et al. 1995; Linton 2000b). As described below, several attempts have been made to develop screening methods such as questionnaires.

A thorough review of screening procedures for back pain has concluded that screening is truly feasible (Waddell et al. 2003). This report found numerous instruments that have been developed for screening purposes. Although these differ considerably, the most efficient can identify about 85% of those who will develop a persistent back pain disability problem. The authors point out that while this percentage is far above guessing, it still involves considerable imprecision in the clinic. However, such imprecision is not unusual in clinical screening in a variety of medical areas, even when biological tests are employed (Waddell et al. 2003; Sheridan and Winogrond 1987). Another important feature concerns the guiding of interventions. While some relatively simple data on age, sex, and education level may be fairly good predictors of receiving disability payments for work incapacity, they tell us little about which preventive interventions might be initiated (Waddell et al. 2003). Let us examine further two instruments designed in part to predict future problems, and in part to focus on important intervention targets.

The first is an instrument developed for use with those suffering work-related upper extremity disorders (Feuerstein et al. 2000). This questionnaire contains items about symptoms, physical function, ergonomics, psychosocial work environment, work demands, social support, and individual psychosocial measures. Outcome was measured three times during the course of a year and consisted of a composite of symptoms, function, mental health, and lost workdays. The sensitivity and specificity of this screening instrument to predict poor outcome 12 months later was 81% and 83%, respectively. This finding suggests that those developing problems might be identified early on. The specificity and sensitivity levels are similar to other instruments in this area and suggest that while they are not precise instruments, they might significantly improve screening procedures.

My colleagues and I have developed the Örebro Musculoskeletal Pain Screening Questionnaire as a clinical tool that focuses on psychological factors and enhances early identification of problem cases (Linton and Halldén 1998; Boersma and Linton 2002). It is a complement to standard medical examinations and provides information concerning the likelihood that a patient will develop disability. It consists of 25 statements or assertions that patients rate on 0–10 point Likert scales. This instrument is self-administered, and most patients complete it within 7 or 8 minutes. A trained health-care provider can score and evaluate it in a couple of minutes. The questionnaire provides an overall score from which risk may be roughly judged as well as ratings on each item. We found it to have satisfactory test-retest reliability (0.83) and validity in a study of 142 patients where the outcome was absenteeism due to sickness (Linton and Halldén 1998). With a cut-off total score of 105, the specificity was found to be 0.75 and the sensitivity 0.88. Several additional studies have shown that this questionnaire is reliable and valid (Linton and Halldén 1998; Hurley et al. 2000, 2001; Boersma and Linton 2002; Linquist et al. 2002; Linton and Boersma 2003). Importantly, the results are also designed to enhance communication with the patient (Boersma and Linton 2002).

EARLY INTERVENTIONS

Once we have identified patients who are at risk of developing persistent problems, the next step is to provide appropriate interventions. Unfortunately, there appears to be a tendency in the health care system to provide "medical" interventions even when psychological factors are identified, perhaps because staff members are trained in medical procedures, but not in providing more psychologically oriented help. Worse, if the treatments are not successful, there may be a tendency to simply provide more of the same treatment, with clinicians increasing the dose of the treatment rather than entertaining new methods. It is logical that if the problem has a psychological aspect, then the intervention might also include a psychological component. Fortunately, health care providers can learn to provide many of these techniques.

COMMUNICATION

Because so many feelings, beliefs, and behaviors are relevant in the interactions patients have with health care professionals, good, clear communication seems to be an imperative method for treating pain and preventing persistent problems. The time pressures of the clinic make this a true challenge, but research indicates that poor communication, be it on the part of the patient or health care provider, may contribute to the development of problems. For example, a recent study of chronic pain patients admitted to a rehabilitation program found that only 32% could provide an accurate cause of their problem, while 20% gave a cause that did not coincide with their diagnosis according to medical records, and the remainder did not know the cause (Geisser and Roth 1998). Furthermore, expectations about the course of the problem often exist, and the patient's own perception of appropriate behavior and the course of the problem are relatively powerful predictors of future disability (Waddell et al. 1993; Linton and Halldén 1998).

The importance of good doctor-patient communication early on is illustrated by a recent study that demonstrated that people seeking help for acute back pain are in fact quite worried that their pain is the result of a serious injury (Von Korff et al. 1998). Thus, typical patients are in need of reassurance and clear advice about how to continue their daily activities (Waddell et al. 1997; Waddell 1998; Main and Spanswick 2000; Nachemson and Jonsson 2000). Consequently, it is not surprising that treatment "style" is related to outcome for patients with low back pain (Von Korff et al. 1994). Doctors with a style featuring frequent recommendations for bed rest and analgesics as needed had patients with significantly more disability at follow-up than did doctors clearly communicating the need for self-care strategies. In further research using audiotapes of primary care visits, the results showed that many doctors avoided asking about how the pain interfered with activities, even though this is one of the most frequent reasons for patients to seek care (Turner et al. 1998). Thus, it seems that many of the attitudes and beliefs patients develop may be related to encounters with health care providers.

The first meeting with the patient offers a unique opportunity to shape the patient's attitudes and behaviors and to enlist him or her as a partner in treatment. This rapport is central because modern interventions invariably involve self-help efforts such as exercising, practicing relaxation, or taking medications on a specific schedule. Indeed, optimal communication with the patient at the first visit appears to be vital. Waddell and colleagues (1997), for example, reviewed the literature on providing advice for back pain patients. They found that advice for bed rest was counterproductive, while advice to remain active despite the pain produced a significantly better long-term result with regard to pain and disability. Consequently, the first consultation may be an excellent opportunity for sowing the seeds of self-management rather than those of disability development. In the early stages, usually as part of the ordinary clinical routine, preventive methods may be relatively easy to administer, have simple content, and involve a minimum of time. However, as the problem grows, so too does the extent of the prophylactic intervention. While good communication and recommendations may be a valuable method for first visits, more elaborate techniques as well as the input of other professionals may become necessary as the problem progresses.

EARLY PSYCHOLOGICAL TECHNIQUES

Although psychological factors are believed to be central in the development of a chronic back pain problem, there have been relatively few attempts to prevent chronic disability with psychological techniques. Still, if psychological risk factors enhance the development of a chronic problem (Kendall et al. 1998; Linton 2000a,b), then psychological interventions might be of real value. In order to provide a replicable secondary preventive intervention from a psychological perspective, our clinic developed a program that builds on experiences from earlier programs provided for chronic pain patients (Compas et al. 1998; Morley et al. 1999; Linton 2000c; van Tulder et al. 2000). However, we focused on the risk factors identified in the screening assessment and the developmental process described above. Thus, the intervention has, from the beginning, been focused on *prevention of persistent pain and disability* and not simply on pain treatment. The intervention encompasses a six-session structured program in which participants meet in groups of 6 to 10 people, once a week for 2 hours. This section describes the application of a cognitive-behavioral approach developed in our clinic as a secondary prevention measure.

GOALS

The intervention has several goals, but the overriding aim is for participants to develop their own coping program. We ask participants to learn and apply all the skills presented during the course so that a tailored program that bests suits each person's needs may be developed.

From a provider's point of view we hope to prevent pain-related disability and absenteeism and minimize the need for health care services, in addition to improving quality of life so that the patient feels and functions better. We address factors such as pain intensity, stress levels, and participation in everyday activities. We realize that back pain is recurrent and therefore we do not intend to eliminate it, but rather to decrease recurrences and reduce their impact.

CONTENT

Sessions were organized to activate participants and promote coping. Each session began with a short review of homework. Subsequently, the therapist introduced the topic for the session and provided information for a maximum of 15 minutes. Participants received a case description together with problems concerning the case that were to be solved with the help of a partner. Solutions were presented in the group and discussed. Subsequently, the therapist introduced new coping skills, and participants practiced them. All participants were asked to apply all of the skills learned in their everyday life to gain some experience. Finally, the session was reviewed, underscoring what the participants had learned and reviewing what the homework assignment would be. Homework assignments were tailored to each participant's needs. Strengths and weaknesses of the session were brought up to provide continual quality assessment for the group and the therapist.

Each session focused on a particular area of relevance, and participants developed a personal coping program. Sessions covered how patients might control pain intensity or participate in activities. In addition, topics centered on problems encountered at work, at home, and during leisure activities. Various coping skills were taught that could be applied to real-life situations. These included pain control measures such as relaxation and distraction. However, many skills were oriented toward activity and function, including problem-solving skills, learning about graded activity, and social and stress management skills. Finally, participants developed their personal coping program based on the techniques they believed were most effective for their problem. The last two sessions focused on finalizing this program and dealing with possible flare-ups and setbacks.

STRATEGIES FOR BEHAVIORAL CHANGE

An important question is how an intervention can change cognitions, emotions, and behavior. Indeed, the courses we offer require the participant to alter current cognitions and behaviors. For example, beliefs about the relationship between pain and activity ("The more I do, the more it will hurt") or beliefs about stress ("I must do everything asked of me and exactly on time") may need to be revised. Likewise, behaviors may need to be changed, perhaps by increasing activity levels or by being able to say "no" to certain demands. The question becomes *how* this goal might be accomplished. Our program employs several strategies.

First, the program is designed to actively engage the participant. Rather than a passive "school" approach, active participation is prompted and then reinforced. In discussions, for example, each participant is asked individually to provide input. Problem-solving exercises are tackled in pairs to promote discussion, and each pair reports the results. Above all, each person is given the charge of developing his or her own personal coping program.

Second, restricted amounts of information are used to provide examples of appropriate coping behaviors. This part of the session is used to model appropriate behaviors as well as to challenge common beliefs.

A third strategy involves behavioral tests. This key method incorporates the power of learning through experience. In this technique a patient's beliefs or behaviors are examined, and then a test is performed to see if the belief is true. By asking patients to test each skill, we encourage them to learn to assess its possible value and provide a basis for them to select the skills necessary for their personal coping program.

Problem solving is a fourth strategy utilized throughout to promote engagement and enhance skill maintenance. This skill is honed in a special problem-based learning module, and it is employed whenever patients describe a "problem" or hindrance.

Fifth, the group leader is taught to shape new thoughts and behaviors by reinforcing successive approximations of good coping behavior. Positive reinforcement, for example in the form of encouragement, is contingently provided when participants correctly approximate a goal behavior. Thus, gradual change is encouraged.

To maximize engagement and skill maintenance, another strategy is to enhance each patient's self-efficacy, that is, the patient's belief that he or she can influence the pain and its course. This is a logical goal because many patients have low self-efficacy levels and do not believe that they can change their health behavior. For example, we might ask patients who have successfully completed a homework assignment, such as practicing relaxation and noting a decrease in pain, to share the "secret" of their success with the entire group.

Finally, enjoyment is used to enhance learning, engagement, skill maintenance, and pleasure. It is an important strategy to ensure that all participants feel they have learned something during each session. People should have the opportunity to laugh and to receive social support. Encouragement should be contingently delivered in a rich schedule so that participants may feel good about their accomplishments.

OUTCOMES

Although early, preventive methods are relatively new to the field, some attempts at evaluation have been promising. For example, Von Korff and colleagues (1998) reported the results of one of the first studies of the effects of a psychological intervention given in groups to help patients specifically deal with psychological aspects in the hope of preventing future problems. The intervention was based on lay-led groups for arthritic pain and focused on self-care (Von Korff 1999). Trained lay leaders assisted participants in a well-organized four-session program including problem-solving skills, activity management, and educational videos. An evaluation was conducted on 255 patients about 8 weeks after a primary care visit for back pain. Participants were randomized to the cognitive-behavioral group or a control group. At the 1-year follow-up the cognitive-behavioral group had significantly reduced worry and disability relative to the treatment-as-usual control. Participants in the lay-led group also had a significantly more positive view toward self-care, but there was no significant difference with regard to pain intensity or medication use. Results were comparable in two other reports using similar methods (Saunders et al. 1999; Moore et al. 2000).

My colleagues and I have tested our own program, described above, in four randomized controlled trials. The first test of utility compared this approach to treatment as usual (Linton and Andersson 2000). Participants suffered acute or subacute pain and perceived that they had a risk of developing a chronic problem, but had not been off work more than 3 months during the past year. Those fulfilling these criteria (243 participants) were randomly assigned to one of three groups. The first two groups received usual treatment plus one of two forms of self-help information for back pain. The third group received the cognitive-behavioral group intervention described above. Results at the 1-year follow-up indicated a preventive effect of the psychological intervention. While all three groups reported benefits including reduced pain intensity, the groups only receiving information were nine times more likely to take long-term sick leave than the cognitive-behavioral intervention group. The group intervention also produced a significant decrease in perceived risk, as well as significantly fewer physician and physical therapy visits compared to the comparison groups. Thus, long-term disability and health care use were "prevented" in the cognitive-behavioral group.

The second test was similar to the first, but focused on a group of non-patients from the general population (Linton and Ryberg 2001), so it may be considered a very early intervention. The 253 participants reported four or more episodes of relatively intense spinal pain during the preceding year, but had not been off work more than 30 days. Participants were randomly assigned to the cognitive-behavioral group or to a treatment-as-usual comparison group. At the 1-year follow-up, results showed that the cognitive-behavioral group, relative to the comparison group, had significantly better outcomes on fear avoidance, number of pain-free days, and amount of sick leave. In fact, the risk for long-term sick leave during the follow-up in the cognitive-behavioral group was one-third that of the treatment-as-usual comparison group.

In a third test the early cognitive-behavioral intervention was combined with return-to-work skills training for patients off work because of their pain

(Marhold et al. 2001). In brief, the results demonstrated that participants on short-term sick leave (mean 3 months) had significantly less absenteeism at the 1-year follow-up relative to a treatment-as-usual control group.

Finally, the fourth test focused on incorporating the cognitive-behavioral groups into a primary care setting (Linton et al., in press). Given that physical therapy is a frequent treatment for back pain, we were interested in seeing whether the psychological and physical therapy modules might be combined. The physical therapy methods employed were of a preventive nature and were based primarily on exercise. Thus, we compared a standardized, guideline-based treatment as usual with cognitive-behavioral therapy, either alone or combined with physical therapy, by randomizing 185 patients seeking help for back pain to these three groups. The results showed that the two groups receiving cognitive-behavioral interventions had fewer days off work for back pain during the 12-month follow-up than did the minimal-treatment group. The risk for developing long-term sick disability leave was more than five times greater in the guideline-based treatment-as-usual group as in the other two groups receiving the cognitive-behavioral intervention. However, there was no difference in sick leave between the two groups receiving cognitive-behavioral therapy alone and with physical therapy.

CONCLUSIONS

This chapter has highlighted psychological variables including behaviors, emotions, and cognitions in the development of a persistent pain problem. Psychological factors are intricately related to this development and appear to enhance or catalyze the problem. A psychological model of pain development may help us to understand this process better. Importantly, while most models are static, the developmental process is quite dynamic. The recurrent nature of musculoskeletal pain provides ample opportunities for learning to occur. Recent data suggest that the process of chronification is highly individual, but normally involves a gradual change in lifestyle. These changes are propelled by certain critical events. The role of the injury and the experience of the pain itself are vital. The experience of the pain interacts with other psychological variables influencing our emotions, cognitions, and behaviors. Thus, when an injury occurs, psychological factors interact with other variables to shape the course of development.

This analysis of the development of chronic pain has several implications for prevention. It suggests that our knowledge about psychological processes may be utilized in the early identification of patients who are likely to develop problems, as well as in the design of preventive interventions. Improving the content of the first visit with the patient, for example, may have considerable preventive consequences. Moreover, providing psychologically oriented early interventions for those patients with a psychological risk profile might also have preventive results. Future efforts should be directed at developing a sound theory concerning the development of chronic pain. As this theory develops, additional investigations will be needed to test the new preventive methods that it may suggest.

REFERENCES

Boersma K, Linton SJ. Early assessment of psychological factors: the Örebro Screening Questionnaire for Pain. In: Linton SJ (Ed). *New Avenues for the Prevention of Pain,* Vol. 1. Amsterdam: Elsevier, 2002, pp 205–213.

Bongers PM, de Winter CR, Kompier MA, Hildebrandt VH. Psychosocial factors at work and musculoskeletal disease. *Scand J Work Environ Health* 1993; 19(5):297–312.

Burton AK, Battié MC, Main CJ. The relative importance of biomechanical and psychosocial factors in low back injuries. In: Karwowski W, Marras W (Eds). *The Occupational Ergonomics Handbook.* Boca Raton, FL: CRC Press, 1999, pp 1127–1138.

Compas BE, Haaga DAF, Keefe FJ, Leitenberg H, Williams DA. A sampling of empirically supported psychological treatments from health psychology: smoking, chronic pain, cancer, and bulimia nervosa. *J Consult Clin Psychol* 1998; 66:89–112.

Crombie IK, Davies JTP. Requirements for epidemiological studies. In: Crombie IK, Croft PR, Linton SJ, LeResche L, Von Korff M (Eds). *Epidemiology of Pain.* Seattle: IASP Press, 1999, pp 17–24.

Crombie IK, Croft PR, Linton SJ, LeResche L, Von Korff M. *Epidemiology of Pain.* Seattle: IASP Press, 1999.

Feuerstein M, Huang GD, Haufler AJ, Miller JK. Development of a screen for predicting clinical outcomes in patients with work-related upper extremity disorders. *J Occup Environ Med* 2000; 42(7):749–761.

Fordyce WE. *Behavioral Methods for Chronic Pain and Illness.* St. Louis: Mosby, 1976.

Frymoyer JW. Predicting disability from low back pain. *Clin Orthop* 1992; 279:101–109.

Gatchel RJ. Psychological disorders and chronic pain: cause and effect relationships. In: Gatchel RJ, Turk DC (Eds). *Psychological Approaches to Pain Management: A Practitioner's Handbook,* Vol. 1. New York: Guilford Press, 1996, pp 33–54.

Gatchel RJ, Polatin PB, Kinney RK. Predicting outcome of chronic back pain using clinical predictors of psychopathology: a prospective analysis. *Health Psychol* 1995,14(5):415–420.

Geisser ME, Roth RS. Knowledge of and agreement with chronic pain diagnosis: relation to affective distress, pain beliefs and coping, pain intensity, and disability. *J Occup Rehabil* 1998; 8(1):73–88.

Hoogendoorn WE, van Poppel MNM, Bongers PM, Koes BW, Bouter LM. Systematic review of psychosocial factors at work and in the personal situation as risk factors for back pain. *Spine* 2000; 25(16):2114–2125.

Hurley D, Dusoir T, McDonough S, et al. Biopsychosocial screening questionnaire for patients with low back pain: preliminary report of utility in physiotherapy practice in Northern Ireland. *Clin J Pain* 2000; 16(3):214–228.

Hurley D, Dusoir T, McDonough S, Moore A, Baxter G. How effective is the Acute Low Back Pain Screening Questionnaire for predicting 1-year follow-up in patients with low back pain? *Clin J Pain* 2001; 17:256–263.

Keefe FJ, Kopel S, Gordon SB. *A Practical Guide to Behavioral Assessment.* New York: Springer, 1978.

Keefe FJ, Dunsmore J, Burnett R. Behavioral and cognitive-behavioral approaches to chronic pain: recent advances and future directions. *J Consult Clin Psychol* 1992; 54:776–783.

Kendall NAS, Linton SJ, Main C. Psychosocial yellow flags for acute low back pain: "Yellow Flags" as an analogue to "Red Flags." *Eur J Pain* 1998; 2(1):87–89.

Linquist L, Ektor-Andersen J, Örbaek P. Prediction of vocational dysfunction due to musculoskeletal symptoms by screening for psychosocial factors at primary care setting. *Abstracts: 10th World Congress on Pain.* Seattle: IASP Press, 2002, p 345.

Linton SJ. Prevention with special reference to chronic musculoskeletal disorders. In: Gatchel RJ, Turk DC (Eds). *Psychosocial Factors in Pain,* Vol. 1. New York: Guilford Press, 1999, pp 374–389.

Linton SJ. Psychologic risk factors for neck and back pain. In: Nachemsom A, Jonsson E (Eds). *Neck and Back Pain: The Scientific Evidence of Causes, Diagnosis, and Treatment.* Philadelphia: Lippincott, Williams, and Wilkins, 2000a, pp 57–78.

Linton SJ. A review of psychological risk factors in back and neck pain. *Spine* 2000b; 25(9):1148–1156.

Linton SJ. Utility of cognitive-behavioral psychological treatments. In: Nachemson A, Jonsson E (Eds). *Neck and Back Pain: The Scientific Evidence of Causes, Diagnosis, and Treatment.* Philadelphia: Lippincott, Williams, and Wilkins, 2000c, pp 361–381.

Linton SJ. Occupational psychological factors increase the risk for back pain: a systematic review. *J Occup Rehabil* 2001; 11(1):53–66.

Linton SJ. Why does chronic pain develop? A behavioral approach. In: Linton SJ (Ed). *New Avenues for the Prevention of Chronic Musculoskeletal Pain and Disability.* Amsterdam: Elsevier Science, 2002, pp 67–82.

Linton SJ, Andersson T. Can chronic disability be prevented? A randomized trial of a cognitive-behavior intervention and two forms of information for patients with spinal pain. *Spine* 2000; 25(21):2825–2831.

Linton SJ, Boersma K. Early identification of patients at risk of developing a persistent back problem: the predictive validity of the Örebro Musculoskeletal Pain Questionnaire. *Clin J Pain* 2003; 19:80–86.

Linton SJ, Götestam KG. Controlling pain reports through operant conditioning: a laboratory demonstration. *Percept Motor Skills* 1985; 60:427–437.

Linton SJ, Halldén K. Risk factors and the natural course of acute and recurrent musculoskeletal pain: developing a screening instrument. In: Jensen TS, Turner JA, Wiesenfeld-Hallin Z (Eds). *Proceedings of the 8th World Congress on Pain,* Progress in Pain Research and Management, Vol. 8. Seattle: IASP Press, 1997, pp 527–536.

Linton SJ, Halldén K. Can we screen for problematic back pain? A screening questionnaire for predicting outcome in acute and subacute back pain. *Clin J Pain* 1998; 14(3):209–215.

Linton SJ, Ryberg M. A cognitive-behavioral group intervention as prevention for persistent neck and back pain in a non-patient population: a randomized controlled trial. *Pain* 2001; 90:83–90.

Linton SJ, Melin L, Götestam KG. Behavioral analysis of chronic pain and its management. *Prog Behav Mod* 1984; 18:1–42.

Linton SJ, Boersma K, Jansson M, Svärd L, Botvalde M. The effects of cognitive-behavioral and physical therapy preventive interventions on pain related sick leave: a randomized controlled trial. *Clin J Pain*; in press.

Main CJ, Spanswick CC. *Pain Management: An Interdisciplinary Approach.* Edinburgh: Churchill Livingstone, 2000.

Marhold C, Linton SJ, Melin L. Cognitive behavioral return-to-work program: effects on pain patients with a history of long-term versus short-term sick leave. *Pain* 2001; 91:155–163.

Marhold C, Linton SJ, Melin L. Identification of obstacles for chronic pain patients to return to work: evaluation of a questionnaire. *J Occup Rehabil* 2002; 12(2):65–75.

McBeth J, Macfarlane GJ. The prevalence of regional and widespread musculoskeletal pain symptoms. In: Linton SJ (Ed). *New Avenues for the Prevention of Chronic Musculoskeletal Pain and Disability*. Amsterdam: Elsevier Science, 2002, pp 7–22.

Moore JE, Von Korff M, Cherkin D, Saunders K, Lorig K. A randomized trial of a cognitive-behavioral program for enhancing back pain self care in a primary care setting. *Pain* 2000; 88:145–153.

Morley S, Eccleston C, Williams A. Systematic review and meta-analysis of randomised controlled trials of cognitive behaviour therapy and behaviour therapy for chronic pain in adults, excluding headache. *Pain* 1999; 80(1–2):1–13.

Nachemson AL. Newest knowledge of low back pain. *Clin Orthop* 1992; 279:8–20.

Nachemson A, Jonsson E (Eds). *Neck and Back Pain: The Scientific Evidence of Causes, Diagnosis, and Treatment*. Philadelphia: Lippincott, Williams and Wilkins, 2000.

National Research Council. *Musculoskeletal Disorders and the Workplace*. Washington, DC: National Academy Press, 2001.

Philips HC, Grant L. The evolution of chronic back pain problems: a longitudinal study. *Behav Res Ther* 1991; 29:435–441.

Pincus T, Burton AK, Vogel S, Field AP. A systematic review of psychological factors as predictors of chronicity/disability in prospective cohorts of low back pain. *Spine* 2002; 27(5):E109–120.

Reid S, Haugh LD, Hazard RG, Tripathi M. Occupational low back pain: recovery curves and factors associated with disability. *J Occup Rehabil* 1997; 7(1):1–14.

Rossignol H, Suissa S, Abenhaim L. The evolution of compensated occupational spinal injuries. *Spine* 1992; 17:1043–1047.

Saunders KW, Von Korff M, Pruitt SD, Moore JE. Prediction of physician visits and prescription medicine use for back pain. *Pain* 1999; 83(2):369–377.

Shaw WS, Feuerstein M, Huang GD. Secondary prevention and the workplace. In: Linton SJ (Ed). *New Avenues for the Prevention of Chronic Musculoskeletal Pain and Disability*. Amsterdam: Elsevier, 2002, pp 215–235.

Sheridan DP, Winogrond IR. *The Preventive Approach to Patient Care*. Amsterdam: Elsevier, 1987.

Skevington SM. *Psychology of Pain*. London: Wiley, 1995.

Turk DC. Biopsychosocial perspective on chronic pain. In: Gatchel RJ, Turk DC (Eds). *Psychological Approaches to Pain Management: A Practitioner's Handbook*. New York: Guilford Press, 1996, pp 3–32.

Turk DC. The role of demographic and psychosocial factors in transition from acute to chronic pain. In: Jensen TS, Turner JA, Wiesenfeld-Hallin Z (Eds). *Proceedings of the 8th World Congress on Pain*, Progress in Pain Research and Management, Vol. 8. Seattle: IASP Press, 1997, pp 185–213.

Turk DC, Flor H. Chronic pain: a biobehavioral perspective. In: Gatchel RJ, Turk DC (Eds). *Psychosocial Factors in Pain: Critical Perspectives*, Vol. 1. New York: Guilford Press, 1999, pp 18–34.

Turk DC, Meichenbaum D, Genest M. *Pain and Behavioral Medicine: A Cognitive-Behavioral Perspective*. New York: Guilford Press, 1983.

Turner J, LeResche L, von Korff M, Ehrlich K. Primary care back pain patient characteristics, visit content, and short-term outcomes. *Spine* 1998; 23:463–469.

van den Hoogen HJM, Koes BW, Devillé W, van Eijk JTM, Bouter LM. The prognosis of low back pain in general practice. *Spine* 1997; 22(13):1515–1521.

van den Hoogen HJM, Koes BW, van Eijk TM, Bouter LM, Devillé W. On the course of low back pain in general practice: a one year follow up study. *Ann Rheum Dis* 1998; 57:13–19.

van Tulder MW, Ostelo R, Vlaeyen JWS, et al. Behavioral treatment for chronic low back pain: a systematic review within the framework of the Cochrane Back Review Group. *Spine* 2000; 25(20):2688–2699.

Vlaeyen JWS, Linton SJ. Fear-avoidance and its consequences in chronic musculoskeletal pain: a state of the art. *Pain* 2000; 85:317–332.

Von Korff M. Perspectives on management of back pain in primary care. In: Gebhart GF, Hammond DL, Jensen TS (Eds). *Proceedings of the 7th World Congress on Pain,* Progress in Pain Research and Management, Vol. 2. Seattle: IASP Press, 1994, pp 97–110.

Von Korff M. Pain management in primary care: an individualized stepped/care approach. In: Gatchel RJ, Turk DC (Eds). *Psychosocial Factors in Pain,* 1st ed. New York: Guilford Press, 1999, pp 360–373.

Von Korff M, Barlow W, Cherkin D, Deyo RA. Effects of practice style in managing back pain. *Ann Intern Med* 1994; 121(3):187–195.

Von Korff M, Moore JE, Lorig K, et al. A randomized trial of a lay-led self-management group intervention for back pain patients in primary care. *Spine* 1998; 23:2608–2615.

Vällfors B. Acute, subacute and chronic low back pain. *Scand J Rehabil Med* 1985; (Suppl 11):1–98.

Waddell G. Low back pain: a twentieth century health care enigma. *Spine* 1996; 21(24):2820–2825.

Waddell G. *The Back Pain Revolution.* Edinburgh: Churchill Livingstone, 1998.

Waddell G, Newton M, Henderson I, Somerville D, Main CJ. A Fear-Avoidance Beliefs Questionnaire (FABQ) and the role of fear-avoidance beliefs in chronic low back pain and disability. *Pain* 1993; 52:157–168.

Waddell G, Feder G, Lewis M. Systematic reviews of bed rest and advice to stay active for acute low back pain. *Br J Gen Pract* 1997; 47:647–652.

Waddell G, Kurton AK, Main CJ. *Screening to Identify People at Risk of Long-Term Incapacity for Work: A Conceptual and Scientific Review.* London: Royal Society of Medicine Press, 2003.

Correspondence to: Steven J. Linton, PhD, Department of Occupational and Environmental Medicine, Örebro University Hospital, Örebro 70185, Sweden. Email: steven.linton@orebroll.se.

Part III

Modulation of Pain by Placebos

Psychological Methods of Pain Control: Basic Science and Clinical Perspectives, Progress in Pain Research and Management, Vol. 29, edited by Donald D. Price and M. Catherine Bushnell, IASP Press, Seattle, © 2004.

8

Neural Mechanisms of Placebo-Induced Analgesia

Antonella Pollo and Fabrizio Benedetti

Department of Neuroscience, Clinical and Applied Physiology Program, University of Turin Medical School, Turin, Italy

SUPRASPINAL MODULATION OF PAIN: THE PLACEBO EFFECT AS A MODEL

The nociceptive input coming from a damaged tissue and traveling through the spinal cord up to the brain is not always experienced in the same way. A complex modulation that occurs at the supraspinal level may either increase or decrease the nociceptive information, thus increasing or decreasing the global experience of pain. Many psychological factors are responsible for this modulation. For example, attention, emotions, mood, stress, expectation, anticipation, distraction, anxiety, depression, and fear all modulate the global experience of pain, although the underlying mechanisms are poorly understood in most of these cases. In recent years, the placebo effect, and in particular placebo analgesia, has emerged as an interesting model to illustrate the physiological and neurobiological mechanisms through which this complex psychological modulation occurs. Of course, an understanding of the placebo effect can only explain some of these factors, such as expectation and anticipation. Nonetheless, investigation of the placebo effect has yielded new insights into the biological mechanisms that link complex mental activity to different body functions. This chapter is a brief overview of what we know today about the neural mechanisms underlying the placebo effect. We will demonstrate that the placebo effect can no longer be considered a tiresome necessity in clinical research, where the efficacy of a new therapy must be validated by a placebo trial, but that it is worthy of scientific inquiry and can give us important information on the intricate mechanisms that link mind, brain, and body.

IDENTIFYING A PLACEBO EFFECT

By definition, the placebo effect is the effect that follows the administration of an inert medical treatment (the placebo), be it pharmacological or
not. The investigation of the placebo effect is full of pitfalls and drawbacks
because in order to demonstrate a placebo effect, the investigators must rule
out several other phenomena. In fact, the placebo agent itself is not always
the cause of the effect that is observed, and this point represents a source of
confusion and dangerous misconceptions. For example, most painful conditions show a spontaneous temporal variation that is known as *natural history* (Fields and Levine 1984; Fields 2004). If a subject takes a placebo just
before the discomfort starts decreasing, he or she may believe that the placebo is effective, although that decrease would have occurred anyway. Clearly,
this is not a placebo effect but a spontaneous remission that leads to a
misinterpretation of the cause-and-effect relationship (Fig. 1A). Another example is related to regression to the mean, a statistical phenomenon. If
individuals tend to receive their initial clinical assessment when their pain is
near its greatest intensity, then their pain level is likely to be lower when
they return for a second pain assessment (Davis 2002). In this case also, the
improvement cannot be attributed to any intervention they might have undergone (Fig. 1B). A further source of confusion is represented by the fact
that a particular type of error made by the patient, a false-positive error, may
explain the placebo effect in some circumstances. This approach, known as
signal detection theory, is based on the occurrence of errors in the detection
of ambiguous signals (Allan and Siegel 2002). For example, a patient may
erroneously detect symptomatic relief (a false-positive) in response to an
inert treatment. The ambiguity of symptom intensity may also lead to biases
following verbal suggestion of benefit (Fig. 1C). It also sometimes happens
that a co-intervention is responsible for the reduction of a symptom (Fig.
1D). Imagine the mechanical stimulation produced by the insertion of a
needle to inject an inert solution. The painful insertion itself may produce
analgesia in a different part of the body, thus leading to misinterpretations.
All these examples show that, although an improvement may occur after the
administration of a placebo, the placebo is not necessarily the cause of the
effect that is observed.

Given that all these sources of confusion are sometimes difficult to
identify, clinical trials do not represent a good model for studying the mechanisms underlying the placebo effect. Indeed, many results obtained in the
clinical trial setting differ from those obtained in the laboratory setting (Vase
et al. 2002). In fact, most of our knowledge on the psychological and physiological mechanisms of the placebo effect come from situations where strictly

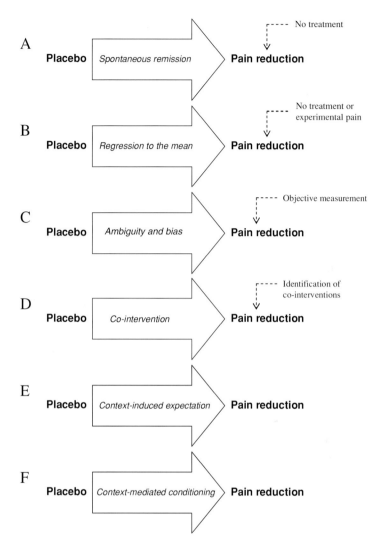

Fig. 1. The pain reduction observed after the administration of a placebo is not always due to the placebo itself. (A) Pain reduction is not due to the placebo itself but to spontaneous remission, which can be revealed by means of a no-treatment group. (B) The observed pain reduction can be due to the statistical phenomenon of regression to the mean, which can be controlled by using either a no-treatment group or an experimental pain model. (C) A report of decreased pain may also be due to detection ambiguities and biases, which can be overcome by means of objective physiological measurements. (D) Co-interventions, such as the mechanical stimulation due to needle insertion, may also be the cause of pain reduction. These can be identified by carefully choosing the appropriate experimental model. (E) and (F) These are the real placebo effects, where the very nature of the causal relationship between placebo and pain reduction is psychological. In fact, the context around the therapy can produce expectations of analgesia or can mediate conditioning mechanisms.

controlled conditions are adopted (Harrington 1997; Guess et al. 2002; Vase et al. 2002). Fig. 1A shows that in the laboratory setting or sometimes in the controlled clinical setting it is possible to test dependent measures such as pain intensity in a no-treatment (natural history) group compared with a placebo group. In this way, the spontaneous remission of the symptom can be identified. The difference between what happens to the symptom in the no-treatment group and the placebo group represents the real placebo effect. In the laboratory setting other confounding variables can be controlled as well. For example, the statistical phenomenon of regression to the mean can be overcome by using either a no-treatment group or an experimental pain model in which pain intensity can be controlled (Fig. 1B). Likewise, symptom detection ambiguity and subjects' biases can be overcome through the measurement of objective physiological parameters (Fig. 1C), as will be described throughout this chapter. It is sometimes more difficult to identify possible effects of co-interventions. In this case, it is necessary to choose the appropriate experimental model that takes different variables and co-interventions into account (Fig. 1D).

It is generally assumed that the term *placebo effect* is different from *placebo response*. The former term has been used to refer to any improvement in the condition of a group of subjects who have received a placebo treatment. Conversely, the latter refers to the change in an individual caused by a placebo manipulation. However, these two terms are often used interchangeably. Needless to say, what is interesting is the placebo response, which represents the psychological and/or physiological response of a subject to the inert treatment. Unfortunately, it is not easy to identify a placebo response in a single individual, and many control subjects are sometimes necessary to rule out spontaneous remissions, biases, and symptom detection ambiguities. Imagine a situation in which a subject reports a pain reduction from 6 to 5 points after the administration of a placebo. Is this decrease a placebo response, a spontaneous fluctuation, or rather a bias? There is no way to differentiate between these phenomena unless other control subjects are tested. For this reason, the placebo effect is better described as a group effect, and indeed, most studies on placebo mechanisms consider the mean reduction of a symptom in a group of subjects after placebo administration. However, in a few instances the natural history of a symptom is straightforward and guarantees a safe identification of the placebo response in a single individual. For example, postoperative pain either increases over time or is constant. Therefore, it is safe to assume that a reduction of postoperative pain after placebo administration is probably not due to a spontaneous fluctuation. It is also important to emphasize that this approach must also be used for drugs and in general for any medical treatment that is to be tested.

Given all these considerations, a placebo effect can be considered real only when the placebo is the cause of the effect that is observed. A controlled experimental approach has revealed several psychological and physiological mechanisms (Amanzio and Benedetti 1999; Benedetti et al. 1999b, 2003; Price 2000, 2002). The mechanisms underlying the causal connection between placebos and placebo effects can be either conscious anticipatory processes or unconscious mechanisms of conditioning (Fig. 1E, F). These mechanisms are further described by Vase and colleagues in Chapter 10. However, some crucial points need to be emphasized here in order to better elucidate the physiological and neurobiological mechanisms.

THE PLACEBO EFFECT IS A CONTEXT EFFECT

The term *placebo effect,* with its connotations of deception, lying, and quackery, has always been a source of confusion and misconceptions. This point has been stressed by Moerman (1979, 2002a,b) and by Moerman and Jonas (2002), who have proposed replacing the term *placebo response* with *meaning response* to clarify that the crucial factor is not so much the inert treatment (the placebo) per se as it is the context and the meaning surrounding the medical treatment. In other words, the therapeutic context has a meaning that induces expectations, which in turn shape experience and behavior, as emphasized by Kirsch (1985, 1990, 1999). According to Moerman, the term *placebo effect* deflects our attention from what is really important (meaning and meaning-induced expectations), and aims it at what is not (the inert pills and, in general, the inert medical treatments).

The concept of the placebo effect as a context effect has been stressed by several authors (Di Blasi et al. 2001; Benedetti 2002). According to the context and the context-induced expectations, placebos may also produce negative outcomes. To distinguish the pleasing from the noxious effects of placebo, several authors have introduced and elaborated the term *nocebo* (Kennedy 1961; Kissel and Barrucand 1964; Hahn 1985, 1997). If the meaning of the context is reversed in the opposite direction, a nocebo effect can be obtained. For example, Benedetti et al. (1997) obtained a nocebo effect (pain increase) by administering an inert saline solution (known to have no algesic effect) to patients with mild pain and telling them that the injection contains a substance that increases pain. In this case, the negative meaning of the verbal instructions induced negative expectations.

The role of symbolic meaning was also emphasized by Brody (1980), who defined the placebo effect as a change in a patient's illness attributable to the symbolic import of a treatment rather than a specific pharmacological or physiological property. Very recently, Brody (2000) defined the placebo effect as a change in the body, or the body-mind unit, that occurs as a result of the symbolic significance attributed to an event or object in the healing environment. This definition is embedded in the notion that symbols induce expectations of an outcome, thus emphasizing the crucial role of meaning (Moerman 2002a,b) and expectation (Kirsch 1999).

The context around a therapy may not only act through meaning, expectation, and conscious anticipatory processes. Some lines of evidence indicate that, at least in some circumstances, the placebo response is a conditioned response due to repeated associations between a conditioned stimulus (e.g., the shape and color of aspirin pills) and an unconditioned stimulus (the active substance of aspirin) (Gleidman et al. 1957; Herrnstein 1962; Wickramasekera 1980; Siegel 1985, 2002; Voudouris et al. 1989, 1990; Ader 1997). In this case, it is the context itself that is the conditioned stimulus (the shape and color of pills, the syringes, the environment of the hospital, and such like). However, even in a typical conditioning procedure, a conditioned placebo response is in fact mediated by expectancy (Montgomery and Kirsch 1997). In other words, conditioning leads to the expectation that a given event will follow another event, and this occurs on the basis of the information that the conditioned stimulus provides about the unconditioned stimulus (Reiss 1980; Rescorla 1988).

A recent study has clearly shown that some physiological functions are affected by placebos through anticipatory conscious processes, whereas some other functions are related to an unconscious mechanism of conditioning (Benedetti et al. 2003). For example, verbally induced expectations of either analgesia or hyperalgesia completely abolish the effects of a conditioning procedure in experimentally induced pain. By contrast, verbally induced expectations of either an increase or decrease of growth hormone and cortisol have no effect on the secretion of these hormones. However, if preconditioning is performed with sumatriptan, a $5\text{-HT}_{1B/1D}$ agonist that stimulates growth hormone and inhibits cortisol secretion, a significant increase of growth hormone and decrease of cortisol plasma concentrations occurs after placebo administration, even when opposite verbal suggestions are given. These findings indicate that verbally induced expectations have no effect on hormonal secretion, whereas they do affect pain. It appears that placebo responses are mediated by conditioning when unconscious physiological functions such as hormonal secretion are involved, whereas they are mediated by expectation when conscious physiological processes, like pain, come into play, even though a conditioning procedure is carried out. The placebo effect thus seems to be a phenomenon that can be learned either consciously or unconsciously, depending on the system that is involved.

The placebo effect can thus be considered a context effect. Different contextual cues, such as the doctor's words, the hospital environment, the smell of the drug, and the sight of complex machines, influence the therapeutic outcome. The context may affect the outcome through expectations and conscious anticipatory processes (Fig. 1E), or the context itself can be a conditioned stimulus that, after repeated associations with an unconditioned stimulus, can elicit conditioned placebo responses (Fig. 1F).

THE NEURAL LINK BETWEEN PLACEBO ADMINISTRATION AND PAIN REDUCTION

Pain is the field in which most of the placebo research has been performed. An important step was made in understanding the mechanisms of placebo-induced effects in the clinical setting when Levine et al. (1978) provided evidence that placebo-induced analgesia is mediated by endogenous opioids. Other studies subsequently further confirmed this exciting and provocative hypothesis (Grevert et al. 1983; Levine and Gordon 1984; Benedetti 1996) (Fig. 2). In addition, cholecystokinin was found to have an inhibitory role in placebo-induced analgesia because cholecystokinin antagonists are capable of potentiating the placebo analgesic effect (Benedetti et al. 1995; Benedetti 1996). Cholecystokinin is an anti-opioid peptide that antagonizes endogenous opioid neuropeptides (Benedetti 1997) (Fig. 2). Thus, placebo analgesic responses appear to result from a balance between endogenous opioids and endogenous cholecystokinin.

Fields and Levine (1984) were the first to hypothesize that the placebo response may be subdivided into opioid and non-opioid components. In particular, Fields and Levine's suggestion was that different physical, psychological, and environmental situations could affect the endogenous opioid systems differently. This concept is further supported by the finding that the placebo effect is not always mediated by endogenous opioids (Gracely et al. 1983). Thus, the question is: What are the conditions necessary for the activation of the opioid systems? This problem was addressed by Amanzio and Benedetti (1999), who showed that both expectation and a conditioning procedure can result in placebo analgesia. The former is capable of activating opioid systems whereas the latter activates specific subsystems (Fig. 2). In fact, if the placebo response is induced by means of strong expectation cues, it can be blocked by the opioid antagonist naloxone. Conversely, if the placebo response is induced by means of prior conditioning with a non-opioid drug, it is naloxone-insensitive.

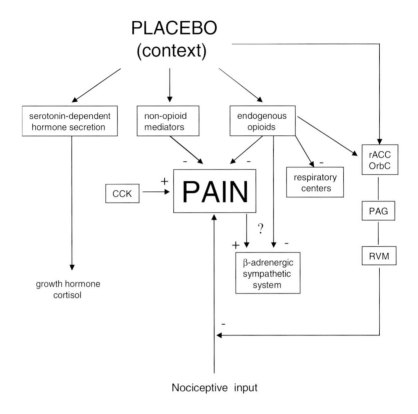

Fig. 2. Cascade of events that may occur during a placebo procedure, in which the context around the therapy may act through either conscious anticipatory mechanisms or unconscious conditioning. Pain may be inhibited by a descending inhibitory network involving the rostral anterior cingulate cortex (rACC), the orbitofrontal cortex (OrbC), the periaqueductal gray (PAG), and the rostral ventromedial medulla (RVM). Endogenous opioids may inhibit pain through this descending network or other mechanisms. The respiratory centers may be inhibited by opioid mechanisms as well. The β-adrenergic sympathetic system is also inhibited during placebo analgesia, although the underlying mechanism is not known; it may involve reduction of the pain itself, direct action of endogenous opioids, or both. Non-opioid mechanisms are also involved. Cholecystokinin (CCK) counteracts the effects of the endogenous opioids, thus antagonizing placebo analgesia. Placebos can also act on serotonin-dependent hormone secretion, mimicking the effect of the antimigraine drug sumatriptan.

We now know that specific placebo analgesic responses can be obtained in different parts of the body (Montgomery and Kirsch 1996; Price et al. 1999) and that these responses are naloxone-reversible (Benedetti et al. 1999b). If four noxious stimuli are applied to the hands and feet and a placebo cream is applied to one hand only, pain is reduced only on the hand where the placebo cream had been applied. This highly specific effect is blocked by naloxone, suggesting that the placebo-activated endogenous opioid systems have a precise and somatotopic organization (Benedetti et al. 1999b). An additional study supporting the involvement of endogenous opioids in placebo analgesia was performed by Lipman et al. (1990) in chronic pain patients. These authors found that patients who responded to a placebo administration showed higher concentrations of peak β-endorphin in the cerebrospinal fluid compared with those who did not respond to the placebo.

A likely candidate for the mediation of placebo-induced analgesia is an opioid neuronal network in the cerebral cortex and the brainstem (Fields and Price 1997; Fields and Basbaum 1999; Price 1999). This opioid network belongs to a descending pain-modulating pathway that, either directly or indirectly, connects the cerebral cortex to the brainstem. In particular, the anterior cingulate cortex (ACC) and the orbitofrontal cortex (OrbC) project to the periaqueductal gray (PAG), which in turn modulates the activity of the rostral ventromedial medulla (RVM). The ACC and the PAG, together with some other nuclei in the brainstem (e.g., the parabrachial nuclei), are rich in opioid receptors and could play an important role in placebo-induced analgesia. In fact, context-related cognitive cues could activate this opioid network in the cerebral cortex and the brainstem. This hypothesis was supported by a recent brain imaging study that used positron emission tomography (PET) (Petrovic et al. 2002). These authors found that the very same brain regions in the cerebral cortex and in the brainstem are affected both by a placebo and by the rapidly acting opioid agonist remifentanil, thus indicating a related mechanism in placebo-induced and opioid-induced analgesia. In particular, the administration of a placebo induced the activation of the rostral ACC (rACC) and the OrbC. Moreover, there was a significant covariation in activity between the rACC and the lower pons/medulla, and a subsignificant covariation between the rACC and the PAG, suggesting that the descending rACC/PAG/RVM pain-modulating circuit is involved in placebo analgesia (Fig. 2), as previously hypothesized by Fields and Price (1997).

THE EFFECTS OF PLACEBO-ACTIVATED ENDOGENOUS OPIOIDS ON DIFFERENT SYSTEMS

Placebo-activated endogenous opioids also produce a typical side effect of opioids, respiratory depression (Benedetti et al. 1998; Benedetti et al. 1999a). After repeated administrations of analgesic doses of buprenorphine in the postoperative phase, which induces a mild decrease of ventilation, a placebo is capable of mimicking the same respiratory depressant response. This respiratory placebo response can be completely blocked by naloxone, indicating that it is mediated by endogenous opioids. Thus, placebo-activated opioid systems act not only on pain mechanisms, but also on the respiratory centers (Fig. 2).

The involvement of other systems during placebo analgesia is further supported by recent work in which the sympathetic and parasympathetic control of the heart was analyzed during placebo analgesia (Pollo et al. 2003). In the clinical setting, the placebo analgesic response to a phasic noxious stimulus was accompanied by a reduced heart rate response. In order to investigate this effect from a pharmacological viewpoint, the same effect was reproduced in the laboratory setting by using tonic noxious stimulation. Naloxone completely antagonized both placebo analgesia and the concomitant reduced heart rate response, whereas the β-blocker propranolol antagonized the placebo heart rate reduction but not placebo analgesia. By contrast, both placebo responses were present during muscarinic blockade with atropine, indicating no involvement of the parasympathetic system. A spectral analysis of the heart rate variability performed to identify the sympathetic and parasympathetic components showed that the β-adrenergic, low-frequency component was reduced during placebo analgesia, an effect that was reversed by naloxone. These findings indicate that opioid-mediated placebo analgesia also affects the cardiovascular system. At least two possible mechanisms may reduce sympathetic activity during placebo analgesia (Fig. 2). First, sympathetic activity might be reduced as a consequence of pain reduction. Second, placebo-activated endogenous opioids might inhibit the sympathetic system directly. Further research is needed to differentiate between these two mechanisms.

NON-OPIOID MECHANISMS OF PLACEBO AND NOCEBO

As described above, when a placebo is given after repeated administrations of sumatriptan, growth hormone increases and cortisol decreases (Benedetti et al. 2003). Although we cannot yet state definitively that these placebo responses are mediated by serotonin, at least we can assert that a placebo procedure by means of sumatriptan conditioning may affect serotonin-dependent hormone secretion (Fig. 2). These new findings may help investigate non-opioid mechanisms in placebo analgesia.

The verbal instructions that induce expectations may have a meaning that either encourages hope and trust or promotes fear and stress (Hahn 1985, 1997; Benedetti and Amanzio 1997; Moerman 2002a,b). In a study performed in postoperative patients (Benedetti et al. 1997), negative expectations were induced by injecting an inert substance (saline solution) along with the instructions that pain was going to increase in a few minutes. In fact, pain did increase, but this increase could be prevented by adding a cholecystokinin (CCK) antagonist, proglumide, to the saline solution. This finding indicates that expectation-induced hyperalgesia of these patients was mediated, at least in part, by CCK. However, the effects of proglumide were not antagonized by naloxone, even at high doses, showing that endogenous opioids were not involved. Given that CCK plays a role in anxiety and negative expectations themselves are anxiogenic, these results suggest that proglumide acted on a CCK-dependent increase of anxiety during the verbally induced negative expectations.

Although further research is needed in order to confirm these findings, knowledge of these mechanisms is particularly important in light of the model suggested by Hahn (1985, 1997). In fact, in his anthropological analysis on the sociocultural creation of sickness and healing, Hahn proposes a model of the placebo-nocebo phenomenon, in which positive and hopeful beliefs and expectations produce therapeutic effects, whereas negative and fearful ones produce pathological outcomes. Likewise, according to Moerman's meaning response (Moerman 2002a,b; Moerman and Jonas 2002), there are positive and negative meanings that, in turn, induce positive and negative expectations. Nocebo hyperalgesia is likely to be mediated, at least in part, by a state of anxiety that anticipates a noxious and dangerous event (Benedetti and Amanzio 1997; Benedetti et al. 1997).

THE PLACEBO EFFECT IN CONDITIONS OTHER THAN PAIN

The release of endogenous substances following a placebo procedure is a phenomenon that is not confined to the field of pain, but is also present in motor disorders, such as Parkinson's disease. As occurs with pain, patients are given an inert substance (placebo) and are told that it is an anti-parkinsonian drug that produces an improvement in their motor performance. Patients with Parkinson's disease respond to placebos quite well (Shetty et al. 1999; Goetz et al. 2000). A recent study used PET to assess the competition between endogenous dopamine and [^{11}C]raclopride for D_2/D_3 dopamine receptors, a method that allows identification of endogenous dopamine release (de la Fuente-Fernandez et al. 2001). This study shows that placebo-induced expectation of motor improvement activates endogenous dopamine in the nigrostriatal pathway of patients with Parkinson's disease, that is, in the very same circuit that is damaged in the disease.

In addition, Pollo et al. (2002) showed that different and opposite expectations of bad and good motor performance modulated the therapeutic effect of subthalamic nucleus stimulation in Parkinsonian patients who had undergone long-term implantation of electrodes for deep brain stimulation. By analyzing the effect of subthalamic stimulation on the velocity of movement of the right hand, we found the hand movement to be faster when the patients expected good motor performance. The expectation of good performance was induced through a placebo-like procedure, thus indicating that placebo-induced expectations have an influence on the outcome of the treatment. All these effects occurred within minutes, suggesting that expectations induce neural changes very quickly.

All these data, taken together, indicate that placebo-induced expectations are capable of inducing the release of endogenous substances in very specific brain regions, such as the cortex and brainstem in analgesia or the striatum in Parkinson's disease. De la Fuente-Fernandez and Stoessl (2002) argue that the expectation-induced release of dopamine in Parkinson's disease is related to reward mechanisms. According to these authors, dopamine release by expectation of reward, in this case the expectation of clinical benefit, could represent a common biochemical substrate in many pathological situations, an interesting hypothesis that needs experimental confirmation. It is worth noting that there is an important interaction between dopamine and opioid systems, and that endogenous opioids are also involved in reward mechanisms (de la Fuente-Fernandez and Stoessl 2002).

Very recently, the neural mechanisms of placebo treatments have also been studied in depression. Depressed patients who received a placebo treatment showed both electrical and metabolic changes in the brain. In the first case, placebos induced electroencephalographic changes in the prefrontal cortex of patients with major depression, particularly in the right hemisphere (Leuchter et al. 2002). In the second case, changes in brain glucose metabolism were measured by using PET in subjects with unipolar depression. Placebo treatments were associated with metabolic increases in the prefrontal, anterior cingulate, premotor, parietal, posterior insula, and posterior cingulate cortex and with metabolic decreases in the subgenual cingulate cortex, para-hippocampus, and thalamus (Mayberg et al. 2002). Interestingly, these regions also were affected by the selective serotonin reuptake inhibitor fluoxetine, a result that suggests a role for serotonin in placebo-induced antidepressant effects. However, these studies on depression need further research and confirmation because they did not include appropriate control groups.

CONCLUSIONS

Study of the placebo effect has yielded its most fruitful results in the field of pain research. Fig. 2 shows that a complex situation has emerged in recent years. A placebo procedure may have different effects, both on pain mechanisms and on other physiological functions and anatomical structures, such as the respiratory centers, the sympathetic nervous system, and the hormonal system. We are learning about the neural mechanisms of the placebo phenomenon, although a lot of work remains to be done. For example, it appears clear that there is no single placebo effect. Different systems can be involved, which suggests that there is no single mechanism and rule for the occurrence of a placebo response. The challenge for future research will be to unravel the mechanisms through which a complex mental activity, such as the expectation of future events, is capable of affecting different systems and structures. Likewise, a future challenge will be to better understand which biological systems and mechanisms can be affected by conditioning. Therefore, today the placebo effect has passed from the status of a nuisance to be controlled for in clinical trials to a psychobiological phenomenon that requires scientific investigation.

ACKNOWLEDGMENTS

This work was supported by grants from the neuroscience and trigeminal pain projects of the National Research Council, from the Alzheimer's disease project of the Italian Ministry of Health, and from MIUR-FIRB.

REFERENCES

Ader R. The role of conditioning in pharmacotherapy. In: Harrington A (Ed). *The Placebo Effect: An Interdisciplinary Exploration.* Cambridge, MA: Harvard University Press, 1997, pp 138–165.

Allan LG, Siegel S. A signal detection theory analysis of the placebo effect. *Eval Health Prof* 2002; 25:410–420.

Amanzio M, Benedetti F. Neuropharmacological dissection of placebo analgesia: expectation-activated opioid systems versus conditioning-activated specific sub-systems. *J Neurosci* 1999; 19:484–494.

Benedetti F. The opposite effects of the opiate antagonist naloxone and the cholecystokinin antagonist proglumide on placebo analgesia. *Pain* 1996; 64:535–543.

Benedetti F. Cholecystokinin type-A and type-B receptors and their modulation of opioid analgesia. *News Physiol Sci* 1997; 12:263–268.

Benedetti F. How the doctor's words affect the patient's brain. *Eval Health Prof* 2002; 25:369–386.

Benedetti F, Amanzio M. The neurobiology of placebo: from endogenous opioids to cholecystokinin. *Prog Neurobiol* 1997; 52:109–125.

Benedetti F, Amanzio M, Maggi G. Potentiation of placebo analgesia by proglumide. *Lancet*
1995; 346:1231.

Benedetti F, Amanzio M, Casadio C, Oliaro A, Maggi G. Blockade of nocebo hyperalgesia by
the cholecystokinin antagonist proglumide. *Pain* 1997; 70:431–436.

Benedetti F, Amanzio M, Baldi S, et al. The specific effects of prior opioid exposure on placebo
analgesia and placebo respiratory depression. *Pain* 1998; 75:313–319.

Benedetti F, Amanzio M, Baldi S, Casadio C, Maggi G. Inducing placebo respiratory depressant responses in humans via opioid receptors. *Eur J Neurosci* 1999a; 11:625–631.

Benedetti F, Arduino C, Amanzio M. Somatotopic activation of opioid systems by target-
directed expectations of analgesia. *J Neurosci* 1999b; 19:3639–3648.

Benedetti F, Pollo A, Lopiano L, et al. Conscious expectation and unconscious conditioning in
analgesic, motor and hormonal placebo/nocebo responses. *J Neurosci* 2003; 23:4315–
4323.

Brody H. *Placebos and the Philosophy of Medicine: Clinical, Conceptual and Ethical Issues.*
Chicago: University of Chicago Press, 1980.

Brody H. *The Placebo Response.* New York: Harper Collins, 2000.

Davis CE. Regression to the mean or placebo effect? In: Guess HA, Kleinman A, Kusek JW,
Engel LW (Eds). *The Science of the Placebo: Toward an Interdisciplinary Research
Agenda.* London: BMJ Books, 2002, pp 158–166.

de la Fuente-Fernandez R, Stoessl AJ. The biochemical bases for reward: implications for the
placebo effect. *Eval Health Prof* 2002; 25:387–398.

de la Fuente-Fernandez R, Ruth TJ, Sossi V, et al. Expectation and dopamine release: mechanism of the placebo effect in Parkinson's disease. *Science* 2001; 293:1164–1166.

Di Blasi Z, Harkness E, Ernst E, Georgiou A, Kleijnen J. Influence of context effects on health
outcomes: a systematic review. *Lancet* 2001; 357:757–762.

Fields HL. Placebo analgesia. In: Dworkin RH, Breitbart S (Eds). *Psychosocial Aspects of
Pain: A Handbook for Care Providers,* Progress in Pain Research and Management, Vol.
27. Seattle: IASP Press, 2004, pp 623–641.

Fields HL, Basbaum AI. Central nervous system mechanisms of pain modulation. In: Wall PD,
Melzack R (Eds). *Textbook of Pain.* Edinburgh: Churchill Livingstone, 1999, pp 309–329.

Fields HL, Levine JD. Placebo analgesia—a role for endorphins? *Trends Neurosci* 1984;
7:271–273.

Fields HL, Price DD. Toward a neurobiology of placebo analgesia. In: Harrington A (Ed). *The
Placebo Effect: an Interdisciplinary Exploration.* Cambridge, MA: Harvard University
Press, 1997, pp 93–116.

Gleidman LH, Grantt WH, Teitelbaum HA. Some implications of conditional reflex studies for
placebo research. *Am J Psychiatry* 1957; 113:1103–1107.

Goetz CG, Leurgans S, Raman R, Stebbins GT. Objective changes in motor function during
placebo treatment in Parkinson's disease. *Neurology* 2000; 54:710–714.

Gracely RH, Dubner R, Wolskee PJ, Deeter WR. Placebo and naloxone can alter postsurgical
pain by separate mechanisms. *Nature* 1983; 306:264–265.

Grevert P, Albert LH, Goldstein A. Partial antagonism of placebo analgesia by naloxone. *Pain*
1983; 16:129–143.

Guess HA, Kleinman A, Kusek JW, Engel LW (Eds). *The Science of the Placebo: Toward an
Interdisciplinary Research Agenda.* London: BMJ Books, 2002.

Hahn RA. A sociocultural model of illness and healing. In: White L, Tursky B, Schwartz GE
(Eds). *Placebo: Theory, Research, and Mechanisms.* New York: Guilford Press, 1985, pp
167–195.

Hahn RA. The nocebo phenomenon: scope and foundations. In: Harrington A (Ed). *The
Placebo Effect: An Interdisciplinary Exploration,* Cambridge, MA: Harvard University
Press, 1997, pp 56–76.

Harrington A (Ed). *The Placebo Effect: An Interdisciplinary Exploration.* Cambridge, MA: Harvard University Press, 1997.

Herrnstein RJ. Placebo effect in the rat. *Science* 1962; 138:677–678.

Kennedy WP. The nocebo reaction. *Med World* 1961; 91:203–205.

Kirsch I. Response expectancy as a determinant of experience and behavior. *Am Psychol* 1985; 40:1189–1202.

Kirsch I. *Changing Expectations: A Key to Effective Psychotherapy.* Pacific Grove, CA: Brooks-Cole, 1990.

Kirsch I (Ed). *How Expectancies Shape Experience.* Washington, DC: American Psychological Association, 1999.

Kissel P, Barrucand D. *Placebos et Effet Placebo en Medecine.* Paris: Masson, 1964.

Leuchter AF, Cook IA, Witte EA, Morgan M, Abrams M. Changes in brain function of depressed subjects during treatment with placebo. *Am J Psychiatry* 2002; 159:122–129.

Levine JD, Gordon NC. Influence of the method of drug administration on analgesic response. *Nature* 1984; 312:755–756.

Levine JD, Gordon NC, Fields HL. The mechanisms of placebo analgesia. *Lancet* 1978; 2:654–657.

Lipman JJ, Miller BE, Mays KS, et al. Peak β endorphin concentration in cerebrospinal fluid: reduced in chronic pain patients and increased during the placebo response. *Psychopharmacology* 1990; 102:112–116.

Mayberg HS, Silva AJ, Brannan SK, et al. The functional neuroanatomy of the placebo effect. *Am J Psychiatry* 2002; 159:728–737.

Moerman DE. Anthropology of symbolic healing. *Curr Anthropol* 1979; 20:59–80.

Moerman DE. Meaningful dimensions of medical care. In: Guess HA, Kleinman A, Kusek JW, Engel LW (Eds). *The Science of the Placebo: Toward an Interdisciplinary Research Agenda.* London: BMJ Books, 2002a, pp 77–107.

Moerman DE. *Meaning, Medicine and the Placebo Effect.* Cambridge, MA: Cambridge University Press, 2002b.

Moerman DE, Jonas WB. Deconstructing the placebo effect and finding the meaning response. *Ann Int Med* 2002; 136:471–476.

Montgomery GH, Kirsch I. Mechanisms of placebo pain reduction: an empirical investigation. *Psychol Sci* 1996; 7:174–176.

Montgomery GH, Kirsch I. Classical conditioning and the placebo effect. *Pain* 1997; 72:107–113.

Petrovic P, Kalso E, Petersson KM, Ingvar M. Placebo and opioid analgesia—imaging a shared neuronal network. *Science* 2002; 295:1737–1740.

Pollo A, Torre E, Lopiano L, et al. Expectation modulates the response to subthalamic nucleus stimulation in Parkinsonian patients. *Neuroreport* 2002; 13:1383–1386.

Pollo A, Rainero I, Vighetti S, Benedetti F. Placebo analgesia and the heart. *Pain* 2003; 102:125–133.

Price DD. *Psychological Mechanisms of Pain and Analgesia.* Seattle: IASP Press, 1999.

Price DD. Factors that determine the magnitude and presence of placebo analgesia. In: Devor M, Rowbotham MC, Wiesenfeld-Hallin Z (Eds). *Proceedings of the 9th World Congress on Pain,* Progress in Pain Research and Management, Vol. 16. Seattle: IASP Press, 2000, pp 1085–1095.

Price DD. Endogenous opioid and non-opioid pathways as mediators of placebo analgesia. In: Guess HA, Kleinman A, Kusek JW, Engel LW (Eds). *The Science of the Placebo: Toward an Interdisciplinary Research Agenda.* London: BMJ Books, 2002, pp 183–206.

Price DD, Milling LS, Kirsch I, Duff A, Montgomery GH, Nicholls SS. An analysis of factors that contribute to the magnitude of placebo analgesia in an experimental paradigm. *Pain* 1999; 83:147–156.

Reiss S. Pavlovian conditioning and human fear: an expectancy model. *Behav Ther* 1980; 11:380–396.

Rescorla RA. Pavlovian conditioning: it is not what you think it is. *Am Psychol* 1988; 43:151–160.

Shetty N, Friedman JH, Kieburtz K, Marshall FJ, Oakes D. The placebo response in Parkinson's disease. Parkinson Study Group. *Clin Neuropharmacol* 1999; 22:207–212.

Siegel S. Drug-anticipatory responses in animals. In: White L, Tursky B, Schwartz GE. *Placebo: Theory, Research, and Mechanisms.* New York: Guilford Press, 1985, pp 288–305.

Siegel S. Explanatory mechanisms for placebo effects: Pavlovian conditioning. In: Guess HA, Kleinman A, Kusek JW, Engel LW (Eds). *The Science of the Placebo: Toward an Interdisciplinary Research Agenda.* London: BMJ Books, 2002, pp 133–157.

Vase L, Riley JL III, Price DD. A comparison of placebo effects in clinical analgesic trials versus studies of placebo analgesia. *Pain* 2002; 99:443–452.

Voudouris NJ, Peck CL, Coleman G. Conditioned response models of placebo phenomena: further support. *Pain* 1989; 38:109–116.

Voudouris NJ, Peck CL, Coleman G. The role of conditioning and verbal expectancy in the placebo response. *Pain* 1990; 43:121–128.

Wickramasekera I. A conditioned response model of the placebo effect: predictions from the model. *Biofeedback Self-Regul* 1980; 5:5–18.

Correspondence to: Fabrizio Benedetti, MD, Dipartimento di Neuroscienze, Università di Torino, Corso Raffaello 30, 10125 Torino, Italy. Tel: 39-011-6707709; Fax: 39-011-6707708; email: fabrizio.benedetti@unito.it.

Psychological Methods of Pain Control: Basic Science and Clinical Perspectives, Progress in Pain Research and Management, Vol. 29, edited by Donald D. Price and M. Catherine Bushnell, IASP Press, Seattle, © 2004.

9

The Placebo in Clinical Studies and in Medical Practice

Luana Colloca and Fabrizio Benedetti

Department of Neuroscience, Clinical and Applied Physiology Program, University of Turin Medical School, Turin, Italy

THE CLINICAL IMPACT OF THE PLACEBO PHENOMENON

Confusion is common regarding the placebo concept in the clinical set-ting. As we have emphasized in Chapter 8, natural history, regression to the mean, and subjects' biases may mistakenly be taken to represent placebo effects. The real placebo effect is represented by the causal psychological relationship between the placebo intervention and the therapeutic outcome. Therefore, in order to understand the importance of the placebo effect in clinical studies and in medical practice, we must recognize that it is a psy-chosocial effect. A placebo effect occurs after the administration of a pla-cebo, that is, an inert treatment. However, the crucial point is that the inert treatment is nothing but a means to simulate a therapy and thus to make the patient know that something has been administered. This knowledge, in turn, will elicit expectations and beliefs. Another crucial point is that the placebo is not the only means through which such knowledge can be achieved. Many situations, such as the interaction with the therapist, induce expecta-tions and beliefs as well, so that a positive doctor-patient interaction may produce the same positive effects. The psychosocial nature of the placebo effect has been emphasized by Moerman (2002a,b), who proposes replacing the term *placebo response* with the more general term *meaning response* in order to make it clear that the meaning and the symbols associated with a therapy are of crucial importance.

This chapter will discuss the clinical impact of the placebo effect. Par-ticular emphasis will be given to the fact that the impact of the placebo in medical practice is represented by the effect of the patient's psychosocial environment. Thus, it will be necessary to broaden the placebo concept to situations other than the mere administration of a placebo. In other words, understanding the placebo effect in clinical studies and in medical practice means understanding the psychosocial influences surrounding medical treatment.

PLACEBO-CONTROLLED CLINICAL TRIALS

The story of the placebo in clinical studies begins with its use in clinical trials for the validation of new therapies. However, it is important to realize that the story of the placebo in clinical trials is not the story of the placebo effect, but rather that of control groups. In fact, even though myriad clinical trials have used control groups whose subjects have been given a placebo treatment, it is possible to assess the occurrence of real placebo effects in only a very small percentage of them (certainly much less than 1%). Only rarely do clinical trials use a no-treatment group, thereby making it impossible to rule out spontaneous remission. The lack of no-treatment groups in most of the available clinical trials is due to at least two reasons. First, ethical constraints make it very difficult to devise trials in which patients are not treated. Second, clinicians, clinical scientists, and drug companies are only interested in seeing whether the active drug is more effective than the placebo, and they are not interested in the placebo effect itself. Therefore, the remission of a symptom observed in the placebo group of a typical clinical trial is not exclusively the result of a real placebo effect but rather the sum of several factors. These include the placebo effect in combination with other confounding variables such as spontaneous remission, symptom detection ambiguity, and patients' biases (see Chapter 8).

While taking these considerations into account, this chapter does not cover the complex issue of the use of placebo groups in clinical trials. This matter, discussed in the Declaration of Helsinki with its many revisions (see below), has little to do with real placebo effects. It is important to realize that the lively debate around the placebo issue in clinical trials (e.g., Lewis et al. 2002; Michels and Rothman 2003) is not aimed at differentiating spontaneous remissions, regression to the mean, patients' biases, and real placebo responses.

However, in a recent meta-analysis by Hrobjartsson and Gotzsche (2001), 130 trials with placebo and no-treatment groups were identified in different pathological conditions. In general, no difference was found between the two groups for many conditions. Unfortunately, this meta-analysis provides limited information because its conclusions have been criticized on both methodological and conceptual grounds (Ader 2001; Brody and Weismantel

2001; DiNubile 2001; Einarson and Hemels 2001; Greene et al. 2001; Kaptchuk 2001; Kirsch and Scoboria 2001; Kupers 2001; Lilford and Braunholtz 2001; Miller 2001; Shrier 2001; Spiegel et al. 2001; Wickramasekera 2001). Despite its flaws and limitations, Hrobjartsson and Gotzsche's meta-analysis reminds us that the placebo effect is not effective in all diseases, a concept that, after all, has long been known. Interestingly, however, in spite of the generally negative conclusions by the authors, a significant placebo effect was found for pain in 29 clinical trials, which indicates that pain is one of the best conditions in which to study the placebo effect.

In another study aimed at investigating the placebo effect in analgesic studies only, Vase et al. (2002) conducted one meta-analysis that included 23 of the 29 clinical trials identified in the meta-analysis by Hrobjartsson and Gotzsche (2001) and another meta-analysis of 14 studies that investigated placebo analgesia mechanisms. These authors found that the magnitudes of the placebo analgesic effects were higher in studies that investigated placebo analgesic mechanisms compared with clinical trials in which the placebo was used only as a control condition (see also Chapter 10). Vase et al. (2002) suggest that this difference might be due to the different placebo instructions and suggestions given in the clinical trial setting compared to the experimental setting. In fact, whereas clinical trial investigators typically avoid giving oral suggestions of analgesia, investigators of the placebo effect typically emphasize such suggestions. Interestingly, as will be described in detail below, subtle differences in oral suggestions, including assuredness or tentativeness, can produce different outcomes (Kirsch and Weixel 1988; Pollo et al. 2001). Taken together, the two meta-analyses, by Hrobjartsson and Gotzsche (2001) and Vase et al. (2002), teach us that placebo analgesia occurs in both the clinical trial setting and the experimental setting, although it is much more pronounced in the latter.

Although most clinical trials use the placebo-controlled design, other experimental paradigms have been devised. The balanced placebo design is particularly interesting for the purpose of this chapter because it indicates that verbally induced expectations can modulate therapeutic outcome. The balanced placebo design was formulated by Ross et al. (1962) for use in pharmacological studies and has been applied to alcohol research (Marlatt et al. 1973; Epps et al. 1998) and studies on aggression (Lang et al. 1975), sexual arousal (Wilson et al. 1985), mood (Rohsenow and Bachorowski 1984), smoking (Sutton 1991), amphetamine effects (Mitchell et al. 1996), and other conditions. The design involves the manipulation of both verbal instructions and treatments in a four-group trial (Fig. 1). The first group receives a placebo and is told it is a placebo. The second receives a placebo and is told it is the active treatment. The third receives the active treatment

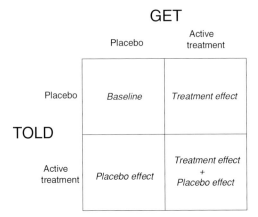

Fig. 1. The balanced placebo design. Different combinations of what the patients get and what they are told allow the investigators to identify the influence of verbal instructions on the active treatment.

and is told it is the active treatment. The fourth receives the active treatment and is told it is a placebo. This paradigm is interesting because it shows that verbal suggestions can modulate therapeutic outcome, both in the placebo group and the active treatment group, thus ruling out, at least in part, effects such as natural history and regression to the mean. In other words, real placebo effects (or psychosocial effects) can be recognized with this protocol, in which even the drug effect can be partially modulated by verbal instructions. Therefore, the balanced placebo design makes us understand that the verbal context plays a very important role. A more recent study confirmed these findings by using the centrally acting muscle relaxant carisoprodol, administered with suggestions that it was either a relaxant or a stimulant (Flaten et al. 1999).

THE PSYCHOSOCIAL CONTEXT OF THE TREATMENT

According to Brody (2000), the placebo effect is a change in the body, or the body-mind unit, that occurs as a result of the symbolic significance attributed to an event or object in the healing environment. A more recent definition, which despite being general helps to clarify the placebo phenomenon, has been proposed by Vase et al. (2002). These authors describe the placebo response as the reduction in a symptom that results from factors related to a subject's perception of the therapeutic intervention. In these two definitions by Brody (2000) and Vase et al. (2002), the role of the therapeutic context emerges as a crucial factor. In other words, the symbolic attribution given to an event and the perception of the therapeutic intervention originate from contextual cues.

The terms "context effect" and "placebo effect" can be used, at least in part, interchangeably, as has been emphasized many times (Di Blasi et al. 2001; Benedetti 2002; see Chapter 8, this volume). We lack full understanding of the role played by the psychosocial context in the effectiveness of the therapy that is being administered or, in the words of Balint (1955), the whole atmosphere associated with the treatment. The psychosocial context is made up of anything that surrounds the patient under treatment, such as doctors, nurses, hospitals, syringes, pills, and machines (Di Blasi et al. 2001). Certainly, doctors and nurses represent an important component of the context because they can transmit a great deal of information to the patient through their words, attitudes, and behavior. However, many other aspects of the context of the patient's care can potentially contribute to either a positive or a negative impact. Turner et al. (1994) emphasized the importance of placebo effects in pain treatment and stressed that the interaction between caregivers and patients can be extremely influential in therapeutic outcomes. Likewise, Thomas (1994) pointed out that a placebo effect can also be produced by a consultation in which no treatment is given. Thus, the classic concept of the placebo as a phenomenon whereby patients are made to feel better after receiving an inert treatment is overly restrictive.

Many clinicians have long known this powerful effect of context and, accordingly, have used the appropriate words and attitudes with their patients. For example, the doctor-patient interaction produces an important emotional impact, as shown by a study investigating the interaction between anesthesiologists and their patients (Egbert et al. 1963, 1964). A study by Egbert et al. (1964) found that postoperative pain was reduced in patients who had been informed about the course of their postoperative pain and were encouraged to overcome it. Moreover, the opioid requirements of these patients were much lower compared with a control group. These important studies compared the outcomes of an analgesic treatment following the anesthesiologist's visit with those following no visit at all, thus emphasizing the important role of the doctor-patient interaction in the global experience of pain. Kaplan et al. (1989) found that blood pressure, blood sugar, functional status, and overall health status were consistently related to specific aspects of physician-patient communication. Although many other studies have demonstrated that the doctor-patient relationship plays an important role in the outcome of illness (Stewart et al. 1979; Starfield et al. 1981; Gracely et al. 1985; Greenfield et al. 1985; Bass et al. 1986; Thomas 1987; Stewart 1995), these effects are often dismissed. Even diagnostic tests, which have nothing to do with therapy, can reduce short-term disability (Sox et al.

1981). In addition, psychosocial treatment may have positive effects in advanced malignant disease (Spiegel et al. 1989), although contrasting data exist (Cassileth et al. 1985).

Thomas (1987) conducted either positive or negative general practice consultations for patients with different kinds of pain, cough, giddiness, nasal congestion, and tiredness. In the positive consultations, the patients were given a firm diagnosis and therapeutic assurance. If no prescription was to be given, they were told that they required none, and if a prescription was to be given, they were told that the therapy would certainly make them better. In the negative consultations, no firm assurance was given. For example, if no prescription was to be given, the following statement was made: "I cannot be certain what your problem is; therefore I will give you no treatment." Conversely, if a prescription was to be given, the patients were told: "I am not sure that the treatment I am going to give you will have an effect." The treatment was a placebo (thiamine hydrochloride) in all cases. Two weeks after consultation there was a significant difference in recovery between the positive and negative groups but not between the treated and untreated groups, thus indicating that the words the doctor used were crucial for recovery.

Another study by Kirsch and Weixel (1988), albeit outside the clinical setting, shows that different verbal contexts produce different outcomes. In this study, regular coffee and decaffeinated coffee were administered following different verbal instructions. In one group the beverages were given according to the usual double-blind design, and subjects knew that either the active or decaffeinated substance was being administered, while in another group decaffeinated coffee was deceptively presented as real coffee. Kirsch and Weixel found that the placebo response was stronger following the deceptive administration than the double-blind paradigm. They concluded that the stronger response was due to the fact that the double-blind administration induces less certain expectations about the outcome.

A similar study was conducted in the clinical setting to investigate the differences between the double-blind and the deceptive paradigm (Pollo et al. 2001). Postoperative patients were treated with buprenorphine, on request, for three consecutive days, and with a basal infusion of saline solution (Fig. 2). However, the symbolic meaning of this infusion varied in three different groups of patients. The first group was told nothing (natural history or no-treatment group), the second was told that the infusion could be either a potent analgesic or a placebo (classic double-blind administration), and the third was told that the infusion was a potent painkiller (deceptive administration). The placebo effect of the saline basal infusion was measured by recording the doses of buprenorphine requested over the 3-day treatment. It

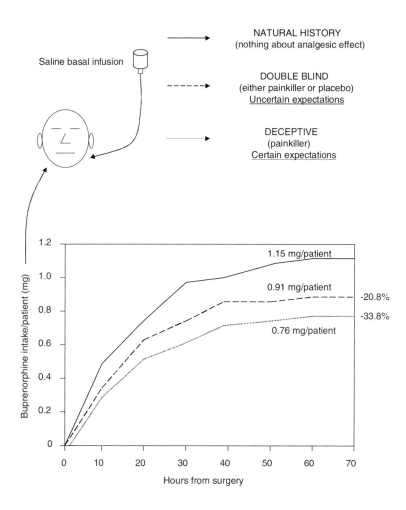

Fig. 2. Experimental design used by Pollo et al. (2001). Postoperative pain patients are treated with buprenorphine on request in combination with a basal infusion of saline solution. However, the symbolic meaning of this saline basal infusion is changed in different groups of patients. Analgesia is represented by buprenorphine consumption. Those patients who are given the saline solution deceptively ("It is a painkiller") show the lowest intake of buprenorphine.

is important to stress once again that the double-blind group received uncertain verbal instructions ("It can be either a placebo or a painkiller. Thus we are not certain that the pain will subside"), whereas the deceptive administration group received certain instructions ("It is a painkiller. Thus pain will subside soon"). Buprenorphine requests decreased in the double-blind group by 20.8% compared with the natural history group, and the reduction in the deceptive administration group was even greater, reaching 33.8%. The time course of pain was the same in the three groups over the 3-day period of treatment, and thus the same analgesic effect was obtained with different doses of buprenorphine. The above studies teach us that subtle differences in the verbal context of the patient may have a significant impact on therapeutic outcome.

OPEN AND HIDDEN THERAPIES

In more recent years, a radically different approach to analyzing placebo effects and psychosocial effects has been implemented. In conventional studies of placebo effects, the placebo component of a medical treatment has been studied by simulating a therapy through the administration of a dummy medical treatment in order to eliminate the specific effects of the therapy itself. In some recent studies, this experimental approach has been changed completely by eliminating the placebo component and maintaining the specific effects of the treatment. In order to eliminate the psychosocial context around a medical treatment, the patient is made completely unaware that a medical therapy is being carried out. In the 1980s, some studies were performed in which drugs were administered by machines through hidden infusions (Levine et al. 1981; Gracely et al. 1983; Levine and Gordon 1984). This hidden procedure is relatively easy to carry out in the postoperative phase, in which a computer-controlled infusion pump can deliver a painkiller automatically, without any doctor or nurse in the room, and with the patient being completely unaware that an analgesic treatment has been started.

In postoperative pain following the extraction of the third molar, Levine et al. (1981) and Levine and Gordon (1984) found that a hidden injection of a 6–8-mg intravenous dose of morphine corresponds to an intravenous injection of saline solution in full view of the patient. In other words, telling the patient that a painkiller is being injected (when it is actually a saline solution) is as potent as 6–8 mg of morphine. These authors concluded that an open injection of morphine in full view of the patient, which represents usual medical practice, is more effective than a hidden one in which the expectation of analgesia is absent.

A careful analysis of the differences between open and hidden injections in the postoperative setting was recently published by Amanzio et al. (2001). The effects of four widely used analgesics (buprenorphine, tramadol, ketorolac, and metamizol) were analyzed by using either open or hidden administrations, as shown in Fig. 3A. A doctor carried out the open administration by telling the patient (at the bedside) that the injection was a powerful analgesic and that the pain would subside in a few minutes. By contrast,

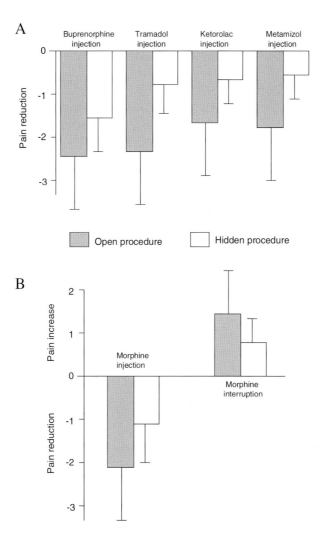

Fig. 3. The open-hidden paradigm. (A) Comparison between open and hidden injections of four widely used analgesics. All the hidden injections were less effective than the open ones. Pain intensity was recorded 30 minutes after the injection (data from Amanzio et al. 2001). (B) A hidden injection of morphine is less effective than an open one (pain was rated 30 minutes after injection). Similarly, a hidden interruption of a morphine treatment induces a slower relapse of pain than an open one. In this case, pain was rated 4 hours after morphine interruption (data from Benedetti et al. 2003).

the hidden injection of the same analgesic dose was performed by an automatic infusion machine without any doctor or nurse in the room so that patients were completely unaware that an analgesic therapy had been started. One analysis determined that the analgesic dose needed to reduce the pain by 50% (AD_{50}) was much higher with hidden infusions than with open ones for all four painkillers. Another analysis found that the time course of post-surgical pain was significantly different between open and hidden injections. In fact, during the first hour after the injection, pain ratings were much higher with a hidden injection than with an open one (Fig. 3A).

In the same study (Amanzio et al. 2001), the difference between open and hidden injections was also investigated in the laboratory setting by using the experimental model of ischemic arm pain in healthy volunteers. As occurred in the clinical setting, a hidden injection of the non-opioid analgesic ketorolac was less effective than an open one. In these controlled experimental conditions, when a 10-mg dose of the opioid antagonist nalox-one was added to an open injection of ketorolac, its effect was reduced to the same level as that produced by a hidden injection of ketorolac. This finding indicates that an open injection in full view of the patient activates endogenous opioid systems that enhance the effects of the injected analge-sic. It is fundamental to remember that ketorolac is a non-opioid drug, thus it does not bind to opioid receptors. Therefore, it is the words the doctor uses at the bedside or the psychosocial context in general that make the difference and activate the endogenous opioid systems. Therefore, the neural mechanisms described in Chapter 8 are also likely to pertain to the routine doctor-patient relationship.

Recently, an extensive study was performed with open and hidden treat-ments in various conditions such as pain, anxiety, Parkinson's disease, ta-chycardia, and bradycardia (Benedetti et al. 2003). As far as pain is con-cerned, this study not only confirmed the previous studies by Levine et al. (1981), Levine and Gordon (1984), and Amanzio et al. (2001), but also revealed important clinical implications of the open-hidden paradigm. In fact, whereas previous studies dealt with the open-hidden administration of an analgesic drug, the study by Benedetti et al. (2003) also investigated the open-hidden interruption of morphine therapy. This study showed that a relapse of pain occurred more quickly and that pain intensity was greater with an open interruption of morphine compared with a hidden interruption, indicating that analgesia was prolonged when patients did not realize that administration of morphine had been interrupted (Fig. 3B). The importance of these findings rests in the paradoxical ethical question that the interrup-tion protocol raises: Is it ethically acceptable to conceal the interruption of a therapy if the hidden interruption is beneficial to the patient? This question will be discussed in the section on ethics. It is important to point out that the same findings for open-hidden administrations and interruptions of medical treatments applied to anxiety, Parkinson's disease, and heart rate changes (Benedetti et al. 2003).

The findings obtained with hidden administrations of medical treatments represent a strong confirmation of the importance of placebo effects in routine medical practice. Because no placebo is given, the difference between an open and hidden injection can not be called a placebo effect. Nevertheless, it strongly indicates the important role of the psychosocial component of a therapy or, as suggested by Price (2001) and Vase et al. (2002), of the patient's perception that a therapy is being received.

THE ETHICAL ISSUE AND GOOD MEDICAL PRACTICE

It goes without saying that positive enhancement of the psychosocial context does not represent an ethical dilemma. A positive therapist-patient interaction and a positive medical environment do not require an ethical discussion and, indeed, they are the essential ingredients of any therapy. Interestingly, the primary reason for lawsuits in the United States is not medical injury itself, but the failure of communication between doctors and their patients. Patients sue their physicians when they feel that they did not care or did not inform them adequately (Levinson 1994). Beckman et al. (1994) identified four types of communication problems: deserting the patient, devaluing patients' views, delivering information poorly, and failing to understand patients' perspectives. Thus, the same communication skills that are capable of reducing the risk of malpractice also lead to better therapeutic outcomes.

The real ethical problem emerges when we manipulate the psychosocial context by means of placebos. At least two questions arise. First, is it ethically acceptable to use placebos in clinical trials? Second, is it ethically acceptable to administer them in routine clinical practice? Although these two questions are similar, they are usually approached differently. The main reason is that the central debate on the use of placebos centers on the clinical trial setting. Although this chapter is not aimed at discussing the methodological-ethical problems of placebo groups in the design of clinical trials, it is important to briefly consider some ethical issues that are also relevant to good medical practice.

IS IT ETHICALLY ACCEPTABLE TO USE
PLACEBOS IN CLINICAL TRIALS?

In the World Medical Association (WMA)'s Declaration of Helsinki, paragraph 29 states: "The benefits, risks, burdens and effectiveness of a new method should be tested against those of the best current prophylactic, diagnostic, and therapeutic methods. This does not exclude the use of placebo, or no treatment, in studies where no proven prophylactic, diagnostic or therapeutic method exists" (World Medical Association 2000).

According to the Declaration of Helsinki, it is unethical to assign patients to receive a placebo when effective treatment does exist. However, the WMA later added a footnote to paragraph 29 stating that a placebo-controlled trial may be ethically acceptable, even if proven therapy is available, "Where for compelling and scientifically sound methodological reasons its use is necessary to determine the efficacy or safety of a prophylactic, diagnostic or therapeutic method" or "Where a prophylactic, diagnostic or therapeutic method is being investigated for a minor condition and the patients who receive placebo will not be subject to any additional risk of serious or irreversible harm" (World Medical Association 2002).

This revision has been criticized on many grounds. For example, Michels and Rothman (2003) consider this clarification to be a step backward in bioethics. The positions of official organizations, such as the U.S. Food and Drug Administration (FDA), the American Medical Association (AMA), the European Committee for Proprietary Medicinal Products (CPMP), and the World Health Organization (WHO), are contrasting. For example, the FDA has always demanded and defended placebo-controlled studies for the development of new pharmaceuticals, even if effective therapy exists (Temple 2002), thus violating the Declaration of Helsinki (Rothman and Michels 1994). In general, the AMA supports the FDA's position, asserting that the existence of an accepted therapy does not necessarily preclude the use of controls (Council on Ethical and Judicial Affairs of the American Medical Association 1996; Michels and Rothman 2003). Conversely, the WHO affirms that placebos are not justified if there is already an approved and accepted drug for the condition that a candidate drug is designed to treat (Council for International Organizations of Medical Sciences 1993). The CPMP takes a somewhat ambiguous position; regarding schizophrenia, it states that in principle placebo-controlled trials will be required to show efficacy of a new product, but it recognizes that suitable alternative designs may be developed (Committee for Proprietary Medicinal Products 1998).

In general, the arguments that are advocated for or against the use of the placebo in clinical studies can be summarized as follows. Placebo defenders sometimes use the utilitarian argument whereby exposing subjects to placebo treatment is justified by the knowledge gained for future patients, whereas placebo opponents reply that ethical obligations to the single individual take precedence over science and society. Placebo defenders also affirm that the approval of the institutional review board and the patient's informed consent are sufficient, whereas placebo opponents contend that most informed consent forms are incomprehensible, thus making the patient unable to judge the experimental situation. Another point raised by many placebo defenders deals with the use of placebos for symptomatic treatments and not for curative therapies. Placebo opponents contend that there is no justification even for minor discomfort. Other scientific and technical arguments in favor of placebo groups focus on the establishment of a reference point by means of placebo groups, the lack of statistical significance tests for equivalence trials (new versus old therapy), and the much larger population required for an equivalence trial compared with a placebo-controlled trial. These technical and methodological issues will not be described in detail here. The gist of the problem is that clinical scientists, biomedical institutions, and even official organizations such as the FDA and WHO interpret ethical guidelines differently. For example, many clinical trials, including those required for FDA approval, do not respect paragraph 29 of the Declaration of Helsinki.

IS IT ETHICALLY ACCEPTABLE TO USE PLACEBOS IN ROUTINE MEDICAL PRACTICE?

The debate on the use of placebos in medical practice is not as lively as that in the clinical trial setting. Of course, the same ethical guidelines described above and the same arguments for and against the use of placebos can be applied to routine clinical practice. A very influential paper was published in the 1970s (Bok 1974). In this article, the administration of a placebo is seen as an unethical procedure because it necessarily involves some degree of deception, thus damaging the institution of medicine and contributing to the erosion of confidence and trust in medical staff and caregivers (see also Bok 2002). The inherent use of deception is justified by Rawlinson (1985) by invoking concepts of paternalism and benevolent deception, in which the physician's purpose is not to deceive but to cure. Rawlinson (1985) goes further by asserting that one of the effects of illness is an undermining of the patient's autonomy, and that it is the physician who must restore this loss, even through the use of benevolent paternalism and deception. Certainly, the use of benevolent deception in routine medical practice requires some rules. For example, it should never be employed for the convenience of the caregiver. It should only be used in cases where substantial evidence indicates that it is necessary. The doctor should determine whether any physical or psychological condition for which other treatments are indicated would be masked by the placebo itself.

On the one hand, we cannot criticize Bok's position (1974, 2002) for several reasons. First, deception must be used appropriately, and it is not easy to devise general ethical regulations for its use. Second, if medical staff is allowed to deceive, then a dangerous precedent is also established for quacks and shamans. On the other hand, deception is often used in medical practice, for example to conceal a stressful situation in a patient who has had a heart attack. So why not use it to conceal a dummy treatment if it works and the patient feels better? Certainly, Bok's concerns about credibility in medicine remain. The discovery of deception can lead to a failure of trust when trust is most needed.

The ethical argument in favor of the use of placebos and deceptions in routine medical practice is strengthened by some studies that show the real positive effects of placebos in some circumstances. Here we will mention only two studies on analgesia. First, in the postoperative trial by Pollo et al. (2001) discussed in detail above, a reduction of narcotic intake of about 30% was obtained by the simultaneous administration of a saline solution that was deceptively stated to be a painkiller. Second, as described above, the hidden interruption of an analgesic in the postoperative phase prolonged the relapse of pain compared with an open interruption (Benedetti et al. 2003). Should we abandon these therapeutic protocols, which involve either deception or lack of information, even though they are beneficial to the patient?

HOW TO RESOLVE THE ETHICAL PROBLEM
OF THE CLINICAL USE OF PLACEBOS

We contend that the ethical issue on the use of placebos in clinical trials and medical practice can be resolved only if the placebo phenomenon is understood at both the psychological and physiological level. To this end, the placebo effect must become a target of investigation. A conference organized by the U.S. National Institutes of Health to discuss placebo attracted clinical scientists, psychologists, neurobiologists, physicians, anthropologists, and humanists (Guess et al. 2002). As Moerman (2002a,b) points out, the term *placebo* has been a misleading concept and a dangerous source of misconceptions. Today we know that rather than a single mechanism underlying the placebo effect there are many mechanisms, depending on the condition, the procedure, and the treatment. As stressed by Hrobjartsson (2002), it might be time to stop using the term *placebo effect* and instead specify which kind of intervention one is referring to. This is particularly important in light of several misunderstandings that have occurred in recent years. For example, we believe that the negative findings of the meta-analysis by Hrobjartsson and Gotzsche (2001) have been exaggerated on both sides.

This meta-analysis shows that real placebo effects are more difficult to detect in the clinical trial setting compared to the experimental setting, as was emphasized by Vase et al. (2002). Therefore, when the placebo effect becomes the target of scientific inquiry, clinical trials do not represent an adequate setting for such an investigation. Also, the positive findings on the placebo effect in pain by Hrobjartsson and Gotzsche (2001) have been dismissed as biases, without any experimental support.

We believe that the extreme positions for and against the clinical use and the importance of the placebo effect derive from our ignorance about a phenomenon that is difficult to investigate. The negative connotation that the term *placebo* has held for many decades is one of the biggest hurdles to understanding its impact in clinical practice. By taking into account the psychophysiological mechanisms described in Chapters 8 and 10, it would be better to replace the term *placebo analgesia* with terms such as *expectation of analgesia, anticipation of analgesia,* and *conditioned analgesia.*

Another important point to be resolved deals with the worldwide ethical code represented by the Declaration of Helsinki, through which the patient can be protected from procedures such as placebo administration. We are not bioethicists, although we understand the concerns of our colleagues who work in this field. Nonetheless, we wish to offer some suggestions and procedures that we use in our routine work with patients who receive a placebo treatment for scientific purposes. First, we would like to refer to the verbal instructions proposed by Price (2001), which, we believe, do not involve any kind of deception. When giving a placebo, Price proposes telling the patient: "This agent is known to powerfully reduce pain in some patients." This is an ethically appropriate suggestion that can be used in many clinical contexts without involving deception. In our routine clinical work, we often use these words not for placebo procedures but for analgesic drugs such as acetaminophen and acetylsalicylic acid.

Second, on the basis of previous works by Levine et al. (1981), Gracely et al. (1983), and Levine and Gordon (1984), we have developed an open-hidden administration paradigm to assess the efficacy of a therapy (Amanzio et al. 2001; Benedetti et al. 2003). As described in detail above, a hidden administration of an analgesic agent is less effective than an open one, so that the placebo component of the treatment is represented by the difference between the two: the greater the difference, the greater is the placebo component, and the smaller is the effect of the active treatment. In this way, we administer no placebos and do not violate the Declaration of Helsinki. In fact, when a hidden analgesic injection is used, the best available therapy is being given, according to paragraph 29 of the Declaration. The only difference is that it is not administered by a doctor but by a concealed computer.

Although patients are aware of this, they do not know *when* the drug will be delivered by the computer. Imagine a patient lying in a bed with an intravenous line. The drug can be delivered at the first or fourth or 10th hour, but the patient does not know this temporal sequence. If the drug is really effective, pain reduction should be temporally correlated with drug administration. With this procedure, it is possible to detect placebo effects without the administration of any placebo and with the best therapy available to the patient. Although a hidden procedure is not easy to perform because it requires that the patient be in a bed with an intravenous line connected to a computer-controlled infusion pump, it can be used in some circumstances.

These examples show that, within the limits of ethics, our efforts should be directed toward better understanding of the role of the psychosocial context surrounding the patient who is receiving treatment. We believe that this understanding will lead to both new therapeutic strategies and better patient-provider interaction.

CONCLUSIONS

On the basis of all these considerations, the term *placebo effect* is misleading and a source of dangerous associations such as quackery, deception, and inertness. If we bear in mind that the concept of placebo is embedded in the notion of psychosocial context, all these negative meanings disappear, and the importance of placebo in medical practice clearly emerges. As pain researchers and physicians, we have no certainties about the correct use of placebos for good medical practice, thus we find it difficult to suggest general rules and principles. We simply believe that the ethics of a procedure cannot be resolved if that procedure is not fully understood. A first big step to bridging the gap in our understanding is to study the relationship between the psychosocial context and the therapeutic outcome. This relationship will be explored further in the following chapter.

ACKNOWLEDGMENTS

This work was supported by grants from the neuroscience and trigeminal pain projects of the National Research Council, from the Alzheimer's disease project of the Italian Ministry of Health, and from MIUR-FIRB.

REFERENCES

Ader R. Much ado about nothing. *Adv Mind Body Med* 2001; 17:293–295.

Amanzio M, Pollo A, Maggi G, Benedetti F. Response variability to analgesics: a role for non-specific activation of endogenous opioids. *Pain* 2001; 90:205–215.

Balint M. The doctor, his patient, and the illness. *Lancet* 1955; 1:683–688.

Bass MJ, Buck C, Turner L, et al. The physician's actions and the outcome of illness in family practice. *J Fam Pract* 1986; 23:43–47.

Beckman HB, Markakis KM, Suchman AL, Frankel RM. The doctor-patient relationship and malpractice: lessons from plaintiff depositions. *Arch Intern Med* 1994; 154:1365–1370.

Benedetti F. How the doctor's words affect the patient's brain. *Eval Health Prof* 2002; 25:369–386.

Benedetti F, Maggi G, Lopiano L, et al. Open versus hidden medical treatments: the patient's knowledge about a therapy affects the therapy outcome. *Prevention Treatment* 2003. Available via the Internet:journals.apa.org/prevention/volume6/toc-jun-03.html.

Bok S. The ethics of giving placebos. *Sci Am* 1974; 231:17–23.

Bok S. Ethical issues in use of placebo in medical practice and clinical trials. In: Guess HA, Kleinman A, Kusek JW, Engel LW (Eds). *The Science of the Placebo: Toward an Interdisciplinary Research Agenda*. London: BMJ Books, 2002, pp 63–73.

Brody H. *The Placebo Response*. New York: Harper Collins, 2000.

Brody H, Weismantel D. A challenge to core beliefs. *Adv Mind Body Med* 2001; 17:296–298.

Cassileth BR, Lusk EJ, Miller DS, Brown LL, Miller C. Psychosocial correlates of survival in advanced malignant disease? *N Engl J Med* 1985; 312:1551–1555.

Committee for Proprietary Medicinal Products. *Note for Guidance on the Clinical Investigation of Medicinal Products in the Treatment of Schizophrenia*. London: Committee for Proprietary Medicinal Products, 1998.

Council for International Organizations of Medical Sciences and World Health Organization. *International Ethical Guidelines for Biomedical Research Involving Human Subjects.* Geneva: Council for International Organizations of Medical Sciences, 1993.

Council on Ethical and Judicial Affairs of the American Medical Association. Ethical use of placebo controls in clinical trials. *Proc House of Delegates AMA* 1996; June 23–27:252–259.

Di Blasi Z, Harkness E, Ernst E, Georgiou A, Kleijnen J. Influence of context effects on health outcomes: a systematic review. *Lancet* 2001; 357:757–762.

DiNubile MJ. Letter to the editor. *N Engl J Med* 2001; 345:1278.

Egbert LD, Battit GE, Turndorf H, Beecher HK. The value of the preoperative visit by an anesthetist. *JAMA* 1963; 185:553–555.

Egbert LD, Battit GE, Welch CE, Bartlett MK. Reduction of postoperative pain by encouragement and instruction of patients. *N Engl J Med* 1964; 270:825–827.

Einarson TE, Hemels M. Letter to the editor. *N Engl J Med* 2001; 345:1277.

Epps J, Monk C, Savage S, Marlatt GA. Improving credibility of instruction in the balanced placebo design: a misattribution manipulation. *Addictive Behav* 1998; 23:427–435.

Flaten MA, Simonsen T, Olsen H. Drug-related information generates placebo and nocebo responses that modify the drug response. *Psychosom Med* 1999; 61:250–255.

Gracely RH, Dubner R, Wolskee PJ, Deeter WR. Placebo and naloxone can alter postsurgical pain by separate mechanisms. *Nature* 1983; 306:264–265.

Gracely RH, Dubner R, Deeter WR, Wolskee PJ. Clinicians' expectations influence placebo analgesia. *Lancet* 1985; 1:43.

Greene PJ, Wayne PM, Kerr CE, et al. The powerful placebo: doubting the doubters. *Adv Mind Body Med* 2001; 17:298–307.

Greenfield S, Kaplan S, Ware JE. Expanding patient involvement in care. *Ann Intern Med* 1985; 102:520–528.

Guess HA, Kleinman A, Kusek JW, Engel LW (Eds). *The Science of the Placebo: Toward an Interdisciplinary Research Agenda.* London: BMJ Books, 2002.

Hrobjartsson A. What are the main methodological problems in the estimation of placebo effects? *J Clin Epidemiol* 2002; 55:430–435.

Hrobjartsson A, Gotzsche PC. Is the placebo powerless? *N Engl J Med* 2001; 344:1594–1602.

Kaplan SH, Greenfield S, Ware JE Jr. Assessing the effects of physician-patient interactions on the outcomes of chronic disease. *Med Care* 1989; 27(Suppl 3):S110–S127.

Kaptchuk TJ. Letter to the editor. *N Engl J Med* 2001; 345:1277.

Kirsch I, Scoboria A. Apples, oranges, and placebos: heterogeneity in a meta-analysis of placebo effects. *Adv Mind Body Med* 2001; 17:307–309.

Kirsch I, Weixel LJ. Double-blind versus deceptive administration of a placebo. *Behav Neurosci* 1988; 102:319–323.

Kupers R. Letter to the editor. *N Engl J Med* 2001; 345:1278.

Lang AR, Goecknar DJ, Adesso VJ, Marlatt GA. Effects of alcohol on aggression in male social drinkers. *J Abnorm Psychol* 1975; 84:508–518.

Levine JD, Gordon NC. Influence of the method of drug administration on analgesic response. *Nature* 1984; 312:755–756.

Levine JD, Gordon NC, Smith R, Fields HL. Analgesic responses to morphine and placebo in individuals with postoperative pain. *Pain* 1981; 10:379–389.

Levinson W. Physician-patient communication: a key to malpractice prevention. *JAMA* 1994; 272:1619–1620.

Lewis JA, Jonsson B, Kreutz G, Sampaio C, Van Zwieten-Boot B. Placebo-controlled trials and the Declaration of Helsinki. *Lancet* 2002; 359:1337–1340.

Lilford RJ, Braunholtz DA. Letter to the editor. *N Engl J Med* 2001; 345:1278.

Marlatt GA, Demming B, Reid JB. Loss of control drinking in alcoholics: an experimental analogue. *J Abnorm Psychol* 1973; 81:223–241.

Michels KB, Rothman KJ. Update on unethical use of placebos in randomised trials. *Bioethics* 2003; 17:188–204.

Miller FG. Letter to the editor. *N Engl J Med* 2001; 345:1277.

Mitchell SH, Laurent CL, de Wit H. Interaction of expectancy and the pharmacological effects of d-amphetamine: subjective effects and self-administration. *Psychopharmacology* 1996; 125:371–378.

Moerman DE. Meaningful dimensions of medical care. In: Guess HA, Kleinman A, Kusek JW, Engel LW (Eds). *The Science of the Placebo: Toward an Interdisciplinary Research Agenda.* London: BMJ Books, 2002a, pp 77–107.

Moerman DE. *Meaning, Medicine and the Placebo Effect.* Cambridge, MA: Cambridge University Press, 2002b.

Pollo A, Amanzio M, Arslanian A, et al. Response expectancies in placebo analgesia and their clinical relevance. *Pain* 2001; 93:77–84.

Price DD. Assessing placebo effects without placebo groups: an untapped possibility? *Pain* 2001; 90:201–203.

Rawlinson MC. Truth-telling and paternalism in the clinic: philosophical reflection on the use of placebo in medical practice. In: White L, Tursky B, Schwartz GE (Eds). *Placebo: Theory, Research, and Mechanisms.* New York: Guilford Press, 1985, pp 403–416.

Rohsenow DJ, Bachorowski J. Effects of alcohol and expectancies on verbal aggression in men and women. *J Abnorm Psychol* 1984; 93:418–432.

Ross S, Krugman AD, Lyerly SB, Clyde DJ. Drugs and placebos: a model design. *Psychol Rep* 1962; 10:383–392.

Rothman KJ, Michels KB. The continuing unethical use of placebo controls. *N Engl J Med* 1994; 15:19–38.

Shrier I. Letter to the editor. *N Engl J Med* 2001; 345:1278.

Sox HC, Margulies I, Sox CH. Psychologically mediated effects of diagnostic tests. *Ann Intern Med* 1981; 95:680–685.

Spiegel D, Bloom JR, Kraemer HC, Gottheil E. Effect of psychosocial treatment on survival of patients with metastatic breast cancer. *Lancet* 1989; 2:888–891.

Spiegel D, Kraemer H, Carlson RW. Letter to the editor. *N Engl J Med* 2001; 345:1276.

Starfield B, Wray C, Hess K, et al. The influence of patient-practitioner agreement on outcome of care. *Am J Public Health* 1981; 71:127–132.

Stewart MA. Effective physician-patient communication and health outcomes: a review. *CMAJ* 1995; 152:1423–1433.

Stewart MA, McWhinney IR, Buck CW. The doctor-patient relationship and its effect upon outcome. *J R Coll Gen Pract* 1979; 29:77–82.

Sutton SR. Great expectations: some suggestions for applying the balanced placebo design to nicotine and smoking. *Br J Addict* 1991; 86:659–662.

Temple RJ. Placebo controlled trials and active controlled trials: ethics and inference. In: Guess HA, Kleinman A, Kusek JW, Engel LW (Eds). *The Science of the Placebo: Toward an Interdisciplinary Research Agenda.* London: BMJ Books, 2002, pp 209–226.

Thomas KB. General practice consultations: is there any point in being positive? *BMJ* 1987; 294:1200–1202.

Thomas KB. The placebo in general practice. *Lancet* 1994; 344:1066–1067.

Turner JA, Deyo RA, Loeser JD, Von Korff M, Fordyce WE. The importance of placebo effects in pain treatment and research. *JAMA* 1994; 271:1609–1614.

Vase L, Riley III JL, Price DD. A comparison of placebo effects in clinical analgesic trials versus studies of placebo analgesia. *Pain* 2002; 99:443–452.

Wickramasekera I. The placebo efficacy study: problems with the definition of the placebo and the mechanisms of placebo efficacy. *Adv Mind Body Med* 2001; 17:309–312.

Wilson GT, Niaura RS, Adler JL. Alcohol, selective attention and sexual arousal in men. *J Stud Alcohol* 1985; 46:107–115.

World Medical Association. Declaration of Helsinki. Amended by the 52nd WMA General Assembly, Edinburgh, Scotland, October 2000. *JAMA* 2000; 284:3043–3045.

Word Medical Association. Declaration of Helsinki. Note of clarification on Paragraph 29. Washington, DC, 2002. Available via the Internet: www.wma.net/e/home.html.

Correspondence to: Fabrizio Benedetti, MD, Dipartimento di Neuroscienze, Università di Torino, Corso Raffaello 30, 10125 Torino, Italy. Tel: 39-011-6707709; Fax: 39-011-6707708; email: fabrizio.benedetti@unito.it.

Psychological Methods of Pain Control: Basic Science and Clinical Perspectives, Progress in Pain Research and Management, Vol. 29, edited by Donald D. Price and M. Catherine Bushnell, IASP Press, Seattle, © 2004.

10

The Contribution of Changes in Expected Pain Levels and Desire for Pain Relief to Placebo Analgesia

Lene Vase,[a] Donald D. Price,[b,c] G. Nicholas Verne,[e] and Michael E. Robinson[d]

[a]*Department of Psychology, University of Aarhus, Aarhus, Denmark; Departments of [b]Neuroscience, [c]Oral and Maxillofacial Surgery, and [d]Clinical and Health Psychology, University of Florida, Gainesville, Florida, USA; [e]Department of Gastroenterology, Veterans Administration Hospital, Gainesville, Florida, USA*

In a patient experiencing pain, the *perception* that an effective treatment has been administered may be sufficient to produce significant pain relief. To the extent that the pain relief is due to the perception alone as opposed to an active principle in the treatment, the relief is a placebo analgesic response. Placebo analgesia has been known for a long time, but there is no consensus concerning how this phenomenon should be defined, its general magnitude, or the exact psychophysiological processes involved.

We suggest a differentiation between the "placebo analgesic agent," the "placebo analgesic effect," and the "placebo analgesic response." The placebo analgesic agent refers to all external aspects of the therapeutic intervention that can be perceived by the patient or experimental subject (see Chapter 9). The placebo analgesic effect is the measured difference in pain across an untreated and a placebo-treated group or across an untreated and placebo-treated condition within the same group (as in crossover studies). Using multiple measurements and inferential statistics, this measured difference can be inferred to result from factors related to the perception of the therapeutic interventions as opposed to changes due to natural history. A placebo analgesic response is a reduction in pain in an individual that results from his or her perception of the therapeutic intervention. This response may be considered both a biological and a psychological event. However, it is inferred and not directly observable, because even when a subject's pain is measured during both a single natural history condition and a single placebo condition, one cannot be certain that the lower pain rating in the placebo condition results from the placebo treatment and not from a change in natural history due to recovery or remission. A placebo response could be shown to occur in an individual if multiple measurements were taken during both a highly predictable and stable natural history condition as well as during a placebo condition. It could also be demonstrated in an individual tested during multiple natural history and multiple placebo conditions. The challenge and difficulty of inferring a placebo response in an individual patient are not commonly recognized, as is evident from the relative ease with which authors claim to know about placebo response rates in analgesia studies (Turner et al. 1994).

In this chapter, we discuss the magnitude of placebo analgesia on the basis of current meta-analyses and review factors both external to and within human experience that contribute to this phenomenon. Emphasis will be placed on how placebo analgesic effects can be predicted and interpreted. Finally, we briefly discuss the psychoneurophysiological processes involved in placebo analgesic effects and consider their theoretical and clinical implications.

THE MAGNITUDE OF PLACEBO ANALGESIA

Anecdotal reports of patients being cured by supposedly inert treatments have existed for many years (Harrington 1997). Beecher's (1955) classical meta-analysis, which showed that 35% ± 2.2% of patients across various illnesses and conditions experienced pain relief following placebo treatment, was one of the first attempts to make a systematic review of the magnitude of placebo effects. Beecher's finding led to the impression that a fixed proportion of individuals respond to placebo treatments. Studies during the 1960s and 1970s attempted to determine whether personality factors such as introversion and extroversion predispose individuals to experience a placebo analgesic effect (Shapiro and Morris 1978). However, these early studies suffered from the major limitation that the level of pain in the placebo group was not compared with that in a no-treatment group. Therefore, it was not possible to know whether the pain-relieving effect resulted from perception of the placebo treatment or from factors related to changes in natural history (see Pollo et al. 2001). Thus, these studies were not true assessments of placebo analgesic effects. From the 1970s onward, researchers recognized that it was crucial to incorporate a natural history condition (in clinical studies) or a repeated baseline control condition (in experimental studies) to be able to investigate the factors that contribute to placebo analgesic effects and to deduce their magnitude (Fields 1981). During the 1970s, 1980s, and 1990s several studies reported substantial placebo analgesic effects and showed that external factors such as conditioning and suggestion as well as internal factors such as expected pain levels contribute to the magnitude of placebo analgesia. Also, researchers discovered that administration of the opioid antagonist naloxone may prevent at least some types of placebo analgesic effects. Therefore, release of endogenous opioids may play a role in mediating such effects (Levine et al. 1978; Gracely et al. 1983; Grevert et al. 1983; Levine and Gordon 1984; Benedetti et al. 1995, 1999; Amanzio and Benedetti 1999; Amanzio et al. 2001). However, despite the accumulating indications of these psychophysiological effects, recent review articles have questioned the existence of placebo analgesic effects (Kienle and Kiene 1996, 1997). Hrobjartsson and Gotzsche (2001) conducted a meta-analysis, including 29 studies of placebo analgesia, where the effect of placebo treatment was compared to a natural history condition. The effect size of placebo analgesia, measured as Cohen's d (pooled standardized mean difference), was 0.27. Cohen's d values from 0.2 to 0.5 are considered small, values from 0.5 to 0.8 are considered medium, and values of 0.8 and higher are considered large. Thus, their finding of an effect size of 0.27 reflects a small but significant effect. Because pain reflects a subjective state, Hrobjartsson and Gotzsche (2001) suggested that the small placebo analgesic effect was due to confounding variables such as response bias. Interestingly, most studies included in the meta-analysis used placebo as a control condition for an active treatment (24 out of 29). In these studies, patients are typically informed, via the informed consent form, that they may receive either an active pain-killing agent or an ineffective (placebo) agent. Hence, in such settings patients are likely to expect that there is only a 50% chance of receiving a pain-relieving agent. In most nonresearch clinical settings or in studies of placebo analgesia mechanisms, however, doctors are more likely to give positive suggestions about the treatment's efficacy, and thus patients are more likely to expect to receive a pain-relieving medication.

Therefore, two new meta-analyses were conducted (Vase et al. 2002). The first meta-analysis included studies in which placebo treatments were used as a control condition, most of which were also included in Hrobjartsson and Gotzsche's (2001) meta-analysis. The second meta-analysis included only studies that focused on placebo analgesic mechanisms. Both meta-analyses included both experimental and clinical studies, and all the studies used a no-treatment control condition or a repeated baseline measure. In studies in which placebo treatments were used as a control condition and weak suggestions for pain relief were given, the mean effect size (Cohen's *d*) was 0.15 (ranging from –0.95 to +0.57), even smaller than Hrobjartsson and Gotzsche's finding of 0.27. However, in the studies of placebo mechanisms, where strong suggestions for pain relief were typically given, the effect size was 0.95 (ranging from –0.64 to +2.29). When the effect sizes were weighted for the number of patients in each study, the difference in effect size was even larger. The mean effect size was –0.04 in the first meta-analysis (studies using placebo as a control) and 1.14 in the second meta-analysis (studies in which placebo was the topic of study) (see Table I) (Price et al. 2003). Hence, these meta-analyses indicate that the magnitude of placebo analgesic effects is highly variable and that one of the factors influencing the magnitude may be the type of suggestion given for pain relief.

To further understand the factors that contribute to the variability in the magnitude of placebo analgesia, Vase et al. subdivided the studies of placebo mechanisms into studies in which the placebo analgesic effect was induced by conditioning alone, by suggestion alone, or by conditioning combined with suggestion. In the studies where placebo analgesia was induced by either conditioning alone or suggestion alone, the effect size was 0.83 and 0.85, respectively. However, in the studies where placebo analgesia was induced by a combination of conditioning and suggestion, the effect size was 1.45, almost twice as high as for either factor alone. Therefore, the effect of external manipulations such as conditioning and suggestion appears to be additive, which indicates that placebo analgesic effects are likely to be related to the perception of the placebo agent rather than to the agent itself.

FACTORS THAT CONTRIBUTE TO THE MAGNITUDE OF PLACEBO ANALGESIA

How is it possible to investigate and conceptualize the ways in which perception of a (placebo) treatment may lead to a pain-relieving effect?

Table I

Effect size (Cohen's *d*) of placebo analgesic effects from a meta-analysis of clinical trials and studies of placebo mechanisms

Clinical Trials	Studies of Placebo Mechanisms
Mean *d* = 0.15 (–0.95 to + 0.57)	Mean *d* = 0.95 (–0.64 to 2.29)
Mean weighted *d* = –0.04	Mean weighted *d* = 1.14

Source: Data from Vase et al. (2002).
Note: Clinical trials (*n* = 23) had weak suggestions for pain relief; studies of placebo mechanisms (*n* = 14) had strong suggestions for pain relief.

Amanzio et al. (2001) investigated the contribution of placebo analgesia to the effectiveness of analgesic drugs in a clinical setting using hidden and open injections of traditional drugs such as buprenorphine (see Chapter 9). When these agents were administrated openly by a doctor who gave verbal suggestions for pain relief, the patients needed less medication to reach analgesia than when the drugs were administrated by a hidden machine. The difference in medication between open and hidden injections is likely to directly reflect the placebo analgesic effect. An additional experimental study (Amanzio et al. 2001) showed that the difference between open and hidden injections could be eliminated by hidden injections of naloxone, providing evidence that part of the variability in the response to analgesic drugs is due to opioid-mediated placebo analgesic effects. Therefore, an important goal of future placebo analgesia research is to identify factors that contribute to the perceived efficacy of the therapeutic intervention. Factors associated with open administration or with suggestions that the agent is a powerful painkiller may be especially useful in clarifying how these factors either mediate or moderate placebo analgesic effects. A number of studies have started to specify these factors.

EXTERNAL FACTORS

Conditioning. The perception of pain treatments is likely to be influenced by previous experiences with pain, by the analgesic remedy, and by the clinical setting. Some investigators have proposed that placebo effects are based on Pavlovian conditioning. Wickramasekera (1985) suggested that when a patient receives an agent (the unconditioned stimulus) that leads to analgesia (the unconditioned response), contextual cues such as the hospital, the white coat, or the pill (conditioned stimuli) are likely to be associated with pain relief. These contextual factors, which represent the conditioned stimuli, come to elicit pain relief in the absence of active agents. This hypothesis is supported by crossover studies finding that when placebo is given as the second drug, the magnitude of placebo analgesia follows the graded doses of the active drug (Laska and Sunshine 1973). The first studies to investigate the contribution of conditioning within a design that included a repeated baseline control condition were those of Voudouris and colleagues (1985, 1989, 1990). In their paradigm, subjects were tested in three conditions: pre-test, manipulation, and post-test. In the pre-test session, a noxious electrical stimulus was applied to determine the subjects' threshold. In the manipulation session, an inert cream was applied to the skin, and the stimulus was surreptitiously reduced to suggest that the cream had an analgesic effect. In the post-test session, the placebo "analgesic" cream was applied, and the original stimulus was delivered to the same area of the skin. Compared to a group given the cream with no conditioning, the conditioning group showed significant pain reduction from the cream. This result indicates that a previous pairing of reduced stimulus intensity with an inert agent can result in large analgesic effects when the conditioned stimulus is given alone.

Amanzio and Benedetti (1999) tested the contribution of conditioning in subjects undergoing ischemic arm pain who rated their pain tolerance. On day one, subjects were tested during a no-treatment session, and on days two and three one group of 14 subjects were conditioned with morphine and another group of 14 subjects were conditioned with the non-opioid agent ketorolac. On day four, both groups of subjects received open injections of saline and were told that the agent was an antibiotic, which served to negate any effect of placebo suggestion. Conditioning produced a moderate and statistically reliable placebo effect in these two groups of subjects. When the entire experiment was repeated with an open injection of naloxone instead of an open injection of saline on day four, a placebo analgesic effect was prevented in the group that was conditioned with morphine but not in the group that was conditioned with ketorolac. Hence, the placebo analgesic effect induced by opioid conditioning (morphine) was mediated by endogenous opioids, whereas that induced by non-opioid conditioning (ketorolac) was not.

Suggestion.   Nonverbal and verbal suggestions for pain relief can lead individuals to expect or believe in future responses without questioning. The influence of nonverbal suggestions has indirectly been tested in a study in which the clinician knew that one group of patients would receive a placebo whereas the second group would receive either a placebo or the active analgesic agent fentanyl (Gracely et al. 1985). When *both* groups received placebo, the placebo analgesic effect was significantly higher in the second group. This result indicates that the clinician's belief that a patient may receive a powerful painkiller influences the magnitude of placebo analgesia even when the clinician does not convey this belief verbally or intentionally. The influence of verbal suggestions on pain relief has been investigated in several studies. Using the same paradigm of ischemic tourniquet pain tolerance, Amanzio and Benedetti (1999) also tested whether suggestion in itself was sufficient to produce placebo analgesia. After the no-treatment session on day one, patients were given an open injection of saline and were told that the agent was a powerful painkiller on day two. This placebo treatment produced a small but statistically reliable placebo effect. When the experiment was repeated with an open injection of naloxone instead of an open injection of saline on day two, the placebo analgesic effect was completely prevented, indicating that suggestion induces a placebo analgesic effect that is mediated by endogenous opioids. Recent studies have shown that both direct and indirect suggestions for pain relief lead to large magnitudes of placebo analgesia (Price et al. 1999; Pollo et al. 2001; Vase et al. 2002; see also Chapter 9). Furthermore, several studies have shown that verbal suggestions can reduce pain in highly specific areas of the body, such as the right hand (Montgomery and Kirsch 1996; Benedetti et al. 1999; Price et al. 1999; De Pascalis et al. 2002), and that such specific placebo effects may be mediated by endogenous opioids (Benedetti et al. 1999; Chapter 9).

Most of the studies described above have shown that conditioning in itself or suggestion in itself may lead to placebo analgesic effects. However, in most studies of the placebo effect and especially in most clinical settings, previous exposure to analgesic agents and verbal suggestions for pain relief combine to produce placebo analgesia. In the study by Amanzio and Benedetti (1999), the placebo effect from a combination of morphine conditioning and verbal suggestions was approximately twice as great as that induced by either conditioning or suggestion alone. This large placebo effect was completely prevented by naloxone. Hence, in accordance with the findings of our previously described meta-analyses (Vase et al. 2002), the effect of conditioning and suggestion seems to be additive in placebo analgesia. Also, even though conditioning and suggestion may make separate contributions to placebo analgesic effects, they are likely to activate a common opioid analgesia network. Furthermore, a recent study by Benedetti et al. (2003) indicates that whereas conditioning and suggestion both influence conscious phenomena such as pain by inducing expectations, conditioning without conscious expectations can influence unconscious physiological processes such as hormonal secretion and cardiovascular responses (see Chapter 8).

EXPERIENTIAL FACTORS

Patients are likely to perceive external factors such as conditioning and suggestion differently, and it is therefore important to examine how these environmental influences and factors within the human experience relate to each other during placebo analgesia.

Expectancy and desire. Expectancy is the experienced likelihood of an outcome or an expected effect. Within the context of pain studies it can be measured by asking subjects about the level of pain they expect to experience. Montgomery and Kirsch (1997) conducted one of the first studies in which expected pain levels were directly measured and manipulated. In a design similar to that of Voudouris et al. (1990), subjects were conditioned with reduced stimuli intensity in the presence of an inert cream and were given verbal suggestions for pain relief. Subjects rated expected pain levels immediately after the manipulation trial. As in the Voudouris study, if the subjects did not know about the stimulus manipulation, pain ratings were markedly diminished by the conditioning procedure. However, by performing regression analyses the authors showed that this effect was completely mediated by expected pain levels. Also, expectancy accounted for 49% of the variance in post-manipulation pain ratings. Furthermore, when another group of subjects was informed about the experimental design and learned that the cream was inert, the placebo analgesic effect disappeared. Hence, conscious expectation appears to overrule the effect of conditioning in placebo analgesia. Price and colleagues (1999) further tested the extent to which expectations of pain relief can be graded and related to specific areas of the body. Using a similar paradigm, they applied three "strengths" of placebo cream on the subjects' forearms and provided external manipulations designed to give subjects the belief that that cream A was a strong analgesic, cream B a weak analgesic, and cream C a control agent. After the creams were applied, subjects were conditioned with surreptitiously lowered heat stimuli in areas A (large reduction) and B (small reduction), but not in area C (no reduction). Immediately after these manipulation trials, subjects were asked to rate their expected pain levels for the next series of trials. The conditioning trials led to graded levels of expectancy for the three creams as well as graded magnitudes of placebo analgesia. Thus, after conditioning trials, subjects expected that applications of agents C, B, and A would result in successively less intense pain, as indicated by their ratings of expected pain. During the post-manipulation trials, when identical stimulus intensities were applied to all three areas, subjects rated pain in areas C, B, and A as progressively less intense, thereby demonstrating a graded placebo effect. Expected pain levels accounted for between 25% and 36% of the variance in post-manipulation pain ratings in this study. Because these placebo effects were induced on three immediately adjacent areas of the arm, these results provide further evidence for the somatotopic specificity of the placebo analgesic effect.

Although expectancy seems to be an important psychological mediator of placebo analgesia, it is unlikely to operate alone. Desire, which is the experiential dimension of wanting something to happen or wanting to avoid something happening, is also likely to be involved in placebo analgesia, given that motivation is known to influence perception. The study by Price et al. (1999) was the first study on placebo analgesia to measure and manipulate subjects' level of desire. Desire for the treatment to have a pain-relieving effect was successfully increased in one group by giving them the prospect of receiving a large number of painful stimuli and was decreased in a second group by telling them that only a few stimuli would be presented. However, ratings of desire for pain relief were not significantly associated with the magnitudes of placebo analgesia. One reason that desire for pain relief did not contribute to the magnitude of placebo analgesia in this experimental setting may be that pain was induced via brief heat stimuli. Desire for pain relief is likely to be more of a factor when pain has an uncertain duration or is threatening and thus likely to induce fear or anxiety, as occurs in many instances of clinical pain. Hence, it is important to investigate the contribution of expected pain levels and desire for pain relief in more clinically relevant settings.

Expectancy and memory.   The memory of previous experiences is also likely to influence the experience of pain. In the study by Price et al. (1999) the placebo analgesic effect was assessed based on both *concurrent* ratings of pain obtained immediately after the stimuli were applied and on *retrospective* ratings of pain obtained approximately 2 minutes after the stimuli were applied. The magnitude of placebo analgesic effects was three to four times greater when based on retrospective ratings than when based on concurrent ratings. The main reason for this difference was that subjects remembered their baseline pain intensity as being much greater than it actually was. Similar to placebo analgesic effects assessed concurrently, the remembered placebo effects were strongly correlated with expected pain intensities ($R = 0.5$–0.6). In fact, there was a stronger correlation between expected pain ratings and remembered pain than between expected pain ratings and actual pain. Thus, it is important to measure placebo analgesic effects concurrently because otherwise they may be distorted by remembered pain. Furthermore, remembered pain and expected pain are closely related and seem to interact. These findings were replicated by De Pascalis et al. (2002).

PREDICTING PLACEBO ANALGESIA

To further understand how factors external to and within human experience may relate during placebo analgesia, Verne et al. (2003) and Vase et al. (2003) conducted two almost identical studies. Patients suffering from irritable bowel syndrome (IBS) were exposed to rectal distention by means of a balloon barostat, which is a type of visceral stimulation that simulates their clinical pain. Subjects were tested under the conditions of natural history, rectal placebo, and rectal lidocaine. Pain intensity and unpleasantness were rated immediately after each stimulus. The first study was conducted as a standard clinical trial in which patients were given an informed consent form stating that they "may receive an active pain reducing mediation or an inert placebo agent" (Verne et al. 2003). This study found a significant pain-relieving effect of rectal lidocaine as compared to rectal placebo ($P <$ 0.001) and a significant pain-relieving effect of rectal placebo as compared to the natural history condition. Inspired by Pollo et al.'s (2001) study and the previously presented meta-analyses (Vase et al. 2002), a second study was conducted that was almost identical to the first study. The one difference was that in the second study the patients were told: "The agent you have just been given is known to significantly reduce pain in some patients" at the onset of each treatment condition (rectal placebo or lidocaine) (Vase et al. 2003). A much larger placebo analgesic effect was found in the second study, and the magnitude of placebo analgesia was so high (an effect size 2.0, Cohen's d) that there was no longer a significant difference between the magnitude of rectal lidocaine and rectal placebo (see Fig. 1). Hence, these two studies indicate that by adding an overt suggestion for pain relief it is possible to increase the magnitude of placebo analgesia to a level that matches that of an active agent.

In both studies, patients were asked to rate their expected pain level and desire for pain relief right after the agent was administered and before it had

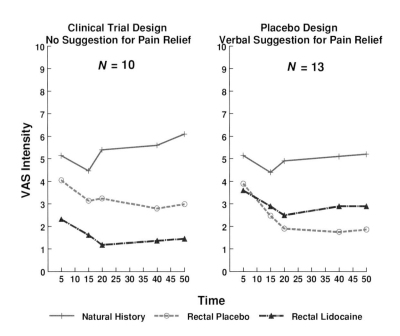

Fig. 1. Comparisons of natural history, rectal placebo, and rectal lidocaine scores on visceral pain intensity ratings on a visual analogue scale (VAS) during a 50-minute session within a clinical trial design, where no suggestions for pain relief are given (left) and within a placebo design with verbal suggestions for pain relief (right).

taken effect. In the second study, which focused on placebo analgesia mechanisms, the combination of expected pain levels and desire for pain relief accounted for 77% of the variance in post-placebo pain ratings (see Table II). In previous studies, expected pain levels have accounted for between 25% and 49% of the variance in post-placebo pain ratings. Thus, it is possible that the *combination* of expected pain level and desire for pain relief accounts for a greater amount of the variance in post-placebo pain ratings than either factor alone. The majority of the contribution came from expected pain level, but the interaction between expected pain level and desire for pain relief also seemed to have contributed (Table II). Interestingly, the combination of expected pain level and desire for pain relief accounted for 81% of the variance in pain ratings during the rectal lidocaine condition (see Table III), thereby supporting the conclusion that placebo factors also strongly contribute to the efficacy of active treatments.

CALCULATING PLACEBO ANALGESIA

Studies of placebo analgesia have thus far examined the placebo effect (the difference between a placebo treatment and no treatment) and the extent to which psychological factors such as expected pain level and desire for pain relief predict the variance in post-placebo pain ratings. While these are important findings, it can be argued that the predictive relationships are not predictions of the placebo effect, but merely predictions of pain ratings in a given condition. In the study presented above (Vase et al. 2003), expected pain ratings from each condition (natural history, rectal placebo, and rectal lidocaine) were all predictive of pain in the respective condition but not optimally informative of the placebo effect. How then is it possible to predict the placebo effect? Given that the placebo effect is the pain reduction from a no-treatment condition to a placebo condition, it can be argued that an equation to predict the placebo effect should use a difference score between ratings in the natural history condition and ratings in the placebo

Table II
The contribution of expectancy and desire
to rectal placebo analgesia

Model	R^2 Change	F	P
Expectancy* + Desire	0.64	9.1	0.006
Expectancy × Desire	0.12	5.0	0.05
Total model	0.77	10.2	0.003

Source: Data from Vase et al. (2003).
* Denotes significant beta weight.

Table III
The contribution of expectancy and desire
to rectal lidocaine analgesia

Model	R^2 Change	F	P
Expectancy* + Desire	0.81	21.5	0.001
Expectancy × Desire	0.006	0.28	0.61
Total model	0.81	13.3	0.001

Source: Data from Vase et al. (2003),
* Denotes significant beta weight.

condition for both the predicted variable (pain ratings) and the predictor variable (e.g., expected pain ratings). Hence, it would be feasible to predict the change from natural history or baseline responding to the placebo condition, and it would then become possible to examine how trait factors, such as personality style or relationship to the health care provider, or more dynamic factors, such as change in expected pain level, predict the pain reduction from no treatment to placebo treatment. Prediction of the difference score between the natural history and placebo condition in an individual should be calculated in the same manner. Similar considerations apply to calculation of nocebo effects.

To determine whether such an approach can reliably predict placebo analgesic effects, we have combined and reanalyzed the data from the two studies presented above (Vase et al. 2003; Verne et al. 2003). The placebo effect (natural history pain intensity minus rectal placebo pain intensity), change in expected pain (natural history pain expectation minus rectal placebo pain expectations), and change in desire for pain relief (natural history desire minus rectal placebo desire) were all calculated for each of 23 subjects. The changes in expectation and desire were entered into a regression equation along with their interaction (centered to reduce multicollinearity), and the placebo effect served as the predicted variable. First, desire change scores and expected pain change scores were entered into the model. This component accounted for 16% of the variance in placebo effects, but alone it was not statistically significant (Table IV). Second, after statistically controlling for this component, a second component, change in desire multiplied by change in expectation, was entered into the regression equation. This component accounted for an additional 22% of the variance in the placebo effect and was statistically significant (Table IV). The entire model accounted for 38% of the variance in the placebo effect. This reanalysis has at least two implications. First, it suggests that the change score approach is a better reflection of placebo analgesic effects and that future studies should, at minimum, include the change score analysis in addition to more standard

Table IV
The contribution of changes in expectancy and
desire to rectal placebo analgesia

Model	R^2 Change	P
Δ Expectancy + Δ Desire	0.16	0.17
Δ Expectancy $\times$ Δ Desire	0.22	0.02
Total model	0.38	0.02

Source: Reanalysis of data of two studies shown in Fig. 1.

analyses. Second, it suggests that the main factor is an interaction between changes in desire and changes in expectation. This interaction is consistent with Price and Barrell's desire-expectation model of emotional feelings (Barrell and Niemeyer 1975; Price and Barrell 1984, 2000; Price et al. 1985, 2001) and with value-expectancy models in general (see references in Price and Barrell 2000). It suggests a consideration of placebo analgesic effects as phenomena that occur within the context of emotions. The following discussion speculates on the possibility that placebo effects are related to mechanisms similar to those mediating other psychological phenomena such as emotions and motivation, learning, and choice behavior.

PLACEBO ANALGESIA AS AN EMOTIONAL RESPONSE

Recent emotional theories have proposed that attention, cognitions, and emotions interact simultaneously in producing conscious states (Damasio 1994; Price and Barrell 2000). Such theories are likely to be relevant for a more coherent understanding of the placebo analgesia phenomenon because attention, cognitive factors, and emotional factors all seem to be involved in the experience of pain in general (Price 1999) and in the experience of placebo analgesia.

THE EMOTION MODEL

A modern formulation of emotional feelings comes from Price, Barrell, and colleagues (Barrell and Niemeyer 1975; Price and Barrell 1984; Price et al. 1985; Price and Barrell 2000; Price et al. 2001). They explain at least some common types of emotional feelings on the basis of two major factors. The first is how much someone *desires* something to happen or not to happen, and the second is his or her level of *expectation* that a desired outcome will happen or has happened. Neither of these two factors is specifically emotional, yet both are integral components of many ordinary emotions such as sadness, anxiety, relief, disappointment, excitement, and satisfaction (Fig. 2).

Price and Barrell tested the two-factor model using both quantitative and qualitative approaches. Psychophysical methods were used to assess the influence of both desirability of an outcome and expectation of its occurrence on the magnitude of emotional feelings. Experiments using both visual analogue and line-production scaling procedures demonstrated that both factors interacted to influence positive and negative emotional feelings. Similar to the placebo effect, the magnitude of positive and negative feeling intensity was shown to be a multiplicative function of both desire for an outcome and its perceived likelihood (expectation) of occurrence. The nature of this interaction also was influenced by whether the goal was to avoid negative consequences (an *avoidance* goal) or to obtain pleasurable or satisfying consequences (an *approach* goal). As can be discerned from Fig. 2, emotional feeling intensity was found to be a positively accelerating function of expectation for *avoidance* goals (Feeling intensity = Desire × Expectation^2 with the curves bending upward to the left), whereas emotional feeling intensity was a negatively accelerating function of expectation for *approach* goals (Feeling intensity = Desire × Expectation$^{0.5}$ with the curves bending downward to the right). These factors and their interrelationships were further used to characterize human emotions such as depression, anxiety, excitement, and satisfaction. For example, as shown by the emotion labels of Fig. 2, anxiety was associated with avoidance goals and with mid-range

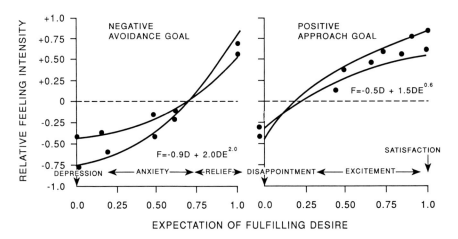

Fig. 2. Relationships of emotional feeling intensities to approach goals (left curves) and avoidance goals (right curves) and to different ranges of expectation. The expectation range of each emotional is shown by double-arrowed horizontal lines. F = magnitude of positive or negative emotional feeling; D = desire for goal; E = level of expectation of goal fulfillment. Reprinted from Price and Fields (1997), with permission.

expectations of avoiding negative outcomes. Feelings of frustration and depression were generally associated with avoidance goals and with low expectations of fulfilling them (Price and Barrell 1984; Price et al. 1985).

APPLYING THE EMOTION MODEL TO PLACEBO ANALGESIA

It may be surprising that interactions between desire and expectation apply to phenomena as seemingly diverse as emotions and placebo analgesic effects. However, interactions between desire and expectation account for magnitudes of positive and negative feelings during hypothetical emotional situations (Price and Barrell 1984) and during real-life emotional feelings (Price et al. 1985). These interactions also can account for direction and strength of choices during instances of decision making (Price et al. 2001). The analysis presented in Table IV extends this list in showing that interactions between changes in desire for relief and changes in expected pain levels account for large and significant amounts of variance in changes in pain that reflect placebo responses.

Paradoxically, the emotion functions shown in Fig. 2 predict that placebo effects, under at least some circumstances, might be enhanced when subjects *decrease* their desire for pain relief. This prediction is illustrated by a hypothetical example in Fig. 3. Suppose that as a result of a placebo

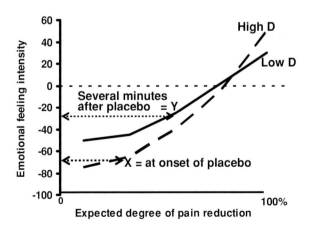

Fig. 3. Hypothetical changes in emotional response associated with an increased placebo response. The emotional feeling curves are based on Fig. 2. "X" represents the emotional feeling intensity near the onset of the placebo treatment, and "Y" represents the emotional feeling intensity several minutes later. A reduction of desire (D) and an increase in expected pain reduction are accompanied by a reduction in negative feeling.

suggestion, a patient expects a small reduction in pain. We can frame this expectation in terms of the patient's degree of expected pain reduction. Thus, an expectation of a 33% pain reduction in combination with a high desire for relief would correspond to the "X" in the dashed curve in Fig. 3. Upon experiencing a small amount of relief near the onset of placebo administration as a result of desired and expected relief, the patient begins to notice that the agent is working and expects further degrees of pain reduction. She also becomes less fearful or anxious, and consequently reduces her desire for pain relief. As time goes by, the patient would be feeling less negative as compared to the onset of treatment as a consequence of an increased expectation of pain reduction and *decreased* desire for pain relief, as indicated by the "Y" on the solid curve in Fig. 3. If placebo responses are driven by these changes in emotional feeling, then the *decreased* desire and *increased* expectations of lower pain intensity would result in a less negative feeling, as shown in Fig. 3. The decline in negative feeling would result in a greater placebo response. According to this explanation, some placebo responses are self-reinforcing and increase over time. This prediction is supported by the results of the two studies shown in Fig. 1. However, this explanation could be tested further by measuring desire for relief and expected pain reduction at two time points, one near the beginning of placebo administration and the other near the time that the placebo effect becomes much larger. We recently conducted such a study, and our preliminary analysis has confirmed our predictions in several ways (L. Vase et al., unpublished manuscript). The study was designed in a manner nearly identical to the one shown in the right panel of Fig. 1 (i.e., enhanced placebo by verbal suggestion). First, consistent with the previous study, the placebo effect increased by 32% over time. Second, consistent with our predictions, expected pain intensity, desire for pain relief, and anxiety ratings significantly decreased from the onset of placebo administration to the period beginning 20 minutes after placebo administration. An even more direct test of our working explanation could consist of having subjects rate their emotional feelings at the onset and several minutes after placebo treatment.

The possible similarity between placebo and emotion mechanisms becomes even more intriguing in the context of approach and avoidance functions of the emotion model (Fig. 2). If placebo effects are dependent on emotion mechanisms, then such responses may differ according to whether the individual's desired and expected therapeutic outcome represents an avoidance or approach goal, a hypothesis that could be further tested. Thus, by changing expectancy, desire, and the type of goal, it may be possible to change the emotional experience and therefore the placebo analgesic response. This situation can be illustrated as follows. The focus on negative consequences during an avoidance goal has the effect that unless the person is close to certainty of avoiding these negative consequences, he or she will feel emotionally negative. This aspect of emotional experience is captured by the positive accelerating curves in the left panel of Fig. 2, which demonstrate that feelings are negative throughout most of the range of expectation in the case of avoidance goals. For example, during the treatment of a visceral pain condition, if the patient is focusing on avoiding devastating consequences of chronic pain and has a moderate (50%) level of uncertainty of avoiding them, he or she is likely to have negative feelings. If expectation of avoiding pain increases to near-certainty, he or she will feel some relief but not intense positive feelings. In fact, the best the patient can feel during a goal of avoiding negative consequences is relief. On the other hand, under conditions in which it is both realistic and appropriate, a clinician may frame a therapeutic outcome in terms of a goal of achieving a more healthy condition (an approach goal). The patient would be more likely to maintain emotional feelings at positive levels over most of the range of expectation (right panel, Fig. 2). Even when expectations of these two scenarios remain uncertain, changing from an avoidance goal (avoiding devastating consequences) to an approach goal (better health) could result in a shift from a negative feeling of anxiety to a more positive feeling. Hence, qualitative changes in type of therapeutic goal combined with expectations of reduced pain may lead to qualitative and quantitative changes in emotional feelings directed toward the therapeutic outcome. This last step may be the one that is most proximal to the placebo effect, a possibility that could be tested. These relationships can be investigated by framing suggestions for approach and avoidance goals and by asking patients to rate their goal, emotional feelings, expected pain levels, and desire for pain relief as well as levels of pain intensity and pain unpleasantness.

Thus, the placebo analgesic effect may at least partly be conceptualized as an emotional response, where the (placebo) treatment sets the patient in a more positive or less negative emotional state. As discussed in Chapter 6, changes toward more positive or less negative emotional feelings are likely to reduce pain unpleasantness and, to some extent, pain intensity. On the other hand, it is possible that desire and expectation are simply factors that are common to both emotions and placebo mechanisms.

PSYCHONEUROPHYSIOLOGICAL PROCESSES INVOLVED IN PLACEBO ANALGESIA

BRAIN IMAGING OF THE PLACEBO EFFECT

One of the most important mechanistic questions about placebo analgesia is whether placebo manipulations really reduce the subjective intensity of pain or simply produce compliance with the suggestions of the investigators. In two functional magnetic resonance imaging (fMRI) experiments published in a single study, Wager et al. (2004) found that placebo analgesia was related to decreased neural activity in pain-processing areas of the brain. Their first study applied electrical shocks to 24 subjects under conditions of baseline and placebo administration. Their second study used heat stimuli applied to skin of the forearm and incorporated a conditioning paradigm similar to that of Voudouris et al. (1990). Pain-related neural activity was reduced during the placebo condition as compared with the baseline condition in both experiments. Furthermore, the same brain areas showed reduced activity in both experiments, including the thalamus, anterior insular cortex, and anterior cingulate cortex (ACC). These placebo-related decreases suggest that the afferent processing of pain is reduced during placebo analgesia, even in brain areas responsible for early levels of pain processing, such as the thalamus. In addition, the magnitudes of these decreases were correlated with reductions in pain ratings. Finally, the same types of decreases occurred regardless of whether the placebo effect was produced by suggestion or by conditioning.

These two experiments contain new important insights into the neural mechanisms of placebo analgesia because they provide strong refutation of the conjecture that placebo responses reflect nothing more than response bias (Hrobjartsson and Gotzsche 2001). They support the hypothesis that various types of placebo manipulations truly diminish the strength of the afferent signal associated with pain.

BRAIN IMAGING OF THE NEURAL EVENTS THAT TRIGGER THE PLACEBO RESPONSE

Another important aspect of Wager et al.'s study was that the authors imaged not only the time period of pain but also that of anticipation of pain. They hypothesized increases in neural activity within brain areas involved in expectation. In support of their hypothesis, they found significant positive correlations ($r = 0.4–0.7$) between increases in brain activity in the anticipatory period and decreases in pain and pain-related neural activity during stimulation within the placebo condition. The brain areas showing positive correlations during the anticipatory phase included the orbitofrontal cortex, dorsolateral prefrontal cortex, rostral ACC (in the second study only), and midbrain periaqueductal gray (PAG). The dorsolateral prefrontal cortex is an area that has been consistently associated with the representation of and maintenance of information needed for cognitive control, consistent with a role in expectation (Miller and Cohen 2001). On the other hand, the orbitofrontal cortex is associated with functioning in the evaluative and reward information relevant to allocation of control, consistent with a role in affective or motivational responses to anticipation of pain (Dias et al. 1997). Such a role is consistent with results showing that desire for relief is a factor in placebo analgesia.

OVERALL BRAIN CIRCUITRY INVOLVED IN PLACEBO ANALGESIA

This chapter has shown that some of the main psychological factors involved in placebo analgesia have been identified. As shown by recent results discussed above and by the discussion presented in Chapter 8, several neurophysiological factors are also starting to be identified. It is thus possible to make a rough outline of the psychoneurophysiological underpinnings of placebo analgesia.

Patients receiving a (placebo) treatment are likely to pay attention to the treatment vehicle and to the nonverbal and verbal suggestions that may go along with it. These contextual cues may be associated with previous pain relief and may thereby condition patients to expect pain relief. Alternatively, the perception of the treatment may lead patients to actively think about previous experiences with pain relief and thus it may evoke specific goals, emotions, and expectations related to pain relief. Expectations of relief would be common to both conditioning and active reflection. These psychological processes are likely to be associated with areas in the brain such as the frontal cortex and the ACC, and they can therefore be conceptualized as being related to *corticolimbic-related circuitry*. Dense opioid receptors have been found in these regions, especially the ACC (Zubieta et al. 2001; Petrovic et al. 2002). Therefore, it is possible that the corticolimbic-related circuitry utilizes endogenous opioids. The prefrontal cortex and the ACC project to the PAG, so the corticolimbic-related circuitry is likely to be functionally related to *brainstem- and spinal-related circuitry* that involves structures such as the PAG, which projects to the rostral ventral medulla. The latter, in turn, projects to the spinal cord, where it may inhibit ascending nociceptive signals (see Chapter 8). Hence, the perception of a (placebo) treatment may lead to expectation and desire for pain relief, which is associated with neural activity in corticolimbic-related circuitry. This circuitry may in itself release endogenous opioids, or it may be related to the brainstem- and spinal-related circuitry that releases endogenous opioids at spinal levels and results in a reduction in pain. On the other hand, evidence also indicates that large *non-opioid* placebo analgesic effects can occur with some types of placebo manipulations, such as conditioning with non-opioid drugs (Amanzio and Benedetti 1999). The extent to which these non-opioid forms of placebo analgesia utilize corticolimbic-related circuitry or brainstem- and spinal-related circuitry is presently unknown. There is evidence for non-opioid reductions of pain at spinal levels in the case of hypnotic analgesia (Chapter 11).

Brain-imaging studies have shown that both the corticolimbic-related circuitry and the brainstem- and spinal-related circuitry may be involved in placebo analgesic effects and that these circuits may utilize endogenous opioids under some conditions. However, it remains to be investigated how patients' ratings of expected pain levels and desire for pain relief relate to the utilization of these circuits and to the release of endogenous opioids. Research directed toward brain circuitry associated with pain relief has a long history (see Chapter 3), and this research has recently been linked to investigations of placebo analgesia. Thus, it would be interesting to see if placebo analgesic effects related to an approach goal are associated with a different modulatory circuitry than those related to an avoidance goal. For example, brain imaging, reflex measures, and measures of endogenous opioid activity could be combined with measures of pain, expectation, desire, and type of goal.

CLINICAL IMPLICATIONS

The research reviewed both in this chapter and in Chapters 8 and 9 shows that placebo analgesia is a phenomenon that causes psychophysiological effects and that placebo analgesic effects are embedded in pain treatments in general. Given the new information about the mechanisms of placebo analgesia reviewed in these chapters, it is important to consider how placebo analgesia can be used in clinical treatments and to examine the ethical considerations involved.

USING INERT AGENTS IN PLACEBO TREATMENT

One potential use of placebo analgesics would consist of a health care provider administering an inert substance without any suggestions or behavioral indications that the agent is effective. However, as placebo analgesia seems to be related to the perception of the treatment, it is unlikely that this type of placebo treatment would have a significant effect. In fact, such a situation is similar to the placebo arm in a clinical trial where no suggestions for pain relief are given. As indicated in the two meta-analyses of placebo analgesia described earlier, effects are generally small under such conditions (Hrobjartsson and Gotzsche 2001; Vase et al. 2002). Hence, administrating inert substances or sham treatments without suggestions for pain relief is ethically problematic because it violates the mandate that patients should receive the best possible treatment under their present circumstances.

Another possibility would be to combine inert substances or sham treatments with suggestions for pain relief. Such a treatment may have an effect, but it is likely to be deceptive and ethically problematic under most circumstances. A common reason for using this type of approach is not to produce analgesia but to determine whether the pain is organic or functional or to discredit the patient's pain report (Goodwin et al. 1979). Given that placebo effects are likely to occur independently of the origin of the pain, such use of placebo treatments is erroneous and unethical. Recent studies have also indicated that this type of placebo administration is used to a large extent to avoid confrontation with the patient (Hrobjartsson and Norup 2003); such use of placebo is very likely to be deceptive and to lead to a poor patient-provider relationship. It is unlikely to facilitate a good treatment effect or to be of any benefit to the patient. Even under circumstances where inert substances or sham treatments are combined with suggestions for pain relief in benevolent ways to help reduce the patient's pain, this use is paternalistic and deceptive (Bok 2002). From the health care provider's perspective it might be justifiable because current knowledge of placebo analgesic mechanisms suggests that the "placebo agent" comprises factors related to suggestions and behaviors of clinicians as well as desires and expectations of patients. However, from the patients' perspective, the agent is more likely to be understood in terms of the properties of the medicine or the treatment being administrated. Therefore, it is possible, perhaps probable, that patients will feel betrayed if they find out that there is no active principle in the agent or the treatment. Hence, such an approach might undermine their trust in the medical personnel and could diminish the efficacy of future treatments. However, it is conceivable that within a good patient-provider relationship, gaining knowledge about the efficacy of placebo-related factors could be received favorably by both patient and provider. This area requires additional research to determine the consequences, from both patient and provider perspectives, of using an efficacious placebo intervention. This line of research could also shed light on the ethical ramifications of not using an effective placebo when one is available.

It may be possible to administer inert substances or sham treatments along with suggestions for pain relief in ethically appropriate ways. One possibility could be to mix inert and active agents on a long-term basis. For example, suppose one-third of the pain medicine capsules prescribed to a patient contained an inert substance. A combination of conditioning and suggestion associated with inert but identical-looking capsules might produce pain relief. Patients could freely choose if they wanted these inert capsules to be part of their treatment. Possible advantages of such an approach might include sparing of side effects and costs. This approach has been suggested for immunosuppressive therapy (Ader 1997). Although this approach might be ethically justifiable, there is no evidence that it would work in the case of pain therapy, and the regulatory agencies are unlikely to support such a complicated approach.

Even when placebo agents are shown to be highly effective in the short term, their continued use in the long term without the patients' knowledge is questionable and ethically suspect. Most critically, patients' eventual discovery that they are receiving an inert agent could be disillusioning and harmful and would lead to a loss of efficacy of the treatment.

ENHANCING PLACEBO COMPONENTS OF ACTIVE TREATMENTS

The approaches just presented relate to an "old" understanding of placebo as an inert agent or a sham treatment. However, as shown in these three chapters on placebo analgesia, it may be more accurate and useful to conceptualize placebo analgesia in terms of the perception of the treatment. When placebo analgesia is seen in this light it becomes clear that suggestions and behavioral indications for pain relief can be interfaced with administration of active agents to enhance the total pain-relieving effect of the treatment. As we have seen, this enhancement can sometimes be considerable (Fig. 1). Under these conditions, patients receive an optimal treatment, and if no deception is involved, it could be ethically acceptable (see also Chapter 9). In fact, it can be argued that enhancing the placebo component of treatment is more effective and therefore more ethical than leaving out this component of therapy. In practice such an approach could be implemented by interfacing standard treatments with attention to patients' thoughts, beliefs, and feelings about the treatment and with attempts to optimize their perception of the treatment. No doubt this sounds like standard practice to many clinicians. However, explicit knowledge about the proximate psychological mediators of placebo analgesia could be helpful in engaging patients in a mindset that is more optimal for therapeutic benefit. For example, by asking patients about their thoughts and emotions in relation to the treatment, clinicians may be able to optimize patients' goals, expectations, and desire for pain relief and thereby enhance the total pain-relieving effect of the treatment. As patients attribute meaning to treatments and to the psychosocial environment in which they are administered (Benedetti 2002; Moerman 2002), clinicians have many opportunities to encourage a perception of the treatment that supports a decrease of pain as opposed to one that may potentially increase the pain.

So far, the few investigations of the use of placebo analgesia in clinical practice have primarily conceptualized placebo as an inert agent (e.g., Hrobjartsson and Norup 2003). It may be more interesting and informative to investigate how the patient's perception of a treatment and the psychosocial context in which it takes place contribute to the total efficacy of the treatment. Previously, the contribution of placebo factors has primarily been investigated by including a separate placebo condition. However, the approach of using open and hidden injections of an analgesic agent shows that it is possible to conceptualize and measure the contribution of the perception of the treatment to the total efficacy of the therapy. Also, if future studies confirm that the combination of expected pain level and desire for relief accounts for most of the variance in placebo analgesic effects, these two factors may constitute additional or alternative means of assessing the contribution of placebo analgesia. Hence, by interfacing standard pain treatments with measurements of expected pain levels and desire for relief it may be possible to assess the contribution of placebo analgesia to the total pain-relieving effect. This interface would be especially important in treatments such as surgery or acupuncture, where the contribution of placebo analgesic factors is difficult to ascertain.

Thus, the research reviewed in these last three chapters on placebo analgesia suggests new ways of empirically investigating the contribution of placebo factors. It also raises questions about the evaluation of efficacy within traditional clinical trials. Large and significant placebo effects are sometimes reported within clinical trials that include natural history, placebo treatment, and active treatment conditions. Thus, it can be debated whether the placebo treatment should be seen as a control condition for which the active treatment must show greater efficacy, or whether the placebo treatment and the active treatment should both be seen as effective interventions that can be tested via equivalence trials. In the latter case, the two treatments must be significantly more effective than natural history but not necessarily significantly different from each other. This approach has important implications because a more refined understanding of placebo analgesia may provide a better understanding of the efficacy of treatments, thereby providing a means of enhancing the pain-relieving effects of many existing therapies.

REFERENCES

Ader R. The role of conditioning in pharmacotherapy. In: Harrington A (Ed). *The Placebo Effect: An Interdisciplinary Exploration.* Cambridge: Harvard University Press, 1997, pp 138–165.

Amanzio M, Benedetti F. Neuropharmacological dissection of placebo analgesia: expectation activated opioid systems versus conditioning-activated specific subsystems. *J Neurosci* 1999; 19:484–494.

Amanzio M, Pollo A, Maggi G, Benedetti F. Response variability to analgesics: a role for non-specific activation of endogenous opioids. *Pain* 2001; 90:205–215.

Barrell JJ, Niemeyer RA. A mathematical formula for the psychological control of suffering. *J Pastoral Counsel* 1975; 10:60–67.

Beecher HK. The powerful placebo. *JAMA* 1955; 159:1602–1606.

Benedetti F. How the doctor's words affect the patient's brain. *Eval Health Prof* 2002; 25(4):369–386.

Benedetti F, Amanzio M, Maggi G. Potentiation of placebo analgesia by proglumide. *Lancet* 1995; 346:1231.

Benedetti F, Arduino C, Amanzio M. Somatotopic activation of opioid systems by target-directed expectations of analgesia. *J Neurosci* 1999; 9:3639–3648.

Benedetti F, Pollo A, Lopiano L, et al. Conscious expectation and unconscious conditioning in analgesic, motor, and hormonal placebo/nocebo responses. *J Neurosci* 2003; 23:4315–4323.

Bok S. Ethical issues in use of placebo in medical practice and clinical trials. In: Guess HA, Kleinman A, Kusek JW, Engel LW (Eds). *The Science of the Placebo: Toward an Interdisciplinary Research Agenda.* London: BMJ books, 2002, pp 63–73.

Damasio A. *Descartes' Error.* New York: Avon Books, 1994.

De Pascalis V, Chiaradia C, Carotenuto E. The contribution of suggestibility and expectation to placebo analgesia phenomenon in an experimental setting. *Pain* 2002; 96:393–402.

Dias R, Robbins TW, Roberts AC. Dissociable forms of inhibitory control within prefrontal cortex with an analogue of the Wisconsin card sorting test: restriction to novel situations and independence from "on-line" processing. *J Neurosci* 1997; 17:9285–9287.

Fields HL, Levine JD. Biology of placebo analgesia. *Am J Med* 1981; 70:745–746.

Garfield SL, Bergin AE (Eds). *Handbook of Psychotherapy and Behaviour Change: An Empirical Analysis,* 2nd ed. New York: Wiley & Sons, 1978, pp 369–409.

Goodwin JS, Goodwin JM, Vogel AV, et al. Knowledge and use of placebos by house officers and nurses. *Ann Intern Med* 1979; 19:106–110.

Gracely RH, Dubner R, Wolskee PJ, Deeter WR. Placebo and naloxone can alter post-surgical pain by separate mechanisms. *Nature* 1983; 306:264–265.

Gracely RH, Dubner R, Deeter WD, Wolskee PJ. Clinicians' expectations influence placebo analgesia. *Lancet* 1985; 5:43.

Grevert P, Albert LH, Goldstein A. Partial antagonism of placebo analgesia by naloxone. *Pain* 1983; 16:129–143.

Harrington A. Introduction. In: Harrington A (Ed). *The Placebo Effect: An Interdisciplinary Exploration.* Boston: Boston University Press, 1997.

Hrobjartsson A, Gotzsche PC. Is the placebo effect powerless? An analysis of clinical trials comparing placebo with no- treatment. *N Engl J Med* 2001; 344:1594–1602.

Hrobjartsson A, Norup M. The use of placebo interventions in medical practice—a national questionnaire survey of Danish clinicians. *Eval Health Prof* 2003; 26(2):153–165.

Kienle GS, Kiene H. Placebo effects and placebo concepts: a critical methodological and conceptual analysis of reports on the magnitude of the placebo effect. *Altern Ther Health Med* 1996; 2:39–54.

Kienle GS, Kiene H. The powerful placebo effect: fact or fiction? *J Clin Epidemiol* 1997; 50:1311–1318.

Laska E, Sunshine A. Anticipation of analgesia: a placebo effect. *Headache* 1973; 13(1):1–11.

Levine JD, Gordon NC. Influence of the method of drug administration on analgesic response. *Nature* 1984; 312:7556.

Levine JD, Gordon NC, Fields H. The mechanisms of placebo analgesia. *Lancet* 1978; 2:654–657.

Miller EK, Cohen JD. An integrative theory of prefrontal function. *Annu Rev Neurosci* 2001; 24:167–187.

Montgomery G, Kirsch I. Mechanisms of placebo pain reduction: an empirical investigation. *Psychol Sci* 1996; 7:174–176.

Montgomery G, Kirsch I. Classical conditioning and the placebo effect. *Pain* 1997; 72:107–113.

Moerman DE. The meaning response and the ethics of avoiding placebos. *Eval Health Prof* 2002; 25(4):399–409.

Petrovic P, Kalso E, Petersson KM, Ingvar M. Placebo and opioid analgesia-imaging a shared neuronal network. *Science* 2002; 295:1737–1740.

Pollo A, Amanzio M, Arslanian A, et al. Response expectancies in placebo analgesia and their clinical relevance. *Pain* 2001; 93:77–84.

Price DD. *Psychological Mechanisms of Pain and Analgesia,* Progress in Pain Research and Management, Vol. 15. Seattle: IASP Press, 1999.

Price DD, Barrell JJ. Some general laws of human emotion: interrelationships between intensities of desire, expectation and emotional feeling. *J Pers* 1984; 52(4):389–409.

Price DD, Barrell JJ. Mechanisms of analgesia produced by hypnosis and placebo suggestions. *Prog Brain Res* 2000; 122:255–271.

Price DD, Barrell JE, Barrell JJ. A quantitative-experiential analysis of human emotions. *Motivation Emotions* 1985; 9:19–38.

Price DD, Milling LS, Kirsch I, et al. An analysis of factors that contribute to the magnitude of placebo analgesia in an experimental paradigm. *Pain* 1999; 83:147–156.

Price DD, Riley J, Barrell JJ. Are lived choices based on emotional processes? *Cogn Emotion* 2001; 15(3):365–379.

Price DD, Riley JL, Vase L. Reliable difference in placebo effects between clinical analgesic trials and studies of placebo analgesia mechanisms. *Pain* 2003; 104:715–716.

Shapiro AK, Morris LA. The placebo effect in healing. In: Garfield SL, Bergin AE (Eds). *Handbook of Psychotherapy and Behavioral Change*. New York: Aldine, 1978.

Turner JA, Deyo RA, Loeser JD, Von Korff M, Fordyce WE. The importance of placebo effects in pain treatment and research. *JAMA* 1994; 271:1609–1614.

Vase L, Riley JL III, Price DD. A comparison of placebo effects in clinical analgesic trials versus studies of placebo analgesia. *Pain* 2002; 99:443–452.

Vase L, Robinson ME, Verne GN, Price DD. The contribution of suggestion, expectancy and desire to placebo effect in irritable bowel syndrome patients. *Pain* 2003; 105:17–25.

Verne GN, Robinson ME, Vase L, Price DD. Reversal of visceral and cutaneous hyperalgesia by local rectal anesthesia in irritable bowel syndrome (IBS) patients. *Pain* 2003; 105:223–230.

Voudouris NJ, Peck CL, Coleman G. Conditioned placebo responses. *J Pers Soc Psychol* 1985; 48:47–53.

Voudouris NJ, Peck CL, Coleman G. Conditioned response models of placebo phenomena: further support. *Pain* 1989; 38:109–116.

Voudouris NJ, Peck CL, Coleman G. The role of conditioning and verbal expectancy in the placebo response. *Pain* 1990; 43:121–128.

Wager TD, Rilling JK, Smith EE, et al. Placebo-induced changes in fMRI in the anticipation and experience of pain. *Science* 2004; 303:1162–1167.

Wickramasekera I. A conditioned response model of the placebo effect: predictions of the model. In: White L, Tursky B, Schwartz GE (Ed). *Placebo: Theory, Research and Mechanisms*. New York: Guilford Press, 1985.

Zubieta J, Smith YR, Bueller JA, et al. Regional mu opioid receptor regulation of sensory and affective dimensions of pain. *Science* 2001; 293:311–315.

Correspondence to: Donald D. Price, PhD, Department of Oral and Maxillofacial Surgery, University of Florida, P.O. Box 100416, Gainesville, FL 32610-0416, USA. Email: dprice@dental.ufl.edu.

Part IV

Modulation of Pain by Hypnosis

Psychological Methods of Pain Control: Basic Science and Clinical Perspectives, Progress in Pain Research and Management, Vol. 29, edited by Donald D. Price and M. Catherine Bushnell, IASP Press, Seattle, © 2004.

11

The Neurophenomenology of Hypnosis and Hypnotic Analgesia

Pierre Rainville[a] and Donald D. Price[b]

[a]Department of Stomatology, Faculty of Dental Medicine, University of Montreal, Montreal, Quebec, Canada; [b]Departments of Oral Surgery and Neuroscience, University of Florida, Gainesville, Florida, USA

The validation of therapeutic and palliative approaches in medicine requires not only the confirmation of their clinical efficacy but also the demonstration of underlying mechanisms that contribute to their integration into the dominant knowledge system within which medical practice is articulated. Reciprocally, when complementary or alternative medical practices are shown to be effective (e.g., for pain relief) and their mechanisms are compatible with mainstream explanatory systems (e.g., physiology), they may contribute to a shift in the body of established medical theory by emphasizing previously neglected factors. In this context, psychological interventions to reduce pain and suffering must be harmonized with the growing knowledge on the physiology, molecular biology, and genetics of nociception. The advent of modern brain-imaging techniques has recently promoted a shift toward the investigation of higher-order brain systems underlying complex psychological mechanisms shown to critically affect pain and suffering. In this chapter, we outline an explanation of hypnotic states that is based on the combination of experiential and functional brain-imaging data. We describe the effects of hypnotic suggestions on the experience of pain and on central and peripheral physiological activity in relation to current knowledge on the psychology of pain and the physiology of the nociceptive system.

HYPNOSIS AND THE BIRTH OF PSYCHOLOGICAL SCIENCE

Scientific research on hypnosis started as early as the end of the 18th century, soon after Franz Anton Mesmer proposed animal magnetism as a universal fluid energy that mediated hypnotic phenomena. Using magnetized metal rods and various procedures to reestablish the "magnetic balance" of his patients, Mesmer developed "rituals" to achieve the desired magnetization. This was the Age of Enlightenment, an epoch that witnessed the birth of modern science. It was not accidental that Mesmer proposed that an invisible force could act on people and affect their physical and mental health. One hundred years earlier, Newton had proposed as the Universal Law of Gravitation an invisible force that irresistibly attracts objects toward each other as a function of their mass and distance. The basic principles of animal magnetism were therefore consistent with the developing physical sciences. Yet Mesmer's theory did not make it into textbooks of medicine. What had gone wrong?

Soon after the publication of Mesmer's theory on animal magnetism, Mesmerism became quite popular, and Louis XVI of France ordered that the practice of Mesmer and his apprentices be examined and that the validity of the underlying principles be evaluated by a royal commission chaired by Benjamin Franklin (Salas and Salas 1996; Laurence 2002). This commission may have been the first scientific task force, its methodological effort an insightful prelude to the emergence of psychological sciences and clinical trials. Mesmer's practice was submitted to a series of experimental tests, comparing the alleged active treatment (contact with magnetized material) to control procedures that lacked the essential ingredient of "magnetization." Subjects submitted to the control treatment did not know that the magnetization could not take place, and therefore these experiments may constitute the first reported assessment of the efficacy of a treatment using a single-blind, placebo-controlled design.

Did Mesmerism pass the scientific test? It did not. Magnetized objects did not account for changes in the patients' conditions, and the report of the Franklin Commission refuted the theory of animal magnetism. However, some patients did show remarkable responses such as fainting, even in what we would now call the control condition. If the contact with magnetized material could not account for the effects observed in some patients, what could? The commissioners concluded their report with the proposition that the subjects' *imagination* was the mechanism by which the changes were produced. Recognizing that imagination might have accounted for the effects observed was a remarkable insight. It is also remarkable that the commission emphasized patients' characteristics of mental activity, rather than an external force or a special ability of the "hypnotizer-magnetizer," as the mediating mechanism. Such an explanation is highly consistent with contemporary theories of hypnosis. Unfortunately, this alternative interpretation provided by the commissioners did not immediately motivate further inquiries into the processes of human imagination and its potential influence on health.

This official debut of a formal description of hypnotic phenomena together with the abrupt end of the theory of animal magnetism reminds us to distinguish an observed phenomenon (the effect) from the theory that attempts to explain its structure, underlying mechanisms, or function. Nothing in the commission's report dismissed the observations of genuine responses of the individual submitted to the procedure. The object of scientific controversy was the formal cause and underlying mechanism. A few hundred years later, theories of hypnosis have evolved within experiential, psychological, social, and physiological frameworks, and important distinctions between the effects of hypnosis and placebo treatments are becoming increasingly well recognized (see Chapter 12). Importantly, those different perspectives on hypnotic phenomena are increasingly considered complementary and have been only tentatively integrated into neuropsychological models. In this chapter, we examine the phenomena of hypnosis from the perspective of the subject undergoing the procedure, using a neurophenomenological approach in order to establish the correspondence between changes in subjective experience and changes in physiological activity. We describe the available evidence in support of the notions that (1) current standardized hypnotic induction methods produce some alteration in the subject's state of consciousness and in corresponding aspects of brain activity, (2) hypnotic suggestions may take various forms and can be tailored to modify specific aspects of subjective experience, (3) hypnotic modulation of specific experiences (e.g., pain) produces changes in brain processes normally underlying those experiences, and (4) hypnosis provides access to modulatory processes that normally escape voluntary control.

HYPNOSIS AS AN ALTERED STATE OF CONSCIOUSNESS

Clinicians interested in the practical applications of hypnosis for the reduction of pain may pay little heed to the debate regarding the status of hypnosis as an altered state of consciousness. However, this notion has the advantage of positioning the problem of hypnosis-related phenomena within the broader context of both philosophical and neurobiological studies of consciousness. The philosopher David Chalmers (2000) has proposed a fundamental distinction between background states of consciousness and content-specific states of consciousness that influence one another but depend upon at least partly segregated neural systems, consistent with the modern neurosciences. A background state of consciousness is the global state of an organism (e.g., attentive, awake, drowsy, asleep, and dreaming) that constrains and regulates the content of consciousness, but it is *not* defined in terms of specific content or perceptual modality. Hypnotic states match this description, because fundamental aspects of subjective experience are modified following the induction of hypnosis, and they can be described in relation to other states of altered consciousness. Consistently, changes in brain activity observed as a result of hypnotic induction involve many networks associated with the regulation of states of consciousness.

AN EXPERIENTIAL PERSPECTIVE ON HYPNOSIS

Price and Barrell (1990) have identified the dimensions of subjective experience that characterize hypnotic states produced by a standard induction procedure (see Fig. 1). The experience of being hypnotized begins with a relaxed condition of mental (and often physical) ease in combination with an absorbed and sustained focus on an object or objects of attention. Thus, initial suggestions for induction of those changes are almost always directed toward these two dimensions (mental ease and absorption). However, a hypnotic state can occur naturally during fascination, watching an absorbing

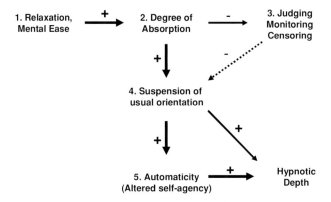

Fig. 1. Experiential model of hypnosis. Hypnotic states are commonly felt and described using the multiple dimensions of subjective experience identified in the model. Positive (+) and negative (–) functional interactions are proposed in which changes in distinct experiential dimensions precede and facilitate changes in other dimensions. Bold arrows represent relations that were confirmed statistically in groups of naive subjects (Price 1996).

movie, or looking at ripples in a stream. It captures us. At first it can be effortful, but with time one proceeds from an *active* form of concentration to a relaxed, *passive* form. Passive attention to one or a few targets contributes to a reduction of orientation as the immediate spatial and temporal environment gradually becomes irrelevant to the experience. At the same time, this relaxation and reduction in range of active attention support a *lack* of monitoring and censoring of that which is allowed into experience. Hence, alternative experiences are facilitated, and inconsistencies are now more tolerable. Contradictory statements, which once arrested attention and caused confusion or disturbance, now no longer do so. The uncensored acceptance of what is being said by the hypnotist is not checked against one's own associations. Consequently, one no longer chooses or validates the correctness of incoming statements. This state allows thinking and meaning-in-itself that is disconnected from active critical reflection. From this way of experiencing, there emerges the sense of *automaticity,* wherein thinking is no longer felt as preceding action but action is felt as preceding thought (an altered feeling of self-agency). Thus, if the hypnotist suggests a bodily action, a sensation, or a lack of sensation (e.g., pain), there is no experience of deliberation or effort on the part of the subject. The subject simply and automatically identifies with the suggested action, sensation, or lack of sensation, as it is suggested. Changes in perception, mental activity, and behavior are simply felt as happening. In this way, the changes experienced during hypnosis *facilitate* the incorporation of suggestions such as analgesia.

Based on these observations, hypnosis can be defined as changes in subjective experience induced by suggestions and characterized by mental ease, absorption, reduction in self-orientation, and automaticity. Notably, those dimensions of experience characterize the experience of one's own mental processes (e.g., mental ease and absorption), a general sense of self-orientation in space and time, and felt intention or lack thereof (a feeling of automaticity, altered sense of self-agency). These experiential data indicate that hypnotic induction modifies several dimensions of the background state of consciousness, thereby altering the usual experience of self or "what it usually feels like to be conscious" (see Rainville and Price 2003). This description is consistent with the proposition that hypnosis is an altered state of consciousness.

THE SIGNATURE OF HYPNOSIS IN THE BRAIN

If hypnosis modifies the background state of consciousness, we would expect changes in brain activity within specific brain networks critically involved in the regulation of consciousness. Those neural systems have been at least partly identified by a century of observation in neurology and research in neurophysiology (reviewed in Damasio 1999), and more recently by functional brain imaging in normal humans (e.g., Kinomura et al. 1996; Fiset et al. 1999). To take just a few examples, a lesion in the dorsal part of the brainstem produces coma, many brainstem nuclei are critical for the regulation of the sleep-wake cycle and dreaming (Steriade and McCarley 1990; Steriade et al. 1993), and specific nuclei of the brainstem (i.e., the locus ceruleus) are critically involved in the regulation of attention (Aston-Jones et al. 1999). Brainstem nuclei further affect thalamocortical oscillations at certain frequencies, a mechanism proposed to be essential for conscious perceptual awareness (e.g., Llinas et al. 1998; Herculano-Houzel et al. 1999). Finally, the posterior parietal and cingulate cortices are critically involved in the spatiotemporal regulation of orientation and attention processes directed toward different sensory modalities or conceptual knowledge (Posner and Dehaene 1994). Many of these subcortical and cortical structures are also directly or indirectly involved in the representation of the body and in the regulation of homeostasis as fundamental aspects of self-representation, self-regulation, and consciousness (Damasio 1999; Parvizi and Damasio 2001). How does hypnosis affect activity within those networks?

A series of functional brain-imaging studies has recently helped clarify the specific brain systems involved in the production of hypnotic states. Rainville et al. (1999b) measured regional cerebral blood flow (rCBF) using positron emission tomography (PET) to examine changes in brain activity between normal waking and hypnotic states. In descriptions of these and other neuroimaging studies discussed in this chapter, rCBF refers to an indirect, yet well-validated, measure of neural activity because increases and decreases in rCBF are respectively correlated with increases and decreases in regional metabolism. The latter, in turn, are associated with directly measured changes in neuron action potentials (Malonek and Grinvald 1996; Vanzetta and Grinvald 1999; Lindauer and Dirnagl 2000). Hypnotic states are associated with higher levels of rCBF in anterior cingulate regions and in occipital cortical areas (see also Maquet et al. 1999; Faymonville et al. 2000). In a subsequent study, Rainville et al. (2002) asked subjects to rate their subjective level of mental relaxation and absorption in the normal control state and in the hypnotic state. As predicted by the experiential model of hypnosis, increases were reported in both mental relaxation and absorption following hypnotic induction, and those increases in self-ratings were significantly correlated with hypnotic susceptibility scores. Changes in mental relaxation and absorption were also associated with changes in partly distinct brain networks involved in the regulation of consciousness, as illustrated in Fig. 2.

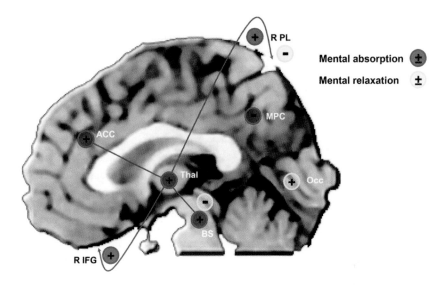

Fig. 2. Effects of hypnotic relaxation (yellow) and absorption (red) on brain activity. Increases in hypnotic relaxation are associated with rCBF increases in the occipital cortex (Occ) and with decreases in the mesencephalic tegmentum of the brainstem (BS) and the right parietal lobule (R PL). In contrast, increases in self-reports of mental absorption during hypnosis are associated with increases (+) in regional cerebral blood flow (rCBF) within a coordinated network of brain structures (connected by red lines) involved in attention and including the pontomesencephalic brainstem (BS), the medial thalamus (Thal), and the anterior cingulate cortex (ACC), as well as the inferior frontal (R IFG) and the parietal lobule (R PL) of the right hemisphere. Additional decreases in rCBF in the medial parietal cortex (MPC) are associated with absorption (Rainville et al. 2002; Rainville and Price 2003).

HYPNOTIC RELAXATION AND ABSORPTION MODIFY CORTICAL DYNAMICS

During normal wakefulness, the cerebral cortex is under both excitatory and inhibitory influences that are mediated in part by cholinergic and noradrenergic brainstem projections. The influence of some inhibitory mechanisms is thought to increase gradually in active attention, vigilance, and arousal and is thought be at its minimum during slow-wave sleep (Kawashima et al. 1995; Hofle et al. 1997; Paus et al. 1997; Paus 2000). For example, actively directing attention toward the auditory modality produces a decrease in rCBF within the visual cortices, a phenomenon called cross-modality suppression that reduces the availability of visual information during auditory processing (Paus et al. 1997). However, this inhibition gradually *decreases* as subjects shift from a high to a low level of vigilance, or from active to passive forms of attention, resulting in a gradual increase in rCBF in the visual cortices. During the shift from an active to a more passive form of attention during the induction of hypnosis, we would expect to observe some decrease in this cross-modality inhibitory mechanism.

The induction of hypnotic states produces changes in brain activity that are consistent with a decrease in cross-modal inhibition. We have observed significant increases in mental relaxation that were specifically associated with a decrease in rCBF in the brainstem tegmentum during hypnosis, consistent with a decrease in vigilance and arousal during hypnotic states (Rainville et al. 2002). In support of this interpretation, hypnosis was also accompanied by a reduction in cortical arousal (increase in slow EEG activity) that was associated with an *increase* in occipital rCBF. This net increase in occipital rCBF may reflect a reduction in inhibitory processes normally affecting cortical activity at moderate to high levels of arousal and vigilance during normal wakefulness. A similar increase in occipital rCBF was found during meditative states (Lou et al. 1999). A general decrease in inhibitory activity could therefore contribute to the general increase in occipital rCBF observed in hypnosis (Maquet et al. 1999; Rainville et al. 1999b).

This gradual release from inhibition may be expressed in a cognitive model by a reduction in "cross-representation suppression," a mechanism that normally exerts inhibitory control over competing alternative representations that are unattended or are inconsistent with the target. Thus, the neural changes associated with mental relaxation during hypnosis are consistent with a reduction in the inhibition of competing mental and neural representations. These changes are likely to relate to the reduction in monitoring or censoring, as previously described in the phenomenological account of hypnotic states. Consistent with that account, the uncensored acceptance of suggested experiential content may thereby facilitate the incorporation of suggested alternative sensations and feelings, such as those related to hypnotic analgesia.

In contrast to the effect of mental relaxation, increases in mental absorption were specifically associated with increases in rCBF in the pontomesencephalic brainstem, medial thalamus, rostral anterior cingulate cortex, and right frontal and parietal cortices (Fig. 2). This pattern of activity precisely maps onto the distributed brain network underlying attention processes (Posner and Dehaene 1994). The involvement of the brain attention processes in hypnosis has been proposed earlier in EEG studies. Activity in the theta range (4–8 Hz) has been associated with both attention and hypnosis (reviewed in Ray 1997; Sabourin et al. 1991; Crawford and Gruzelier 1992; Graffin et al. 1995). Attention processes involve the selective enhancement of a target representation and the selection of relevant processes (e.g., Posner and Dehaene 1994; Botvinick et al. 1999; Carter et al. 2000; Paus 2000). In the model proposed in Fig. 3, the induction of hypnosis produces an increase

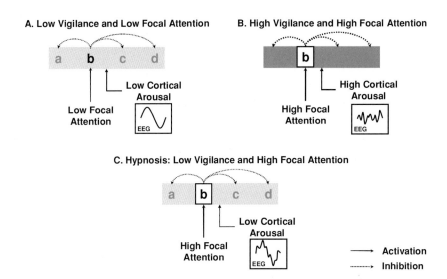

Fig. 3. Involvement of vigilance and attention processes in hypnosis. (A) In normal states of low vigilance and low attention (e.g., relaxed, sleepy, or drowsy), there is characteristic global slow-wave EEG activity, (Low Cortical Arousal; inset), weak activation of the target representation (Low Focal Attention to b), and a weak inhibition of alternative representations (dotted lines from b to a, c, and d). This state is accompanied by a sense of mental ease with only weak attentional focus, often leading to spontaneous and uncontrolled shifts between seemingly unrelated representations (as in daydreaming). (B) In contrast, when attention is focused in normal, highly vigilant states, the EEG is globally desynchronized (High Cortical Arousal; inset), and there is both a strong activation of the target representation and a strong inhibition of alternative competing representations ("cross-representational suppression"). This state may have a highly controlled attentional focus. (C) During hypnosis, there is some EEG activity in the slow-wave range (relatively Low Cortical Arousal; inset) combined with a *strong* activation of the target representations and a *weak* inhibition of alternative competing representations. This state is accompanied by a sense of mental ease with a feeling of high mental absorption that may lead to smooth, fluid shifts between representations that would normally compete (e.g., in panel B).

in focal attention enhancing the activation of the target experience (b) and creates an increased feeling of absorption. At the same time, there is a *reduction* in the suppression of competing experiences (a, c, and d) that is associated with an increase in hypnotic relaxation and a reduction in vigilance and arousal. This effect results in a net increase in the sense of mental flexibility and in the availability of alternative experiences (a, c, and d) introduced by the incoming hypnotic suggestions.

These effects of hypnotic relaxation and absorption are consistent with the proposition that brain mechanisms underlying the regulation of consciousness are involved in producing hypnotic states. Attention mechanisms contribute to those changes, but the complex pattern of brain activation implies that other mechanisms are also at play. More specifically, hypnotic relaxation and mental ease may facilitate the incorporation of suggestions by reducing the competition between alternative experiences. However, the experiential model described above and recent studies of hypnotic analgesia also indicate that, although attention processes undoubtedly contribute to hypnosis, they are insufficient to fully account for hypnosis and hypnotic analgesia, as we will see below.

HYPNOSIS AND THE ALTERATION OF SELF-AGENCY

The experiential model shown in Fig. 1 predicts that the increases in hypnotic relaxation, mental ease, and mental absorption contribute to a suspension of usual self-orientation that further contributes to the sense of automaticity that characterizes an altered sense of self-agency. Changes in brain activity observed by Rainville et al. (2002) in relation to hypnotic relaxation and absorption implicate parietal areas (see Fig. 2) involved in orientation responses to novel stimuli in the environment and attention to spatial or temporal aspects of stimuli (Coull and Nobre 1998; Nobre 2001). Those changes in parietal activity may further contribute to the changes in self-agency experienced in hypnosis.

Although the hypnotized subjects are the critical players in the actualization of hypnotic suggestions, they typically experience automaticity, in which an active movement (e.g., moving the arm) may be felt as if it were happening by itself or under the influence of an imagined external cause (e.g., a heavy weight pulling down the hand). Similarly, changes in sensory experiences (e.g., hypnotic analgesia or hallucination) may be felt as simply happening automatically or as if they were real properties of external objects rather than as being caused by self-generated, imaginative, cognitive processes.

Functional brain imaging studies have begun to explore the neural correlates of agency and are suggesting that the anterior insula and the posterior parietal cortex may be critical for the attribution of agency to the self or to an external source (Ruby and Decety 2001; Chaminade and Decety 2002; Farrer and Frith 2002; Farrer et al. 2003). A recent study has examined specifically the altered sense of agency in response to hypnotic suggestions for passive movement of the arm (Blakemore et al. 2003). In this study, the experimenter gave hypnotic suggestions to six highly hypnotizable subjects, suggesting that their left hand and forearm would be moved rhythmically by a pulley (a "deluded" passive movement), while their brain was being scanned using PET. This condition was contrasted to a voluntary active movement and a "real" passive movement (in which the arm was really moved by a pulley). Results suggested stronger activity in the parietal operculum and in the cerebellum associated with the deluded passive movement and the real passive movement compared to the voluntary active movement. Based on a theoretical model of intentional action illustrated in Fig. 4A, Blakemore and Frith (2003) concluded that self-generated actions normally involve efferent signals from the frontal cortices both to the output motor system and to the sensory systems of the parietal cortex. The latter corollary signal allows the parietal sensory and association systems to anticipate the sensory changes produced by the motor command generated intentionally. A feeling of self-agency is produced when the sensory feedback matches the corollary discharge. When a match occurs, the parietal activation normally resulting from the sensory feedback is dramatically reduced. In contrast, there is robust parietal activity and no feeling of self-agency when the sensory feedback is perceived without the matching corollary discharge (no anticipatory signal) coming from the frontal control system. This is also the case in the real passive movement condition when the arm is moved by an external agent. This model offers several possible interpretations of the altered sense of self-agency experienced in the deluded passive movement condition. There may be a failure to generate the corollary anticipatory signal, a failure of communication between the frontal and parietal systems, a modification of the processing of the corollary signal in the parietal cortices, or a failure to adequately compare the sensory feedback with the corollary signal. Regardless of the exact neural mechanisms, the absence of a matching corollary discharge may be accompanied by a loss of sense of self-agency and hence a gain of the sense of automaticity.

Woody and Szechtman (2000) proposed a slightly different interpretation of hypnotic hallucination in which the representation of the self is actively modified in response to hypnotic suggestions, *as if* the self were being modified by an external agent. In a study on auditory hallucination, these authors observed that the felt clarity and externality of the hallucinated auditory percept under hypnosis is correlated with the activity of the medial prefrontal cortex (Szechtman et al. 1998). According to their interpretation, hypnotic hallucinations not only produce changes in specific sensory cortices consistent with the specific content of the suggestions (here the auditory cortices) but also alter self-representation and brain activity (here in the medial prefrontal cortex) as if the experience had been triggered by an external agent.

The interpretation of Blakemore and Frith (2003) and that of Woody and Szechtman (2000) both involve modification of the representation of self. However, the former implies an indirect modification of the self because of a failure to update self-representation with respect to the top-down mechanisms involved in the production of a movement or, by extension, the

A. Self-agency during movement   **B. Self-agency in mental imagery**

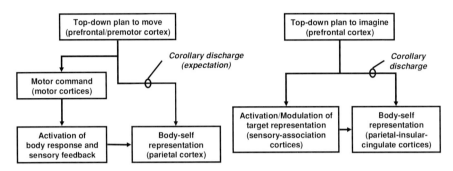

Comparison process:
Match = sense of self-agency
Mismatch = no sense of self-agency

Fig. 4. The feeling of automaticity experienced in hypnosis is the consequence of an alteration of self-agency; i.e., the self is no longer felt as the causal agent of behavioral or mental actions. *Self-generated* behaviors (e.g., a movement in A) or mental actions (e.g., mental imagery in B) are normally characterized by the experience that they are intentionally produced. This sense of self-agency has been suggested to reflect the existence of two separate processing pathways in the generation of voluntary movements (A). The two pathways originate in the executive control system (involving the prefrontal cortices) and provide both an efferent signal (a plan to move) to the motor system and a corollary discharge to the parietal cortex. The motor system then produces the intended movement. The sensory feedback associated with the movement reaches brain areas involved in the representation of the position of the body in relation to external space (i.e., the parietal cortex). The corollary discharge sent from the executive system to the parietal cortex is conceptualized as an anticipatory signal that "prepares" the parietal cortex to receive afferent feedback from the body, according to the motor plan (expectation). When the feedback message matches the corollary discharge, there is a sense of self-agency and little resulting activation of the parietal cortex. In contrast, when the feedback message does not match the corollary discharge, there is a reduced sense of self-agency and a robust activation of the parietal cortex. Consistent with these observations, hypnotic delusion of movement may be explained by a failure in this process that leads to a mismatch between the sensory feedback and the corollary discharge. We propose here to generalize the proposed model to imaginative processes (B). Voluntary mental imagery in an alert individual generally involves some sense of self-agency over the mental content activated. Brain areas critically involved in the representation of the body and self (e.g., parietal, insular, and cingulate cortices) may also receive a corollary discharge in the expectation of bodily changes that would normally accompany the mental image evoked. When this happens, we feel that the changes are self-generated, and the somatic consequences of the images on the body may be attenuated. In hypnosis, mental images may be evoked without a sense of self-agency because of a failure of the corollary discharge to produce the expected changes in self-representation. The mental image thereby gains a quality of external reality (e.g., hypnotic hallucination). During hypnotic analgesia, the processing of nociceptive signals is altered by top-down processes according to the experience imagined, but the failure to update the representation of self as the generator of those changes may facilitate the reduction of pain automatically.

activation of a mental image (see Fig. 4). In this case, the movement or mental image is produced without the self-awareness of being the agent of the effect. In contrast, Woody and Szechtman (2000) propose that the representation of the self is directly modified as a result of the suggestions, so that the movement or mental image evoked by the hypnotic suggestions is accompanied by a sense of externality. Future studies are necessary to evaluate those alternative interpretations of the neural mechanisms for the altered sense of agency. However, the data and the theoretical models available clearly point to the involvement of prefrontal or posterior parietal systems and their interactions in producing and modulating feelings of self-agency.

NEUROPHENOMENOLOGY OF HYPNOSIS

The above discussion on the neural correlates of hypnosis is based on the combination of experiential and functional brain-imaging data. The information available is consistent with the interpretation of hypnosis as an altered state of consciousness in which basic dimensions of conscious experience are modified with changes in neural systems underlying self-representation and self-regulation. These changes further imply that hypnotic states facilitate the incorporation of suggestions by modifying the interplay between brain mechanisms involved in the regulation of vigilance, arousal, and attention, thereby facilitating the access to alternative experiences. The available data on the brain correlates of the sense of automaticity experienced during hypnosis are highly consistent with current theoretical models of the neural basis of intentional acts and the experience of self-agency. Although these interpretations have been proposed in studies performed in various contexts (delusion of passive movement and auditory hallucination), it is likely that their conclusions can be generalized to most hypnotic contexts, including those of hypnotic analgesia, because they examine critical dimensions of hypnotic phenomenology. We will now examine the implications of these interpretations for the understanding of hypnotic analgesia and describe the physiological correlates of pain relief by hypnosis.

HYPNOTIC ANALGESIA

In this section, we will first discuss the different forms of hypnotic suggestions for analgesia and the factors that contribute to analgesic efficacy. We will specifically examine the conditions that facilitate the incorporation of specific suggestions to alter the experience of pain and their relationship with the neurophenomenology of hypnotic states.

HYPNOTIC SUGGESTIONS FOR ANALGESIA

Hypnotic analgesia can be produced using a variety of suggestions that can be categorized along different axes based on the style of the suggestion, the processes involved, and their specific target. The style of the suggestions can be permissive, allowing for alternative and even opposite experiences (e.g., "you may feel only warmth or coolness"), or restrictive, specifying the experience to be felt. Suggestion style may also be direct (e.g., "The sensation you once experienced as painful will be experienced as only warmth or coolness") or indirect (e.g., "I wonder if you will notice whether the sensation you once experienced as painful will be experienced as just warmth or coolness"). Limited evidence indicates that more people may benefit from indirect or permissive suggestions (Price and Barber 1987; Price and Barrell 1990). These different styles are described in more detail in Chapter 12. To our knowledge, no study has specifically compared the physiological effects associated with those various styles of suggestions for analgesia.

The hypnotic suggestions for altering pain may also be described in terms of the psychological processes involved. One type provides dissociative imagery by suggesting experiences that are disconnected from the felt sense of the body. An example would be a suggestion to imagine oneself "floating out of the body and up in the air," combined with the implicit or explicit suggestion that the pain belongs to the body and not to the one who experiences being somewhere else. Common to suggestions for dissociation is the intention for subjects not to feel parts of their bodies that would otherwise be painful or to experience themselves in another location and context altogether. Another type is focused analgesia that is intended to replace sensations of pain with others such as numbness or warmth or with the complete absence of sensation. In complete contrast to dissociative analgesia, focused analgesia requires increased attention to the body area that is in pain combined with a replaced sensation in that area. Examples might include suggestions to focus on sensations in the hand and to experience all sensations of the hand as if it were in a large glove. Focused analgesia generally implies a specific body part, while dissociative imagery may involve the whole body or a specific part of the body. A third type of suggestion involves the reinterpretation of the meaning of the sensory experience. In this case, the significance of the experience for the integrity of the body is reduced or completely abolished so that pain sensations are no longer associated with feelings of threat. De Pascalis et al. (1999; also see De Pascalis et al. 2001) compared analgesic effects produced by experimental conditions of deep relaxation, dissociated imagery, focused analgesia, and placebo in contrast to a waking control condition (Fig. 5). Of the four experimental conditions, deep relaxation, dissociated imagery, and focused analgesia produced statistically significant reductions on all pain-related measures. These results have several implications. Hypnotic analgesia cannot be simply reduced to the effect of relaxation or to a nonspecific reduction of distress. Hypnosis may be more effective than at least some types of placebo manipulations. Finally, hypnotic analgesia does not require that attention be redirected away from the pain. In fact, analgesia was found to be stronger when the subjects specifically attended to the stimulated area in the condition of focused analgesia.

Hypnotic suggestions for analgesia may further vary according to the specific dimensions of pain targeted or affected by the suggestions. The experience of pain includes sensory-discriminative and affective-motivational

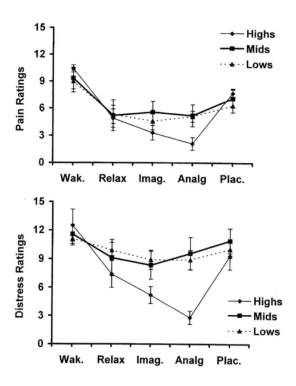

Fig. 5. Pain sensory and distress ratings in response to noxious electrical stimulation delivered to the wrist in normal subjects with high (Highs), moderate (Mids), or low (Lows) hypnotic susceptibility. Both pain sensory and distress ratings decreased significantly in response to hypnotic suggestions for relaxation (Relax), dissociative imagery (Imag.), and focused analgesia (Analg), compared to the baseline wakefulness (Wak.) and placebo (Plac.) conditions. Greater pain reductions were observed in more susceptible subjects (Highs) and during focused analgesia. No significant placebo analgesia was observed in any of the three groups (De Pascalis et al. 2001).

dimensions, each comprising several subdimensions that can be modified more or less directly and effectively by hypnotic suggestions for analgesia. In the experiment by De Pascalis et al. (2001) illustrated in Fig. 5, hypnotic analgesia was reflected in ratings of both pain and distress, suggesting parallel modulation of the sensory and affective dimensions of pain. This finding implies that hypnotic analgesia may not simply blunt the emotional responses integral to pain while preserving all sensory aspects of the experience. Price (1999) has proposed an additional distinction between primary and secondary affective stages of pain processing (see also Chapter 2). The primary stage corresponds to the immediate unpleasantness/aversiveness of the pain and is intimately dependent upon the basic sense of threat integral to all pain experiences. The secondary stage of pain affect encompasses the emotions associated with the pain condition that characterize the more general sense of suffering (e.g., despair) associated with the broader meaning of the pain (e.g., disability). According to this model, hypnotic suggestions may, at least in principle, affect different dimensions of the experience of pain or their determinants, including pain sensation (e.g., pain intensity), the basic sense of threat and the primary pain affect (e.g., pain unpleasantness), or the more general meaning of the pain and the associated cognitive responses (e.g., expectation of relief) and emotional feelings (e.g., anger, sadness). Some suggestions are designed to specifically alter the quality or intensity of painful sensations so that they become less intense or absent altogether. Pain affect could be modulated by suggestions for reinterpreting sensations as neutral or pleasant rather than unpleasant or by suggestions for reducing or eliminating the sense of threat or harm associated with the sensations. Furthermore, hypnotic suggestions may be developed to attenuate negative emotions associated with pain. The therapist may directly suggest positive emotional feelings or propose alternative interpretations of the meaning of pain (see Chapter 12). Hypnotic suggestions may therefore be tailored according to the specific aspects of the pain that one wants to relieve.

The effects of hypnotic analgesia on pain sensation and pain affect were examined more specifically in a series of experimental studies conducted to separate the different stages of pain processing. The paradigm took advantage of the flexibility of hypnotic suggestions to examine the functional relation between different aspects of pain experience (Rainville et al. 1999a). In all experimental conditions, normal volunteers rated the intensity and the unpleasantness of the pain produced by the immersion of the hand in hot water for one minute. In one experiment, hypnotic suggestions were designed to target pain sensation using suggestions such as: "You may be surprised to notice how much less intense the sensation is than you might have expected it to be, how it tends to feel only warm. ... As time passes, you can turn down the dial of your sensation, much like turning down the volume dial on a stereo." In another experiment, suggestions targeted pain affect using wording such as: "During the stimulation, a sensation of well-being will just sweep through all your hand and arm ... your experience will seem surprisingly more agreeable ... surprisingly more comfortable ... surprisingly more restful than you might have expected. When you feel the onset of the stimulus, you can feel an onset of well-being quickly spreading into your hand ... your arm ... into your whole body ... and all through your experience." In addition, all experiments included additional conditions in which hypnotic suggestions were given to *increase* pain (sensation or affect). Importantly, suggestions for analgesia included explicit references to the area stimulated (the hand), and no suggestions were given for dissociation. These instructions could therefore be described as suggestions for focused analgesia with some reinterpretation of the sensory or affective aspect of the experience. Modulatory effects were confirmed in the target pain dimension, and additional modulation of pain unpleasantness was observed in the condition of pain sensation modulation (Fig. 6). These results clearly demonstrate that it is the specific content of the hypnotic suggestions that determines which dimension of pain is modulated. In addition, the results supported Price's theoretical model in which pain affect is at least partly determined by pain sensation intensity (Price 1999).

Another aspect of pain-related experiences that can be targeted more or less specifically by hypnotic suggestions is the secondary affect, or the emotions associated with pain and their determinants (e.g., the context and meaning of pain). Strong or persistent negative emotions related to pain (e.g., anxiety, anger, depression) may be experienced when the pain is anticipated, is uncontrolled, or is associated with disability. Controlled clinical studies evaluating the efficacy of hypnotic procedures to control pain typically include measures of anxiety (see the review by Patterson and Jensen 2003). For example, significant reductions of pain-related and treatment-related anxiety have resulted from hypnotic procedures in the treatment of burn pain (Frenay et al. 2001), during lumbar puncture and bone narrow aspiration in pediatric oncology patients (Zeltzer and LeBaron 1982; Liossi and Hatira 1999, 2003), and both before (Enqvist and Fischer 1997) and during surgical procedures (Faymonville et al. 1997; Lang et al. 2000; Ghoneim et al. 2000). However, in clinical trials, anxiety measures are simply another outcome measure, and the goal is not to assess the mechanisms by which hypnosis affects pain and pain-related emotions. In that context, the effects of hypnosis on more complex or extended pain-related emotions, such as pain-related depression, frustration, and anger, may be a secondary

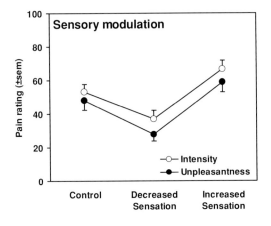

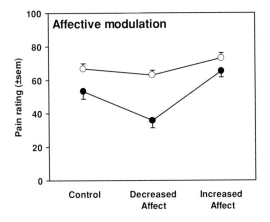

Fig. 6. Ratings of pain experienced during the immersion of the hand in hot water following hypnotic suggestions directed at the sensory and affective dimensions of pain. Suggestions for pain sensation modulation (upper panel) produce parallel changes in ratings of pain sensation intensity and unpleasantness. In contrast, suggestions for the reinterpretation of pain with increased and decreased sense of threat and discomfort (lower panel) produce specific changes in pain unpleasantness that largely exceed the changes in pain sensation intensity compared to a baseline condition (Rainville et al. 1999a).

consequence of pain relief itself as the intensity and immediate unpleasantness of the pain contribute to these secondary pain-related emotions (Price 1999). However, in some conditions, the reduction of anxiety and other negative emotions may also have a reciprocal beneficial effect on pain relief.

We have recently started to examine experimentally the impact of hypnotic suggestions specifically designed to alter pain-related emotions on pain sensation intensity, pain unpleasantness, and pain-related physiological responses in normal volunteers (see Chapter 6; Huynh Bao and Rainville

2003). Our findings support the clinical observation that pain-related nega-tive emotions are associated with some increase in pain sensation intensity and with a robust increase in pain unpleasantness. In a clinical context, hypnotic suggestions may be designed more or less specifically to control those aspects of emotional distress that are most relevant to the patients. However, therapists must take into account the context of each patient's individual phenomenology of pain, as emphasized in Chapter 12.

SOME FACTORS THAT CONTRIBUTE TO THE EFFICACY OF HYPNOTIC ANALGESIA

The specific type of hypnotic suggestion used may influence the effi-cacy of hypnotic analgesia, as illustrated by the strongest effect observed in response to focused analgesia in the studies by De Pascalis et al. (1999, 2001), as described above. However, further experimental studies are needed to examine whether this result is specific to the type of pain used (in this case, electric shocks) and whether different types of pain may be relieved more effectively using different types of suggestions. Furthermore, there may be some individual variations in preference, willingness, or aptitude to respond to different types of suggestions such as dissociation or focused analgesia.

The main factor that indisputably influences the efficacy of hypnotic analgesia is hypnotizability or hypnotic susceptibility (Hilgard and Hilgard 1994). Standardized measures have been developed in which series of sug-gestions are administered that require increasing levels of hypnotic engage-ment. A score of hypnotic responsiveness is obtained based on a subject's behavioral responses to those hypnotic challenges. The demonstration of a significant relationship between this standardized hypnotic responsiveness score and the effect of interest is a cornerstone of hypnosis research and has been argued to be necessary to support hypnosis-related interpretations. Sig-nificant correlations between hypnotizability and hypnotic analgesia have been reported by Price and Barber (1987), Kiernan et al. (1995), Rainville et al. (1999a), De Pascalis et al. (1999, 2001), and a number of other hypnosis researchers (e.g., see Hilgard and Hilgard 1994). For example, as can be seen in Fig. 5, subjects with higher levels of hypnotizability ("Highs") expe-rienced superior analgesia, especially in the condition of focused analgesia. However, it is also clear from Fig. 5 that individuals with low hypnotic scores also benefited from suggestions for hypnotic relaxation, hypnotic dissocia-tion, and focused analgesia. Price and Barber (1987) also reported that those with lower levels of hypnotic susceptibility ("Lows") could experience some reduction of the affective aspects of pain more readily than pain sensation intensity, although this finding was not apparent in the results of De Pascalis et al. (1999, 2001). In the study by Rainville et al. (1999a), hypnotizability was correlated most strongly with changes in pain sensation intensity in the pain sensation modulation experiment and with pain unpleasantness in the experiment on pain affect modulation. This finding implies that the effect of hypnotizability manifests itself most clearly in relation to the primary dimension of experience that the hypnotic suggestions target. Similarly, analgesia was found to correlate positively with hypnotic scores at a site targeted by the suggestions for focused analgesia compared to other sites that were not targeted (Benhaiem et al. 2001). Whether analgesic effects observed in Lows should be considered hypnotic effects and whether Highs rely on different psychological and neural mechanisms to achieve hypnotic states and analgesia are important theoretical questions, but they should not prevent patients from receiving the potential benefit of hypnotic analgesic procedures.

HOW DO HYPNOTIZABILITY AND HYPNOTIC STATES AFFECT ANALGESIC EFFICACY?

Hypnotizability is an interesting factor that appears to be independent of other individual psychological variables such as cognitive abilities or personality (Nordenstrom et al. 2002). However, there is one factor that has been repeatedly associated with hypnotic responsiveness, and that is the ability and propensity to experience deep mental absorption (Nadon et al. 1987; Radtke and Stam 1991; Balthazard and Woody 1992). Mental absorption has been described as a state of total attention that fully engages one's representational resources and results in imperviousness to distracting events (Tellegen and Atkinson 1974). We have proposed, above, that hypnotic relaxation and absorption are associated with important changes in brain activity that may facilitate shifts in experience suggested by hypnotic suggestions. Common to all types of suggestions for analgesia is the reference to experiences that are proposed implicitly or explicitly as alternatives to the experience of pain. A nociceptive stimulus may activate ascending nociceptive pathways and the corresponding network of subcortical and cortical structures associated with the experience of pain, whereas top-down processes activated by hypnotic suggestions of analgesia diminish nociceptive signals, thereby modulating activity in pain-related neural systems. Hypnotic states may therefore contribute to the efficacy of hypnotic analgesia by reducing the cross-representational suppression normally exerted by nociceptive inputs, allowing a modification of the associated experience by top-down processes.

The contribution of hypnotic relaxation and absorption to hypnotic anal-gesia can be examined in the data collected in one of our brain-imaging studies of the hypnotic modulation of pain (Hofbauer et al. 2001; Rainville et al. 2002). In that study, subjects rated their level of hypnotic relaxation and absorption as well as the pain experienced during the immersion of their hand in hot water. Subjects were tested in the prehypnotic state, in the hypnotic state, and in the hypnotic state with suggestions to increase or decrease pain sensory intensity. Table I reports the correlations between hypnotizability, self-ratings of mental relaxation and absorption, and the magnitude of pain modulation in the experimental conditions. Based on these correlation analyses, the levels of mental relaxation and absorption were associated with hypnotizability during the hypnotic state but not in the prehypnotic state, consistent with the notion that the increase in mental relaxation and absorption in response to the induction procedure is a hyp-notic phenomenon. Second, pain modulation was also positively related to hypnotizability, as discussed above (Fig. 7A). However, significant correla-tions were also observed between pain modulation and hypnotic relaxation and absorption (Fig. 7B). Furthermore, partial correlation analyses indicated that the positive relation between pain modulation and hypnotizability de-creased to a level that did not reach significance after hypnotic relaxation or

Table I

Nonparametric correlation between self-ratings of hypnotic relaxation, hypnotic absorption, individual levels of hypnotizability, and degree of pain modulation in control and hypnotic states before and after suggestions for pain modulation

	Mental Relaxation	Mental Absorption	Pain Modulation
Prehypnotic State			
Hypnotizability	0.27, n.s.	0.15, n.s.	n.a.
Mental relaxation		0.72*	n.a.
Hypnotic State			
Hypnotizability	0.80**	0.65*	n.a.
Mental relaxation		0.70*	n.a.
Hypnotic State with Suggestions to Modulate Pain			
Hypnotizability	0.82**	0.71*	0.83**
Mental relaxation		0.91***	0.80**
Mental absorption			0.73*
Hypnotizability (partial correlation controlling for relaxation)			0.49, n.s.
Hypnotizability (partial correlation controlling for absorption)			0.64, n.s.

Note: * $P < 0.05$; ** $P < 0.01$; *** $P < 0.001$; n.a. = not applicable; n.s. = not significant.

absorption was accounted for (see Table I). This result implies that the moderating effect of hypnotizability levels on hypnotic analgesia may be partly mediated by the level of hypnotic relaxation and absorption reached during the hypnotic procedure. Additional factors may include changes in self-agency and feelings of automaticity, which were not specifically assessed in that study. Although conclusions based on post hoc correlative analyses should be considered provisional, those effects are consistent with the proposed model in which hypnotizability is an individual characteristic that predisposes the subjects to experience hypnotic states characterized by deep mental relaxation and absorption, which, in turn, facilitate the incorporation of suggestions to alter the experience of pain.

HYPNOTIC ANALGESIA AFFECTS PAIN-RELATED ACTIVITY IN THE BRAIN

Several psychophysiological studies have provided evidence that hypnotic analgesia can modulate central nociceptive processes. Evidence for a significant effect of hypnotic analgesia on the amplitude of late positive

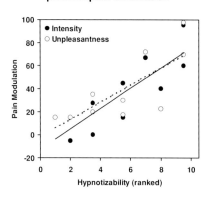
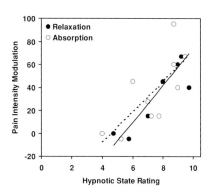

Fig. 7. Effects of hypnotizability and hypnotic states on pain modulation. (A) Individuals that are more responsive to the hypnotic procedure show greater changes in pain intensity and pain unpleasantness in response to hypnotic suggestions for pain modulation. Here, hypnotizability was assessed independently with the Stanford Hypnotic Susceptibility Scale Form A, and suggestions were given for pain sensation modulation (as in the upper panel in Fig. 6). (B) Self-ratings of mental relaxation and mental absorption also predict the magnitude of pain-modulatory effects. The moderating effect of hypnotizability on the magnitude of pain modulation is at least partly mediated by those changes in relaxation and absorption (see Table I). Data are from Hofbauer et al. (2001) and Rainville et al. (2002).

brain potentials evoked by brief noxious stimuli (electric shocks or laser heat pulses) has been observed consistently (Arendt-Nielsen et al. 1990; Zachariae and Bjerring 1994; Crawford et al. 1998; De Pascalis et al. 1999, 2001), although some negative results have also been reported (Meier et al. 1993). For example, in the study by De Pascalis et al. (2001) described above, focused analgesia not only produced the strongest analgesic effect, but also led to a reduction in the amplitude of brain potentials over the parietal cortex evoked about 300 ms after stimulus onset. However, because the classical evoked potential studies remain anatomically imprecise and because late brain potentials are commonly associated with cognitive rather than sensory processes, the interpretation of those findings has been difficult.

Two PET brain-imaging studies, the first by Rainville et al. (1997) and the second by Hofbauer et al. (2001), helped to clarify brain structures differentially involved in hypnotically induced reductions in pain affect and pain sensation intensity. The results of these two studies are summarized in Figs. 6 and 8. In both studies, subjects rated pain sensation intensity and pain unpleasantness of moderately painful immersion of the left hand in a 47°C water bath. Importantly, cortical activity was examined specifically in the contralateral primary (S1) and secondary (S2) somatosensory cortices, the insular cortex, and the anterior cingulate cortex (ACC) because these areas receive ascending nociceptive afferents and are consistently activated in functional brain imaging studies of pain (e.g., Peyron et al. 2000). Two experimental conditions of the first study included one in which hypnotic suggestions were given to *enhance* pain unpleasantness and another in which suggestions were given to *decrease* pain unpleasantness. Suggestions also were given in both conditions to the effect that, unlike pain unpleasantness, pain sensation would not change. Suggestions for enhancement of unpleasantness increased magnitudes of pain unpleasantness ratings and neural activity in the ACC (area 24) relative to the condition that provided suggestions for decreased unpleasantness. Furthermore, pain unpleasantness ratings were significantly correlated to ACC activity precisely at the site of pain-related activity in the hypnotic modulation conditions. Confirmatory evidence of the involvement of the ACC in hypnotic analgesia comes from Faymonville et al. (2000). In that study, significant changes in pain were observed in response to hypnotic analgesia but not mental imagery compared to a control condition, and the hypnotic modulation of pain was significantly associated with changes in ACC activity. However, the study did not test the specificity of the association with pain unpleasantness. Rainville et al. (1997) further reported that pain-related activity in S1, like subjects' mean ratings of pain sensation intensity, was not statistically different across

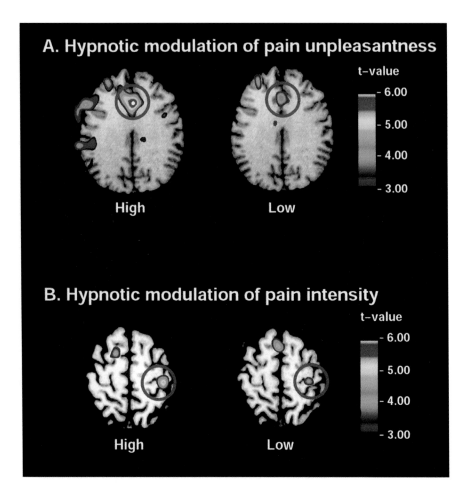

Fig. 8. Results of two PET studies demonstrating changes in brain activity within pain-related areas during the hypnotic modulation of pain affect (A) and pain sensation intensity (B). The specific increase (High) or decrease (Low) in pain unpleasantness modulates pain-related activity in the anterior cingulate cortex (ACC; red circles in A). In contrast, the increase (High) or decrease (Low) in pain sensation intensity modulates mainly the activity in the primary somatosensory cortex (S1; red circles in B).

the two experimental conditions in which pain affect was modulated. A second study used hypnotic suggestions to modify the intensity of pain sensation. In this experiment, the suggestions were effective in producing parallel changes in ratings of pain sensation intensity and neural activity in S1 (Hofbauer et al. 2001). The combination of those results provides compelling evidence that hypnotic suggestions could target sensory or affective dimensions of pain and associated brain structures. The second study shows that the modulation of ACC activity in the first study was not simply the result of nonspecific cognitive factors associated with hypnosis but was integral to the affective dimension of the pain experience.

The modulation of pain-related activity in cortical areas receiving ascending nociceptive signals critically involved in pain strongly validates the hypnotic procedure by demonstrating a significant modulation of brain activity that has previously been shown to be involved in pain. In addition to those changes specifically found in pain-related areas, suggestions for pain modulation (combined suggestions for pain increase and decrease) also produced widespread increases in activity in the lateral and medial prefrontal cortices including the dorsal aspect of the ACC (area 32), as well as in the parietal cortices, the brainstem, and the left ventral striatum (Rainville et al. 1999b). Interestingly, the activation found in the frontal and parietal cortices in response to hypnotic suggestions for increases and decreases in pain are consistent with the activation observed in the medial prefrontal cortex during hypnotic auditory hallucination (Szechtman et al. 1998), and with activation of the lateral parietal cortex during hypnotic delusion of movement (Blakemore et al. 2003), as discussed above. This pattern of activity is highly consistent with the observation that hypnotic suggestions, including those for analgesia, are actualized without a sense of self-agency (Fig. 1). These changes may also reflect the activation of modulatory circuits that affected pain-related areas directly through corticocortical connections or indirectly through descending projections affecting thalamic or brainstem nuclei. A recent reanalysis of the data collected by Faymonville et al. (2000) suggested that the ACC interacts with many other cortical and subcortical structures of the cerebral network involved in pain perception, including the insular cortices, the rostral ACC, the right prefrontal cortices, the striatum, the thalamus, and the brainstem (Faymonville et al. 2003). In that study, coactivation of the brainstem with the ACC has been suggested as reflecting the activation of descending mechanisms involved in the regulation of spinal nociceptive processes. In addition to their contribution to the regulation of ascending nociceptive activity, these mechanisms are likely to influence the nociceptive responses generally observed in the rest of the body.

THE HYPNOTIZED BODY

In addition to changes in brain responses to noxious stimuli produced by hypnotic analgesia, a substantial body of research has examined the effects of hypnotic analgesia on peripheral physiological responses normally associated with pain and dependent upon nociceptive processes at lower levels of the neuraxis. Brain-imaging studies of hypnotic analgesia are thereby complemented by studies that examine whether hypnotic analgesia involves a modulation of reflexive motor and autonomic regulatory processes. Descending mechanisms of this kind have played a central conceptual role in our thinking about pain modulation for over 30 years (see Fig. 9).

A test of whether brain-to-spinal cord mechanisms are at all involved in hypnotic analgesia was conducted by Kiernan et al. (1995), who examined changes in the R-III, a nociceptive spinal reflex, during hypnotic reduction of pain sensation and unpleasantness. The R-III was measured in 15 healthy volunteers who used a visual analogue scale to rate the sensory and affective qualities of an electrical stimulus during conditions of resting wakefulness without suggestions and during hypnosis with suggestions for hypnotic analgesia. A critically important feature of this study was that subjects were blind to the physiological index being measured, and, when later informed that measurements were being made of the R-III flexion reflex, they were

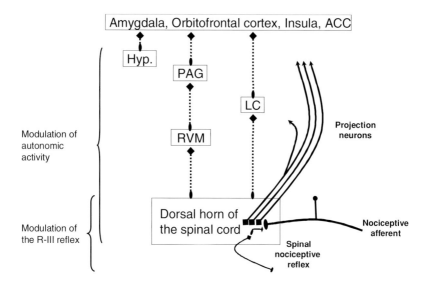

Fig. 9. Potential descending mechanisms (dotted lines) involved in the hypnotic modulation of spinal and autonomic nociceptive responses. Nociceptive afferents activate spinal nociceptive reflexes as well as ascending neurons projecting to various areas of the brain. Descending projections from the amygdala, the orbitofrontal cortex, the anterior insula, and the anterior cingulate cortex (ACC) toward the hypothalamus (Hyp.), the periaqueductal gray area (PAG), and the locus ceruleus (LC) contribute to modulate nociceptive processes in the brainstem and spinal cord. These mechanisms may affect the output of autonomic nuclei of the brainstem and spinal cord as well as spinal nociceptive motor reflexes. The evidence reviewed in this chapter indicates that some of these mechanisms may be involved in the hypnotic modulation of pain.

unable to intentionally reduce the magnitude of this reflex. This hypnotic modulation of a motor reflex that cannot be modified voluntarily is particularly interesting in relation to the altered sense of agency. We speculate that the felt sense of automaticity experienced during hypnosis may facilitate the modulation of involuntary processes and contribute to hypnotic analgesia. Consistent with this proposition, hypnotic sensory analgesia was related to the significant reduction in the R-III ($R^2 = 0.51$, $P < 0.003$). This finding suggests that hypnotic sensory analgesia is at least partly mediated by descending antinociceptive mechanisms that exert control at spinal levels and are not under voluntary control.

Danziger et al. (1998) subsequently conducted a similar study of the R-III reflex and late somatosensory evoked potentials in 18 highly susceptible subjects. The verbally reported pain threshold, the R-III nociceptive flexion reflex, and late somatosensory evoked potentials were investigated in parallel. The hypnotic suggestion of analgesia induced a significant increase in pain threshold in all subjects. All subjects showed substantial changes of 20% or more in the amplitudes of their R-III reflexes during hypnotic analgesia in comparison with control conditions. Although the extent of the increase in pain threshold was similar in all subjects, two distinct patterns of modulation of the R-III reflex were observed during hypnotic analgesia. Among 11 subjects (subgroup 1), a strong inhibition of the reflex was observed, consistent with the results of Kiernan et al. (1995) described above. Among the other seven subjects (subgroup 2), there was a strong facilitation of the reflex. All the subjects in both subgroups displayed similar decreases in the amplitude of late somatosensory evoked cerebral potentials during hypnotic analgesia. These results suggest that different strategies of modulation can be operative during effective hypnotic analgesia and that these are subject-dependent. A decrease of the late somatosensory evoked potential occurred in all subjects, consistent both with a mechanism that inhibits pain-related information from reaching the somatosensory cortex and with a mechanism that reduces subsequent cognitive processing of pain. The relatively nonspecific nature of cortical-evoked potentials does not allow us to distinguish between these two alternatives. The inhibition of somatosensory processing appears to relate to inhibition at spinal levels for some subjects and perhaps at higher levels for others (in whom the spinal flexion reflex is facilitated). The results of Danziger et al. (1998) partially corroborate and extend those of Kiernan et al (1995) by indicating the possibility of at least two general physiological mechanisms of pain inhibition recruited by hypnotic procedures.

In addition to those studies documenting the implication of central mechanisms in hypnotic analgesia, psychophysical studies have demonstrated that hypnotic analgesia may also have positive consequences on peripheral physiological responses associated with pain. Activation of the nociceptive system at various levels of the neuraxis induces a number of autonomic responses (Jänig 1995), and many psychophysiological studies, including those investigating hypnosis, support a positive relationship between pain perception and autonomic responses. For example, both cardiovascular response and pain ratings evoked by experimental ischemia decrease significantly following hypnotic suggestions of analgesia (Lenox 1970). Likewise, lower pain ratings were associated with smaller heart rate increases among hypnotized subjects exposed to the cold pressor test (Hilgard et al. 1974; Hilgard and Hilgard 1994). In the study by De Pascalis et al. (2001) described above, focused analgesia not only produced the strongest analgesic effect and a reduction in brain potential responses, but it also reduced the skin conductance response and heart rate response to the electrical noxious stimuli. These results strongly support the existence of a functional interaction between pain perception and autonomic activation that can be separated from the physical characteristics of the noxious stimulus. Rainville et al. (1999a) found that the increase in stimulus-evoked heart rate was significantly correlated with the change in pain unpleasantness induced by hypnosis, independent of changes in pain intensity, suggesting a direct functional interaction between pain affect and autonomic activation. The rapid changes in peripheral physiological responses to noxious stimuli imply that the central neurophysiological mechanisms engaged during hypnotic analgesia may influence brainstem and spinal systems responsible for autonomic regulation.

There is also some evidence that hypnosis may be used to attenuate inflammatory responses (Zachariae and Bjerring 1990) and stimulate adaptive immune responses (Gruzelier et al. 2001; Gruzelier 2002). However, more studies are needed to assess more specifically the potential effects of hypnotic analgesia on pain-related inflammatory and immune responses.

CONCLUSIONS

The induction of hypnotic states produces changes in subjective experience that are associated with specific changes in brain activity. We have argued that changes characterizing the felt increase in hypnotic relaxation and absorption may help facilitate the integration of hypnotic suggestions by reducing the reciprocal inhibition between competing representations and experiences. Preliminary evidence supports that conclusion. In addition to those experiential changes, the felt sense of automaticity associated with the effects of hypnotic suggestions implies a modification in self-representation and involves brain structures involved in the attribution of self-agency, such as the posterior parietal cortex. These changes in self-agency may also relate to the privileged access, during hypnosis, to physiological mechanisms that usually are not under voluntary control, such as motor and autonomic reflexes. These changes reflect the activation of endogenous circuitry that descends to brainstem and spinal levels, inhibits nociceptive transmission within cells of origin of ascending pathways, and modulates motor and autonomic responses. Variations in the specific physiological processes involved in hypnotic analgesia clearly relate to the type of hypnotic suggestions used, as demonstrated by the differential brain responses observed when suggestions are directed to sensory or affective aspects of pain. Future studies should further compare other types of suggestions and evaluate whether individual preferences or aptitude to engage in various forms of hypnotic analgesia may account for the variability in central as well as peripheral physiological responses. More basic research is also needed to assess the potential contribution of different forms of hypnosis to the prevention of chronic pain and to discover the underlying physiological mechanisms.

We have come a long way since Franklin and Lavoisier proposed that the patient's imagination, rather than animal magnetism, explained the effects of hypnosis. However, learning more about the psychological and neural underpinnings of hypnosis still raises many questions about the power of imagination and the potential of hypnotic interventions to regulate physiological processes that are usually conceived as autonomous and out of our voluntary control. Paradoxically, it is the abandonment of our subjective sense of self-control during hypnosis that may provide this privileged access to those involuntary physiological processes.

REFERENCES

Arendt-Nielsen L, Zachariae R, Bjerring P. Quantitative evaluation of hypnotically suggested hyperaesthesia and analgesia by painful laser stimulation. *Pain* 1990; 42:243–251.

Aston-Jones G, Rajkowski J, Cohen J. Role of locus coeruleus in attention and behavioral flexibility. *Biol Psychiatry* 1999; 46:1309–1320.

Balthazard CG, Woody EZ. The spectral analysis of hypnotic performance with respect to "absorption." *Int J Clin Exp Hypn* 1992; 40:21–43.

Benhaiem J-M, Attal N, Chauvin M, Brasseur L, Bouhassira D. Local and remote effects of hypnotic suggestions of analgesia. *Pain* 2001; 89:167–173.

Blakemore SJ, Frith C. Self-awareness and action. *Curr Opin Neurobiol* 2003; 13:219–224.

Blakemore SJ, Oakley DA, Frith CD. Delusions of alien control in the normal brain. *Neuropsychologia* 2003; 41:1058–1067.

Botvinick M, Nystrom LE, Fissel K, Carter CS, Cohen JD. Conflict monitoring versus selection-for-action in anterior cingulate cortex. *Nature* 1999; 402:179–181.

Carter CS, Macdonald AM, Botvinick M, et al. Parsing executive processes: strategic vs. evaluative functions of the anterior cingulate cortex. *Proc Natl Acad Sci USA* 2000; 97:1944–1948.

Chalmers DJ. What is a neural correlate of consciousness? In: Metzinger T (Ed). *Neural Correlates of Consciousness: Empirical and Conceptual Questions*. Cambridge, MA: MIT Press, 2000, pp 17–39.

Chaminade T, Decety J. Leader or follower? Involvement of the inferior parietal lobule in agency. *Neuroreport* 2002; 13:1975–1978.

Coull JT, Nobre AC. Where and when to pay attention: the neural systems for directing attention to spatial locations and to time intervals as revealed by both PET and fMRI. *J Neurosci* 1998; 18:7426–7435.

Crawford HJ, Gruzelier JH. A midstream view of the neuropsychophysiology of hypnosis: recent research and future directions. In: Fromm E, Nash MR (Eds). *Contemporary Hypnosis Research*. New York: Guilford Press, 1992, pp 227–266.

Crawford HJ, Knebel T, Kaplan L, et al. Hypnotic analgesia: 1. somatosensory event-related potential changes to noxious stimuli, and 2. transfer learning to reduce chronic low back pain. *Int J Clin Exp Hypn* 1998; 46:92–132.

Damasio AR. *The Feeling of What Happens: Body and Emotion in the Making of Consciousness*. New York: Harcourt Brace, 1999.

Danziger N, Fournier E, Bouhassira D, et al. Different strategies of modulation can be operative during hypnotic analgesia: a neurophysiological study. *Pain* 1998; 75:85–92.

De Pascalis V, Magurano MR, Bellusci A. Pain perception, somatosensory event-related potentials and skin conductance responses to painful stimuli in high, mid, and low hypnotizable subjects: effects of differential pain reduction strategies. *Pain* 1999; 83:499–508.

De Pascalis V, Magurano MR, Bellusci A, Chen AC. Somatosensory event-related potential and autonomic activity to varying pain reduction cognitive strategies in hypnosis. *Clin Neurophysiol* 2001; 112:1475–1485.

Enqvist B, Fischer K. Preoperative hypnotic techniques reduce consumption of analgesics after surgical removal of third mandibular molars: a brief communication. *Int J Clin Exp Hypn* 1997; 45:102–108.

Farrer C, Frith CD. Experiencing oneself vs another person as being the cause of an action: the neural correlates of the experience of agency. *Neuroimage* 2002; 15:596–603.

Farrer C, Franck N, Georgieff N, et al. Modulating the experience of agency: a positron emission tomography study. *Neuroimage* 2003; 18:324–333.

Faymonville ME, Mambourg PH, Joris J, et al. Psychological approaches during conscious sedation. Hypnosis versus stress reducing strategies: a prospective randomized study. *Pain* 1997; 73:361–367.

Faymonville ME, Laureys S, Degueldre C, et al. Neural mechanisms of antinociceptive effects of hypnosis. *Anesthesiology* 2000; 92:1257–1267.

Faymonville ME, Roediger L, Del Fiore G, et al. Increased cerebral functional connectivity underlying the antinociceptive effects of hypnosis. *Brain Res Cogn Brain Res* 2003; 17:255–262.

Fiset P, Paus T, Daloze T, et al. Brain mechanisms of propofol-induced loss of consciousness in humans: a positron emission tomographic study. *J Neurosci* 1999; 19:5505–5513.

Frenay MC, Faymonville ME, Devlieger S, et al. Psychological approaches during dressing changes of burned patients: a prospective randomised study comparing hypnosis against stress reducing strategy. *Burns* 2001; 27:793–799.

Ghoneim MM, Block RI, Sarasin DS, Davis CS, Marchman JN. Tape-recorded hypnosis instructions as adjuvant in the care of patients scheduled for third molar surgery. *Anesth Analg* 2000; 90:64–68.

Graffin NF, Ray WJ, Lundy R. EEG concomitants of hypnosis and hypnotic susceptibility. *J Abnorm Psychol* 1995; 104:123–131.

Gruzelier JH. A review of the impact of hypnosis, relaxation, guided imagery and individual differences on aspects of immunity and health. *Stress* 2002; 5:147–163.

Gruzelier J, Smith F, Nagy A, Henderson D. Cellular and humoral immunity, mood and exam stress: the influences of self-hypnosis and personality predictors. *Int J Psychophysiol* 2001; 42:55–71.

Herculano-Houzel S, Munk MHJ, Neuenschwander S, Singer W. Precisely synchronized oscillatory firing patterns require electroencephalographic activation. *J Neurosci* 1999; 19:3992–4010.

Hilgard ER, Hilgard JR. *Hypnosis in the Relief of Pain,* revised ed. New York: Brunner/Mazel, 1994.

Hilgard ER, Morgan H, Lange AF. Heart rate changes in pain and hypnosis. *Psychophysiology* 1974; 11:692–702.

Hofbauer RK, Rainville P, Duncan GH, Bushnell MC. Cortical representation of the sensory dimension of pain. *J Neurophysiol* 2001; 86:402–411.

Hofle N, Paus T, Reutens D, et al. Regional cerebral blood flow changes as a function of delta and spindle activity during slow wave sleep in humans. *J Neurosci* 1997; 17:4800–4808.

Huynh Bao QV, Rainville P. Modulation of experimental pain by emotion induced using hypnosis. *Pain Res Manage* 2003; 8 (Suppl B):35B.

Jänig W. The sympathetic nervous system in pain. *Eur J Anaesthesiol* 1995; 12:53–60.

Kawashima R, O'Sullivan BT, Roland PE. Positron-emission tomography studies of cross-modality inhibition in selective attentional tasks: closing the "mind's eye." *Proc Natl Acad Sci USA* 1995; 92:5969–5972.

Kiernan BD, Dane JR, Philips LH, Price DD. Hypnotic analgesia reduces R-III nociceptive reflex: further evidence concerning the multifactorial nature of hypnotic analgesia. *Pain* 1995; 60:39–47.

Kinomura S, Larsson J, Gulyas B, Roland PE. Activation by attention of the human reticular formation and thalamic intralaminar nuclei. *Science* 1996; 271:512–515.

Lang EV, Benotsch EG, Fick LJ, et al. Adjunctive non-pharmacological analgesia for invasive medical procedures: a randomized trial. *Lancet* 2000; 355:1486–1490.

Laurence JR. 1784. *Int J Clin Exp Hypn* 2002; 50:309–319.

Lenox JR. Effect of hypnotic analgesia on verbal report and cardiovascular responses to ischemic pain. *J Abnorm Psychol* 1970; 75:199–206.

Lindauer U, Dirnagl U. Synaptic activity and regional blood flow: physiology and metabolism. In: Casey KL, Bushnell MC (Eds). *Pain Imaging,* Progress in Pain Research and Management, Vol. 18. Seattle: IASP Press, 2000.

Liossi C, Hatira P. Clinical hypnosis versus cognitive behavioral training for pain management with pediatric cancer patients undergoing bone marrow aspirations. *Int J Clin Exp Hypn* 1999; 47:104–116.

Liossi C, Hatira P. Clinical hypnosis in the alleviation of procedure-related pain in pediatric oncology patients. *Int J Clin Exp Hypn* 2003; 51:4–28.

Llinas R, Ribary U, Contreras D, Pedroarena C. The neuronal basis for consciousness. *Philos Trans R Soc Lond B Biol Sci* 1998; 353:1841–1849.

Lou HC, Kjaer T, Friberg L, et al. A ^{15}O-H$_2$O PET study of meditation and the resting state of normal consciousness. *Hum Brain Mapp* 1999; 7:98–105.

Malonek D, Grinvald A. Interaction between electrical activity and cortical microcirculation revealed by imaging spectroscopy: implications for functional brain mapping. *Science* 1996; 272:551–554.

Maquet P, Faymonville ME, Degueldre C, et al. Functional neuroanatomy of hypnotic state. *Biol Psychiatry* 1999; 45:327–333.

Meier W, Klucken M, Soyka D, Bromm B. Hypnotic hypo- and hyperalgesia: divergent effects on pain ratings and pain-related cerebral potentials. *Pain* 1993; 53:175–181.

Nadon R, Laurence JR, Perry C. Multiple predictors of hypnotic susceptibility. *J Pers Soc Psychol* 1987; 53:948–960.

Nobre AC. Orienting attention to instants in time. *Neuropsychologia* 2001; 39:1317–1328.

Nordenstrom BK, Council JR, Meier BP. The "big five" and hypnotic suggestibility. *Int J Clin Exp Hypn* 2002; 50:276–281.

Parvizi J, Damasio A. Consciousness and the brainstem. *Cognition* 2001; 79:135–160.

Patterson DR, Jensen MP. Hypnosis and clinical pain. *Psychol Bull* 2003; 129:495–521.

Paus T. Functional anatomy of arousal and attention systems in the human brain. *Prog Brain Res* 2000; 126:65–77.

Paus T, Zatorre RJ, Hofle N, et al. Time-related changes in neural systems underlying attention and arousal during the performance of an auditory vigilance task. *J Cogn Neurosci* 1997; 9:392–408.

Peyron R, Laurent B, Garcia-Larrea L. Functional imaging of brain responses to pain: a review and meta-analysis. *Neurophysiol Clin* 2000; 30:263–288.

Posner MI, Dehaene S. Attentional networks. *Trends Neurosci* 1994; 17:75–79.

Price DD. Hypnotic analgesia: psychological and neural mechanisms. In: Barber J (Ed). *Hypnosis and Suggestions in the Treatment of Pain*. New York: Norton, 1996, pp 67–84.

Price DD. *Psychological Mechanisms of Pain and Analgesia,* Progress in Pain Research and Management, Vol. 15. Seattle: IASP Press, 1999.

Price DD, Barber J. An analysis of factors that contribute to the efficacy of hypnotic analgesia. *J Abnorm Psychol* 1987; 96:46–51.

Price DD, Barrell JJ. The structure of the hypnotic state: a self-directed experiential study. In: Barrell JJ (Ed). *The Experiential Method: Exploring the Human Experience.* Acton, MA: Copely, 1990, pp 85–97.

Radtke HL, Stam HJ. The relationship between absorption, openness to experience, anhedonia, and susceptibility. *Int J Clin Exp Hypn* 1991; 39:39–56.

Rainville P, Price DD. Hypnosis phenomenology and the neurobiology of consciousness. *Int J Clin Exp Hypn* 2003; 51:105–129.

Rainville P, Duncan GH, Price DD, Carrier B, Bushnell MC. Pain affect encoded in human anterior cingulate but not somatosensory cortex. *Science* 1997; 277: 968–971.

Rainville P, Carrier B, Hofbauer RK, Bushnell MC, Duncan GH. Dissociation of pain sensory and affective dimensions using hypnotic modulation. *Pain* 1999a; 82:159–171.

Rainville P, Hofbauer RK, Paus T, et al. Cerebral mechanisms of hypnotic induction and suggestion. *J Cogn Neurosci* 1999b; 11:110–125.

Rainville P, Hofbauer RK, Bushnell MC, Duncan GH, Price DD. Hypnosis modulates activity in brain structures involved in the regulation of consciousness. *J Cogn Neurosci* 2002; 14:887–901.

Ray WJ. EEG concomitants of hypnotic susceptibility. *Int J Clin Exp Hypn* 1997; 45:301–313.

Ruby P, Decety J. Effect of subjective perspective taking during simulation of action: a PET investigation of agency. *Nat Neurosci* 2001; 4:546–550.

Sabourin ME, Cutcomb SD, Crawford HJ, Pribram K. EEG correlates of hypnotic susceptibility and hypnotic trance: spectral analysis and coherence. *Int J Psychophysiol* 1991; 10.

Salas C, Salas D. The first scientific investigation of the paranormal ever conducted: testing the claims of Mesmerism. *Skeptic* 1996; 4:66–83.

Steriade M, McCarley RW. *Brainstem Control of Wakefulness and Sleep.* New York: Plenum Press, 1990.

Steriade M, McCormick DA, Sejnowski TJ. Thalamocortical oscillations in the sleeping and aroused brain. *Science* 1993; 262:679–685.

Szechtman H, Woody E, Bowers KS, Nahmias C. Where the imaginal appears real: a positron emission tomography study of auditory hallucinations. *Proc Natl Acad Sci USA* 1998; 95:1956–1960.

Tellegen A, Atkinson G. Openness to absorbing and self-altering experiences ("absorption"), a trait related to hypnotic susceptibility. *J Abnorm Psychol* 1974; 83:268–277.

Vanzetta I, Grinvald A. Increased cortical oxidative metabolism due to sensory stimulation: implications for functional brain imaging. *Science* 1999; 286:1555–1558.

Woody E, Szechtman H. Hypnotic hallucinations: towards a biology of epistemology. *Contemp Hypn* 2000; 17:4–14.

Zachariae R, Bjerring P. The effect of hypnotically induced analgesia on flare reaction of the cutaneous histamine prick test. *Arch Dermatol Res* 1990; 282:539–543.

Zachariae R, Bjerring P. Laser-induced pain-related brain potentials and sensory pain ratings in high and low hypnotizable subjects during hypnotic suggestions of relaxation, dissociated imagery, focused analgesia, and placebo. *Int J Clin Exp Hypn* 1994; 42:56–80.

Zeltzer L, LeBaron S. Hypnosis and nonhypnotic techniques for reduction of pain and anxiety during painful procedures in children and adolescents with cancer. *J Pediatr* 1982; 101:1032–1035.

Correspondence to: Pierre Rainville, PhD, Department of Stomatology, Faculty of Dental Medicine, University of Montreal, CP 6128, Montreal, PQ, Canada H3C 3J7. Tel: 514-343-6111; Fax: 514-343-2111; email: pierre.rainville @umontreal.ca.

Psychological Methods of Pain Control: Basic Science and Clinical Perspectives, Progress in Pain Research and Management, Vol. 29, edited by Donald D. Price and M. Catherine Bushnell, IASP Press, Seattle, © 2004.

12

Hypnotic Analgesia: Mechanisms of Action and Clinical Applications

Joseph Barber

Department of Rehabilitation Medicine, University of Washington School of Medicine, Seattle, Washington, USA

Like placebo, hypnosis is a phenomenon largely misunderstood by the public as well as by many clinicians. This misunderstanding is partly due to the long history of unscientific claims about the nature and effects of hypnosis. These claims often lead the credulous to the conclusion that hypnosis is a powerful supernatural phenomenon and the skeptical to the belief that it is merely a trick. The evidence suggests that it is neither of these. However, even among the empirically minded the understanding of hypnosis is not straightforward because it is a highly complex psychological process, not wholly accessible to behavioral analysis alone.

The terms "placebo," "hypnosis," and "suggestion" are often popularly used to convey the same idea: "It's all in your head." They convey the implicit message: "It isn't real." Fortunately, contemporary research can help us to understand the reality of psychological events, including those that result from placebo, hypnosis, and suggestion.

While there is ample evidence that the processes underlying placebo and hypnosis are different, one similarity between them is that the effects of each depend upon suggestion (De Pascalis et al. 2002). In a sense, people tend to underestimate the power of placebo—"Oh, that's only a placebo response"—while overestimating the power of hypnosis. Popular accounts of hypnosis reliably convey erroneous ideas, including claims of powerful influence and magical effect. A persistent image associated with hypnosis is that of a man with a penetrating gaze mysteriously compelling someone (usually an attractive young woman) to behave in dramatically uncharacteristic ways. More, the attractive young woman is defenseless against the power of the hypnotist. This characterization of powerfulness has its roots in the early history of hypnosis, which, unfortunately, was often an amalgam of mysticism, magic, and social psychological manipulation. Although the 18th-century physician Franz Anton Mesmer (1734–1815) initiated the development of what we now understand as the domain of clinical hypnosis, his theory of action was mistaken; he thought that the phenomenon depended upon the transfer of magnetic energy from the clinician to the patient. His fascination with the drama of the process may have been a distraction that prevented him from understanding that its essence was psychological, not magnetic. Kihlstrom (2002) offers a thorough account of the history of hypnosis, including a particularly thoughtful analysis of Mesmer's role.

At the behest of the king of France, in 1783 the Societé Royale created a panel of eminent scientists chaired by Benjamin Franklin to experimentally investigate Mesmer's claims of magnetism. The Franklin Commission concluded that Mesmer's technique had a real effect, but that this effect was due not to magnetism but to the patient's imagination. The commission's investigative work was historic for two reasons: It was perhaps the first instance of formal psychological experimentation, and the experimental results would ultimately lead to the psychological concepts of hypnosis and suggestion.

The subsequent development of the theory and practice of hypnosis in the 19th century focused primarily upon its medical applications, most notably pain relief. In 1843, the British physician James Braid documented the importance of the psychological responsiveness of the patient (in contrast to the belief in the overarching power of the hypnotist, a myth that still exists today). Braid observed that a suggested idea could dramatically alter the patient's experience. He eventually coined the term "hypnotism" to denote the phenomenon. This choice was unfortunate because it wrongly connotes a condition of sleep. Rather, hypnosis is an active, cognitive state of focused absorption in a suggested experience.

In 1850, James Esdaile, a British surgeon working in India, successfully used hypnotic methods to induce anesthesia for a series of major surgical cases (Esdaile 1957). This practical development was met with disbelief but also hope, because it promised an end to the agony and associated high morbidity of surgery. Since Esdaile's initial report, there have been numerous accounts of surgery performed with hypnotic suggestion as the only anesthetic. Almost simultaneous with these initial reports of hypnoanesthesia, however, was the announcement of the successful use of a chemical anesthetic, chloroform, which led to the birth of the science and art of anesthesia, the development of other effective chemical anesthetics, and thus to a waning of interest in hypnoanesthesia.

Toward the end of the 19th century and into the early years of the 20th century, the focus of clinicians interested in hypnotic phenomena was its application in the treatment of psychopathology, principally the symptoms of hysteria and dissociation. However, aside from reports of hypnotic methods used in battlefield hospitals, there were few significant developments in the understanding of hypnotic methods for the relief of pain until the late 1950s. During this period the work of Ernest and Josephine Hilgard inspired a wealth of increasingly sophisticated psychological research into the nature of hypnotic phenomena.

After securing his reputation as a premier scholar of human learning, Ernest Hilgard established the Hypnosis Laboratory at Stanford University in 1957. For the next three decades, that laboratory was a fountainhead of hypnotic research, including especially the investigation of hypnotic analgesia (Weitzenhoffer and Hilgard 1959; Hilgard 1965a,b, 1967, 1969, 1973; Hilgard and Morgan 1975; Hilgard et al. 1975; Hilgard and LeBaron 1984; Hilgard and Hilgard 1994). Martin Orne, directing the Unit for Experimental Psychiatry at the University of Pennsylvania, also began to conduct hypnosis research, including the investigation of hypnotic analgesia (Orne 1976, 1980). One of Orne's unique contributions was the integration of social psychological concepts with behavioral ones. For instance, Orne (1962) asserted that the "demand characteristics of the situation" modified a hypnotized subject's behavior.

These pioneering efforts were the basis for a wide range of subsequent research that has led to the richness of theory and research informing our contemporary understanding of hypnotic analgesia. This understanding, however, is necessarily limited by the constraints of the behavioral paradigm employed in this research. It was the evolution of the phenomenological paradigm that has led to the growth in quality of psychological investigation of hypnotic phenomena.

Peter Sheehan and Kevin McConkey (1982) contributed substantially to our understanding by their introduction of the Experiential Analysis Technique (EAT). Whereas prior research examined a subject's behavior, EAT enabled us to access the internal experience of the hypnotized subject. This technique involves videotaping the hypnotized subject during an experiment. Immediately after the experiment, the subject and experimenter review the videotape, and the subject is asked to comment upon his or her internal experience during salient moments of the experiment. Price and Barrell (1990) used a different technique to apply the phenomenological paradigm to hypnotic investigation. In doing so, they identified five features of the hypnotic experience that tend to be present for most people: (1) a feeling of well-being; (2) an absorbed and sustained focus of attention; (3) an absence of judging, monitoring, and censoring; (4) a lack of orientation toward time, location, and sense of self; and (5) an experience of one's own responses as automatic.

The array of hypnosis research over the past 50 years has greatly enriched our understanding of hypnotic phenomena. One puzzle that remains, though, is the relationship between hypnosis and placebo.

HYPNOSIS AND PLACEBO

The relationship between placebo and hypnosis is not well understood, in part because the mediating factors of placebo analgesia (expectation, desire for relief, and conditioning) have been elucidated to some extent in recent years, whereas those for hypnotic analgesia are largely unaddressed. For example, we know very little about whether hypnotized subjects explicitly expect reductions in pain, and there are good reasons to suspect that unconscious mechanisms are at work during hypnotic analgesia (D.D. Price, personal communication, 2003).

A descriptive definition may be useful at this point: Hypnosis is an altered state of consciousness characterized by a markedly increased receptivity to suggestion, resulting in the possibility for the systematic modification of perception and memory. Nothing in this description suggests that a person has been rendered powerless by the hypnotic condition. On the contrary, the integrity of personality remains unchanged. An individual who is ordinarily vulnerable to the influence of others will continue to be vulnerable in the hypnotic circumstance. Similarly, an individual who is not ordinarily vulnerable to influence will continue to be invulnerable while hypnotized (or, for the same reason, will not experience hypnotic phenomena). For this reason, the effective clinician remains alert for ways to support the patient's sense of safety, to defuse the patient's fears, and to engage the patient's motivation for relief. Although "miracle cures" apparently occur often enough to maintain the superstitious illusion of hypnotic power, it is not likely that a clinician can successfully suggest to a hypnotized patient that his or her symptoms will abruptly vanish. Rather, hypnotic suggestions can be used as psychological leverage to enhance the effectiveness of a clinical intervention. In the therapeutic examples offered later in the chapter, you may notice that the clinician's acknowledgment of the patient's complexity—for instance, his or her pessimism, skepticism, or unrealistic expectation, and, especially, the meaning of the pain to the patient—is reflected in the subtlety and complexity of the suggestions.

With the advent of safe and effective chemical anesthetics, hypnotic analgesia is not needed in the operating room. However, the patient with unremitting or recurrent pain who has not responded to curative intervention may well benefit from hypnosis. Laboratory and clinical research efforts have highlighted the value of hypnotic procedures as both primary and adjunctive clinical interventions. This chapter focuses on how these interventions, as well as interventions involving nonhypnotic suggestion, can be used in the clinical management of acute or chronic recurrent pain. Technical accounts of hypnotic interventions and of the relevant research appear in Barber and Adrian (1982), Hilgard and LeBaron (1984), Lynn and Rhue (1991), Fromm and Nash (1992), Hilgard and Hilgard (1994), and Barber (1996).

THE BIOLOGY AND PSYCHOLOGY OF HYPNOSIS

Because hypnosis is often mistakenly considered a magical or occult phenomenon, it is worth remembering that hypnotic phenomena are, in fact, psychological phenomena and therefore are fundamentally explicable by psychological theory and principles. As Kihlstrom (1998) reminds us, "Nothing about hypnosis changes the way the mind works." How, then, are we to understand phenomena that cut across the spectrum of experience, including amnesia, analgesia, and hallucination? Although there remains the challenge of explaining hypnotic phenomena within a single, integrated psychological theory, over the past 20 years two primary explanatory schema have risen to prominence: (1) Ernest Hilgard's neodissociation theory, with variations suggested by Kenneth Bowers, John Kihlstrom, and Eric Woody; and (2) variants of a sociocognitive theory that is primarily the work of Theodore Barber, William Coe, Irving Kirsch, Steven Lynn, Theodore Sarbin, and Nicholas Spanos.

NEODISSOCIATION THEORY

Dissociation theory, which originated in the late 19th century, offers an explanation of various psychopathologies, most notably hysterical disorders, and provides the essential concept of "a division between two streams of consciousness ... with only one of these streams accessible" to conscious awareness (Kirsch and Lynn 1998).

As it happens, hypnotic suggestion is effective both in altering the symptoms of hysterical patients (including sensory alterations, such as blindness, deafness, and anesthesias, as well as motor symptoms, such as paralysis and mutism) and in creating similar symptoms among normal human subjects. Consequently, there seems to be a logical connection between dissociative processes and hypnotic processes. Building upon the dissociation theory proposed by psychiatrist Pierre Janet (1901) nearly a century earlier, Ernest

Hilgard offered what he termed a "neodissociation" interpretation of hypnotic analgesia (1973). The neodissociation perspective reflects the recognition that some behaviors are not consciously intended, initiated, or controlled. "Dissociated control" in everyday life is particularly well revealed in
various mental lapses (think of a "slip of the tongue"), but is also the basis
for hypnotic responsiveness (Bowers 1990; Miller and Bowers 1993): "Such
dissociated control of thought and behavior depends on a hierarchical model
of mind, which assumes ... that different cognitive control systems can
operate in relative independence of each other" (Bowers and Davidson 1991,
p. 135).

The neodissociation model proposes that the hypnotic process creates a
temporary functional separation between certain cognitive control structures,
resulting in the corollary separation of awareness. For example, Hilgard
suggests that the hypnotized patient comfortably undergoing a painful procedure is able to do so because of the separation—the dissociation—between the cognitive structures responsible for the perception of pain and the
central control structures responsible for the individual's conscious awareness. Because a central feature of all hypnotic phenomena is the experience
of automaticity—that the thought or behavior occurs without effort or, perhaps, even intention—Hilgard's explanation applies to hypnotic phenomena
in general, not only hypnotic analgesia. Moreover, his explanation also accounts for nonhypnotic dissociative processes.

SOCIOCOGNITIVE THEORIES

It is well known that social psychological variables affect individual
psychological variables in a variety of circumstances. Orne's classic research (1959, 1962) demonstrated that hypnotic experience is modified by
social variables. This recognition of the relevance of social psychology to
the understanding of hypnotic processes has led some to propose that it is
social variables that are primarily involved in hypnotic phenomena (Spanos
1991). Spanos writes: "Thus, from my perspective, successful hypnotic responding to suggestions ... reflects goal-directed actions by subjects who, in
coordinated fashion, generate experiences and enact behaviors in order to
meet what they tacitly understand to be the requirements of the test situation" (1991, p. 325).

Sarbin and Coe (1972) have referred to these socially directed experiences as "role playing," emphasizing the tacit social agreement among those
involved to behave "as if" an alteration in experience is occurring. Variations of contemporary sociocognitive theory of hypnotic processes have
been described by Spanos (1991), Kirsch (1991), and Kirsch and Lynn (1998).

The neodissociation theory of divided consciousness and sociocognitive theories both focus upon mechanisms that create alterations in awareness, but while neodissociation theories emphasize a temporary splitting (dissociating) of consciousness, sociocognitive theorists emphasize ordinary conscious processes; these do not include perceptions and cognitions that are out of ordinary awareness. Kirsch (1991), for instance, theorizes that it is an individual's belief and expectation that determine the hypnotic experience. Typical hypnotic responses can easily be altered by providing subjects with expectancy-altering information. This view suggests, for example, that an individual's expectation of analgesia is self-confirming. It is this expectation that reduces the pain.

No one theory has fully accounted for the range of hypnotic phenomena, and all contemporary theories are necessarily tentative. It is likely that any successful theory that emerges will take into account both social processes and an individual's psychological processes. Although the sociocognitive and neodissociation models each contribute to our understanding of hypnotic processes, my view is that the neodissociation perspective is of greater clinical utility. It is supported by a substantial accumulation of data from both basic and clinical research (Orne 1959, 1962, 1980; Hilgard 1967, 1969, 1975; Goldstein and Hilgard 1975; Mayer et al. 1976; Barber 1977, 1980; Barber and Mayer 1977; Finer and Terenius 1981; Deltito 1984; Hilgard and LeBaron 1984; Fricton and Roth 1985; Gfeller et al. 1987; Price and Barber 1987; Olness and Gardner 1988; DeBenedittis et al. 1989; Arendt-Nielsen et al. 1990; Bowers 1990, 1992; Kurtz and Bienias 1990; Bowers and Davidson 1991; Adams and Stenn 1992; Hall et al. 1992; Kihlstrom 1992; Meier et al. 1993; Miller and Bowers 1993; Hargadon et al. 1995; Kiernan et al. 1995; Zamansky and Ruehle 1995; Bejenke 1996; Enqvist 1996; Lambert 1996; Rainville et al. 1997, 1999a,b; Eastwood et al. 1998; Szechtman et al. 1998; Zachariae et al. 1998).

It is particularly clear from this research that hypnotic experience is commonly experienced as automatic and involuntary and that lack of awareness of certain thoughts or behaviors is central to the experience. This finding contradicts a central tenet of sociocognitive theory, which is that hypnotized individuals are experiencing no more than that which they expect and intend to experience. The neodissociation perspective offers the most parsimonious psychological explanation of hypnotic analgesia and has sufficient empirical support to warrant both our tentative confidence and further exploration (Arendt-Nielsen et al. 1990; Woody and Bowers 1994; Zamansky and Ruehle 1995; Woody and Sadler 1998).

PSYCHOPHYSICAL AND NEUROPHYSIOLOGICAL INVESTIGATIONS

Psychophysical and neurophysiological evidence also supports the neodissociation perspective. In reviewing this evidence, Price (1996) has identified three components that underlie the processes suggested by Hilgard: (1) selective reduction of the affective dimension of pain, (2) reductions in sensory pain by mechanisms that divert pain from conscious awareness once nociceptive information has reached higher centers, and (3) inhibition of pain signals at the spinal level.

In a particularly ingenious experiment, Kiernan et al. (1995) demonstrated the dissociative quality of hypnotic analgesia. These investigators were the first to suggest the role of inhibitory spinal mechanisms in hypnotic analgesia, identifying specific spinal efferent activity associated with hypnotic analgesia. This finding was later confirmed by Zachariae et al. (1998). It suggests that one of the effects of hypnosis is the downstream inhibition exerted upon spinal pathways, creating changes in the body's periphery. Surprisingly, hypnosis is *not* "only in your head."

A report by Croft et al. (2002) provides evidence for the role of gamma oscillations in the subjective experience of pain. Further, this evidence is consistent with the view that hypnosis involves the dissociation of the prefrontal cortex from other neural functions. At a different level of analysis, Ray et al. (2002) demonstrated that hypnotic analgesia affects the later components of sensory evoked potential.

Evidence for endorphin involvement in analgesia, including acupuncture analgesia (Mayer et al. 1976), led to the hypothesis of a similar role in hypnotic analgesia; several investigations, however, have failed to support this hypothesis (Goldstein and Hilgard 1975; Barber and Mayer 1977; Finer and Terenius 1981). In fact, no evidence has been developed to associate particular neurotransmitters with hypnotic analgesia. Sternbach (1982), for example, did not find evidence to support his hypothesis for acetylcholine's involvement in hypnotic analgesia.

In a series of innovative studies, Rainville et al. (1998, 1999a,b) investigated cerebral blood flow changes that varied with onset and offset of hypnotic analgesia. They reported that their "results provide a new description of the neurobiological basis of hypnosis by demonstrating a specific pattern of cerebral activation underlying the multiple cognitive processes involved in this intervention" (see also Chapter 11). This finding was replicated by Wik et al. (1999). Friederich et al. (2001) and Willoch et al. (2000), using laser-evoked sensory potentials, also confirmed these findings. In my opinion, such brain-imaging studies represent the most promising innovation in the long history of biological investigations of hypnotic processes.

Nonetheless, while the findings from such studies are interesting as technical achievements, it is not clear to what extent this avenue of research can illuminate our understanding of hypnotic processes.

HYPNOTIC RESPONSIVENESS

Scientific observation of hypnotic phenomena over the past 200 years has varied, but one observation most investigators agree upon is that—as with all psychological variables—there are individual differences in response. It is well known that, as with any treatment, patients differ in the degree to which they respond to hypnotic treatment (Hilgard and LeBaron 1984; Hilgard and Hilgard 1994). "Who can be hypnotized?" is a question commonly asked. The question particularly relevant to the clinician considering its use with a patient is: "Under what conditions can hypnotic methods be used to reduce a particular patient's suffering?"

Research exploring this question has determined that variables such as age, intelligence, and personality do not predict hypnotic responsiveness (Hilgard and Hilgard 1994). The only personality trait that is significantly correlated with responsiveness is imaginative absorption—an individual's capacity to have a temporary experience of "believing in" imaginary perceptions (Hilgard 1975).

Experimental investigations intended to identify predictors of hypnotic responsiveness (also referred to variably as hypnotic susceptibility and hypnotizability) have yielded differing results. In the typical study, hypnotic responsiveness is measured by reference to an individual's performance on a standardized test. Such a test creates the opportunity to respond to a hypnotic induction and to several suggestions for classic hypnotic behaviors (e.g., analgesia, amnesia, and hallucination). The number of behaviors the individual demonstrates then becomes the numeric measure of hypnotic responsiveness. Hilgard and Morgan (1975), for example, demonstrated that the correlation between such measures and an individual's ability to hypnotically reduce experimental pain is significant ($r = 0.50$) and accounts for 25% of the variance. However, Hilgard and Morgan also reported that 44% of individuals whose responsiveness scores were low were able to reduce their pain by 10% or more. "This means that the relation between reduction and hypnotic responsiveness is probabilistic, with a greater probability of successful pain reduction for those highly responsive to hypnotic suggestions. The data do not mean that those unresponsive to hypnotic suggestion, as measured by the scales, have no possibility of help through suggestion" (Hilgard and Morgan 1975, p. 68).

A preponderance of laboratory evidence clearly supports the idea that hypnotic responsiveness is a relatively stable trait and that only a minority of individuals can achieve clinically significant hypnotic analgesia (Hilgard 1965a,b, 1969; Hilgard and LeBaron 1984; Hilgard and Hilgard 1994). However, the issue is not as clear as these findings suggest, for evidence also indicates that other variables may help determine the clinical effectiveness of hypnotic treatment (Barber 1977, 1980, 1982, 1991; Alman and Carney 1981; Fricton and Roth 1985; Gfeller et al. 1987).We can infer from these investigations that variables inherent in the clinical context (including the clinician-patient relationship and the patient's felt need for relief) may engender responsiveness to hypnotic treatment in individuals whose responsiveness scores are measurably low. The laboratory research of Gfeller et al. (1987), in particular, confirmed the clinical lore that the clinical relationship is a primary determinant of responsiveness.

Gfeller and his colleagues compared a treatment with little interpersonal training with a treatment designed to augment rapport with the trainer and diminish resistance to responding. Following the intervention, 50% of unresponsive subjects had test scores indicating superior responsiveness to hypnotic suggestion. The performance of control subjects was stable across testing. The importance of rapport was demonstrated by ratings paralleling group differences in hypnotic responding.

In general, the clinical literature reports hypnotic suggestion to be more effective as an analgesic than one would predict from the experimental reports. There is at least one explanation for this disparity between clinical and experimental research findings in relationship to analgesic effects in subjects with low and high responsivity to hypnotic suggestion. Those with high responsivity are better able to reduce the sensory-discriminative component of pain, but those with low responsivity are still sufficiently able to reduce the motivational-affective component (Price and Barber 1987). This may mean that low responders are less capable of dissociating from the sensory-discriminative component, but are nonetheless able to reinterpret the meaning of the experience, thereby reducing the motivational-affective component. If these two components are not each independently measured, it is possible that some patients' measures reflect the sensory component, whereas others' reflect the affective component. Without measuring both variables, it is impossible to determine the validity of each measurement. This distinction may be particularly salient between the hypnosis laboratory (where pain measures tend to emphasize the sensory component by asking "How intense is the sensation?") and the clinic (where pain measures tend to emphasize the affective component, because it is suffering that brings the patient to the clinic).

Such findings may explain why clinicians generally report higher incidences (compared to laboratory reports) of hypnotic analgesia in individuals with various degrees of responsivity. In addition, reporting bias may play a role in generating the discrepancy between findings in the laboratory and the clinic. Experimental subjects are significantly less motivated to experience a hypnotic effect than are clinical patients seeking relief from suffering. There are also significant differences in the behavior and motivation of experimenters and clinicians. Experimental protocols usually require rigid adherence to a well-operationalized, standardized induction and set of suggestions. Rarely is the purpose of an experiment the search for optimum hypnotic effect. However, that is precisely the purpose of the clinical intervention. Effective clinical use of hypnotic suggestion requires an individualized approach not possible in most clinical investigations. In the clinic, a standardized set of procedures is rarely followed, and the clinician, normally focused only on doing what is effective, may vary or repeat procedures until success is obtained. Although this strategy may lead to successful clinical outcomes, it is usually impossible to assess the causal link between treatment and results.

Moreover, as Diamond (1984) suggests, the relationship between the clinician and patient is a powerful determiner of the hypnotic effect (or any clinical effect). The relationship between an experimenter and subject is significantly less personal (sometimes the hypnotic induction is even conveyed by a tape recorder) than the well-developed, intimate, and more potent relationship of a concerned clinician and a suffering patient. Whatever the explanation for the disparity of reported hypnotic effect between experimental and clinical contexts, it is clear that clinical success with hypnotic suggestion requires innovative, personalized, clinically sophisticated procedures. It is difficult to compare such procedures with well-controlled experimental procedures. So, for the moment, the complex question of hypnotic responsiveness remains an open one.

The therapeutic goals in the treatment of acute or recurrent pain are the reduction of suffering and return to good function; hypnotic methods may be suitable to both goals. The primary advantage of hypnotic intervention is that, in a particular case, it may be effective when no other treatments have been. It is less invasive than medical pain management interventions, and it does not produce side effects, such as somnolence or motor retardation, as opioid medications may. Moreover, because suggestions can include those that encourage a healthy outlook and expectation for recovery, the clinician may expect that, in addition to analgesic effects, successful hypnotic intervention will also facilitate the patient's development of this optimistic and salutary outlook.

Unlike other pain management interventions that are done *to* the patient, hypnotic methods require the active psychological engagement with and involvement of the patient. So, in the case of a patient who may be ambivalent about achieving symptom reduction (for example, a patient for whom there are financial disincentives for rehabilitation), this ambivalence may result in only intermittent or temporary response, or by a lack of treatment responsiveness altogether. Adequate evaluation prior to treatment will identify such ambivalence, and treatment plans can be guided by this information.

A distinct advantage of hypnotic methods of pain management is the potential for long-term effectiveness (Jensen and Barber 2000). In this connection, the importance of utilizing posthypnotic suggestions will be discussed later in the chapter, under the heading "Extending Pain Relief."

INDICATIONS/CONTRAINDICATIONS

[A] medicament is not really potent unless it is able to be dangerous on occasions; and it is very difficult to think of any method of treatment which would be efficacious although it could never by any possibility do harm. Pierre Janet, 1860 (Nahum 1965, p. 221)

As Janet observes, the corollary of healing power must be the power to harm. This potential must be acknowledged when we consider hypnotic treatment for a patient. A patient who suffers from acute or recurrent pain may be a likely candidate for hypnotic treatment if the following contraindications are not present: (1) disincentive for relief (e.g., financial or social reward for continued suffering); (2) intellectual impairment (characterized by an inability to attend and to learn); (3) psychological impairment (characterized by blurring of psychological boundaries, poor reality orientation, or severe depression).

Because hypnotic treatment can cause radical alterations in cognitions and behavior—with a concomitant experience of nonvolitionality—concern is sometimes expressed that hypnotic techniques can be harmful. Much effort has been made to settle the question of whether hypnosis can cause an individual to behave in ways that would be harmful. Even though there has been no satisfactory documentation of an instance of harm coming to an individual as a result of clinical hypnotic intervention, this concern is often raised because of the occasionally harmful consequences of the antics performed by subjects of night-club hypnotists. Whereas the behavior demonstrated in such acts can be explained without reference to hypnosis (e.g., compliance with demand characteristics), there is still reason to believe that the psychological changes that can be produced by hypnotic intervention are sufficiently powerful as to warrant its use only by trained clinicians. Hypnotic treatments, like any other clinical tool, can be misapplied, resulting in harm. This caveat is the reason behind the careful training of clinicians, however, not for avoiding the use of powerful clinical tools.

Hypnotic methods can be harmful in two situations. The first is when the clinician lacks an adequate understanding of the patient's psychological needs and capacities. However, adequate training can prepare the clinician to respond appropriately to the patient. The second is when the patient's capacity for coping with deep absorption in fantasy, or with intense emotional contact with the clinician, is insufficient. The clinician can prepare for this eventuality, too, by adequately evaluating the patient prior to treatment. This evaluation would involve a clinical interview as well as formal assessment instruments such as the Minnesota Multiphasic Personality Inventory (MMPI-2). In addition, he or she might include a depression inventory such as the Beck Depression Scale. The purpose of this evaluation is to inform the clinician about the patient's psychological health and provide guidance about the patient's likely response to treatment. The Tellegen Absorption Scale (Tellegen and Atkinson 1974) offers a helpful means for inferring how readily the patient may respond to hypnotic intervention, which requires imaginative absorption. Although the various scales of hypnotic responsiveness are useful in research, I believe their use in the clinical circumstance is inappropriate for two reasons. First, assessment with these scales requires the clinician to challenge the patient in a manner that is inappropriate to the clinical situation; and second, poor performance on such tests may result in unwarranted pessimism by both the clinician and the patient.

The experience of being hypnotized is generally innocuous and often pleasant, yet hypnotic treatment should only be undertaken by someone with sufficient clinical skills, including knowledge of psychological phenomena and psychopathology (NIH 1996). Because hypnotic techniques can be applied across several areas of clinical expertise, it might be a temptation for a clinician trained in one area to use "hypnotherapy" to treat a patient whose problem would otherwise lie outside the clinician's training. For example, a psychologist may be well trained to treat a patient's pain, if the patient has already had an adequate medical evaluation, and if the psychologist is mindful of the medical aspects of the patient's condition. It would not be appropriate for the psychologist to treat a patient's pain without proper medical collaboration. Similarly, a gynecologist may be properly trained to hypnotically treat a patient's pelvic pain, but it would be inappropriate to treat the patient's psychosexual dysfunction with "hypnotherapy." If the patient's

pelvic pain is associated with psychological factors, it is best for the gynecologist to refer the case to someone with appropriate psychological training. One should only treat a problem one is trained to treat. If one is also
trained in the use of hypnotic methods for such a problem, those methods
will probably enhance the treatment. Training in hypnotic methods, alone,
however, is not an alternative for adequate clinical training in general.

CLINICAL TECHNIQUES

Hypnotic treatment requires the patient's cooperation and responsiveness, so it is helpful for the clinician to observe how the patient responds.
For example, the initial social suggestions made to a patient about sitting
comfortably provide an important opportunity to observe how the patient
responds. For example, how literal or confluent is the response? How at ease
is the patient? This is not a hypnotic response, but it offers a clue to subsequent responses. Moreover, the importance of such interactions reminds us
that suggestions alone—in the absence of a hypnotic experience—can substantially augment clinical effectiveness, both by encouraging patient comfort and confidence and by promoting healthy expectations.

The manner in which the clinician introduces the topic of hypnotic
treatment to the patient may either augment or diminish the patient's subsequent responses. The word "hypnosis" tends to have unhelpful connotations
for most people and probably does not convey an accurate idea of the
treatment intended by the clinician. Therefore, it may be most helpful to
discuss the treatment by using more operational terms, thus obviating the
use of the word "hypnosis" altogether. The intention is not to obfuscate or
deceive, but rather to communicate clearly. Of course, if the patient uses the
word "hypnosis," the best response probably requires use of the word. If a
patient has had prior experience with hypnotic treatment—especially if the
experience was satisfying—this experience can be utilized.

Here is an example of what might be said to introduce the topic of
hypnotic treatment, using operational terms: "You probably know that the
relationship between mind and body is a powerful one. Would you like me
to show you how to use the power of your imagination to help you feel
better?" Or: "Let's use your ability to fantasize, now, to help you feel
better." Or: "Mental imagery can be very helpful in retraining your nervous
system so that the nerves that carry the useless information about your pain
will do so less and less in the future." Or: "Your ability to become deeply
absorbed by your imagination can be really helpful to you now. Will you
close your eyes right now, and take a very deep, very relaxing breath, so you

can begin to notice how really relaxed your mind can become?" Each example is intended to convey to patients that they possess the means to increase their comfort. The clinician who uses such "nonhypnotic" language to introduce hypnotic treatment should remember subsequently to use language that is consistent with this introduction.

The three fundamental elements of hypnotic treatment are induction, therapeutic suggestions, and suggestions to end the hypnotic experience.

INDUCTION

Hypnotic induction is the facilitation of the patient's alteration in consciousness from ordinary wakefulness to a state of imaginative absorption that supports the utilization of clinical suggestions. The goal of the induction is to engage the patient's capacity to dissociate. Although there are a few classic induction techniques, the clinician employs whatever induction will most readily facilitate the patient's experience of trust, security, and interest in what the clinician is saying. Instruction in the technique of induction is well beyond the scope of this chapter. However, the literature is replete with such instruction (Bernheim 1957; Haley 1967; Crasilneck and Hall 1975; Frankel 1976; Barber 1977, 1996; Barber and Adrian 1982; Hilgard and LeBaron 1984; Brown and Fromm 1986; Olness and Gardner 1988; Hilgard and Hilgard 1994). In the context of this chapter, however, we can explore the ideas that comprise an effective hypnotic induction.

Because hypnotic treatment requires the active involvement of the patient's imagination, the first goal of the clinician about to embark upon hypnotic induction is that of engaging the patient's interested attention. Often, the clinical context itself—and the patient's wish to be relieved of suffering—will be sufficiently interesting.

The second goal is to help the patient to focus his or her attention—to reduce the range of attention—and then to direct that attention inward, at which point the patient's imagination can begin to emerge as the agent of the ensuing hypnotic process. At this point, suggesting that the patient close his or her eyes has the virtue of both eliciting a cooperative, voluntary response from the patient and eliminating visual sources of distraction, as well as offering another opportunity to observe how the patient responds to a suggestion.

The final goal of the induction process is that of dissociation. It is dissociation that distinguishes the hypnotic experience from the nonhypnotic. Dissociation is the active cognitive compartmentalization of some aspect of experience from conscious awareness. The human experience of dissociation involves a spectrum, from the normal, everyday narrowing of awareness that permits one to concentrate to pathological examples, most notably the

various symptoms of hysteria. In the context of pain management, the hypnotic experience systematically evokes the patient's ability to dissociate
pain and suffering from conscious awareness. Some adults and most children are able to develop a hypnotic experience with little or no facilitation
by the clinician (Hilgard and LeBaron 1984; Olness and Gardner 1988). In
such cases, the clinician can function best by acting as a guide.

The following is an example of a hypnotic induction. It has been highly
abbreviated for purposes of highlighting the essential suggestions (which, in
practice, may often be repeated for emphasis). (1) Engaging the patient's
interest and attention: "Are you ready to begin learning how to use your
imagination to see if you can feel better?" (2) Focusing attention and turning
it inward: "Close your eyes and take a very deep, very comfortable breath
and, now, hold it ... hold it ... That's fine. Now, let it all the way out, and
just notice how easily can feel yourself sink down into a place of very deep
quiet and relaxation." (3) Dissociation: "As you become more and more
aware that each breath contributes to a greater sense of comfort and ease,
you may have already noticed that the sensations you can feel ... all the
feelings you can notice ... are becoming more and more a part of your
experience of comfort and relaxation ... with nothing to bother you, and
nothing to disturb you."

THERAPEUTIC SUGGESTIONS

Once the patient is experiencing dissociation, suggestions can be offered to reach the therapeutic goal—dissociation of the painful symptoms.
Posthypnotic suggestions will be discussed later in the chapter, but it is at
this stage of treatment that they may be communicated. It is helpful to the
clinician to know if the patient is responding to suggestions. Because the
analgesic response takes place only in the patient's imagination and is essentially invisible to the clinician, suggestions for other, overt behaviors
may be helpful, simply to assess the patient's responsiveness. Examples of
therapeutic suggestions will be given later in the chapter.

SUGGESTIONS TO END THE HYPNOTIC EXPERIENCE

Once therapeutic suggestions, including posthypnotic ones, have been
given, the hypnotic experience can be brought to an end. (In the case of
immobile patients, such as those in a burn ward, this step may not be
necessary. Because they are immobile, these patients do not need to return
to an alert, active state.) Normally, the clinician suggests that the patient
will, following the experience, feel alert, rested, curious about the outcome,

and so on. For example: "So now, I'd like you to take one or two very deep, very refreshing, very energizing breaths. As you open your eyes, notice how easy it is for you to quickly feel alert and refreshed. Almost like waking from a very refreshing nap. And ready to be pleasantly surprised."

STRATEGIES FOR CREATING HYPNOTIC ANALGESIA

Just as there is an almost limitless range for creating a hypnotic induction, so, too, the patient's capacity for developing hypnotic analgesia may be accessed by a variety of suggestive strategies. When developing the treatment plan and considering which strategy to use, the clinician should be clear about the goal. In an acute context, for example, the goal may be simply to facilitate the patient's comfort in the moment. In the context of treating recurrent pain, however, the clinician might keep in mind that the goal is to facilitate a reduction of suffering on the part of the patient with a concomitant return to good function (except, of course, in the case of patients with end-stage terminal illness). Although the clinician may elect to follow one of the classic strategies described below, optimal effectiveness may depend upon creativeness guided by the clinician's understanding of the patient's individual needs (e.g., autonomy or dependence, firmness or gentleness, clarity or ambiguity). For instance, does the patient feel more at ease if the clinician relates as an equal partner in the treatment or as an authority? Does the patient respond more readily if the intervention is approached as skills training or as an experience of altered consciousness? To what extent is the patient ambivalent about experiencing a reduction in pain? What consequences might the clinician expect if the patient feels less pain and suffering? Should the reduction in pain be suggested to occur immediately or at a later time? These are a few of the many questions the clinician will consider during the ongoing observation and growing understanding of the patient.

ACUTE PAIN

For the patient who is undergoing a painful procedure, is receiving postoperative care, or is incapacitated by disease or injury, activity and full orientation to the environment are not important. Suggestions for dissociation from severe pain (and from the unpleasantness of the circumstance) can yield substantial levels of comfort. Because the clinical goal is to reduce the patient's suffering, the nature of the pain is irrelevant. What is crucial is the patient's understanding and expectation about the pain. In other words, the meaning of the pain is what distinguishes the intervention from one patient to the next. Patients suffering from postoperative pain, burn pain, dental pain, labor pain, and acute pain from other medical procedures may all benefit from hypnotic intervention.

Here is an example of a suggestion intended to produce such dissociation for a postoperative patient:

> You don't have to stay here in bed, conscious of all the work, all the noise, that goes on here in the hospital. Would you enjoy a kind of vacation from this room? Wouldn't it be pleasant to imagine gently floating through the window and out into the beautiful blue sky of this sun-filled day? And to just float on, to wherever you'd like to be? Almost like living a favorite daydream … just enjoying going wherever you'd like to go, being wherever you'd like to be, leaving your body here in the room to be taken care of. Your mind, your imagination, can take you far away, if you'd like, to a holiday from discomfort, a holiday from boredom, to really enjoy yourself.

CHRONIC PAIN SYNDROMES

Because hypnotic processes take place at the highest level of neural organization, the nature, quality, and location of pain are not essential determinants of success (as would be the case, for example, with a local anesthetic acting on peripheral nerves.) That is, there is no strategy unique to treatment of osteoarthritic pain of the knee rather than the elbow, or of causalgic pain of the arm or of the leg, or of neuropathy of the face or of the foot. Hypnotic treatment can be effectively applied to any pain syndrome, so long as pain relief is in the patient's interest.

The primary variable in choosing a strategy for treating various pain syndromes is the phenomenology of the pain. How the patient experiences the pain and, most especially, what the pain means to the patient are crucial to effective treatment. Does the pain worsen with activity (as might be the case, for example, with osteoarthritis)? Does the pain worsen with certain mood states? Does the pain threaten the patient's life? Does the pain threaten the patient's sense of self? Does the pain remind the patient of the trauma that caused the pain? Does the patient think someone else is responsible for causing the pain (as might be the case with a patient injured by a drunk driver)? If so, does the patient feel victimized by the injury or illness? Does the pain mean to the patient that life can no longer be happy, satisfying, or meaningful? Does the pain mean that the patient can no longer enjoy certain activities? Does the pain mean that the patient expects increasing disability and death? Will the patient receive compensation so long as there is pain? The answer to these questions will guide the clinician's interventions.

INTERIM STRATEGIES

Ordinarily, the patient suffering from recurring pain has had prior experiences of treatment failure, so the clinician may find it helpful to utilize temporary interventions in order to alter the patient's pessimistic expectations and beliefs about pain relief. Once the patient has experienced what may be initially implausible—that is, the modulation of intransigent pain—more ambitious clinical goals may be set. The following are examples of some initial treatment strategies.

Sensory substitution. Just as one's imagination can alter the perceived intensity of pain, so it can also alter the perceived sensory quality, resulting in a reinterpretation of sensations that may be more tolerable. A sensation of intolerable burning, for instance, can be replaced by a sensation of cold. The substituted sensation does not necessarily have to be pleasant, but only more tolerable than the original sensation. Substituting a sensation is probably not the ultimate clinical goal, but it has the following advantages: (1) The patient knows the pain is still present (so the cancer patient, for instance, can be assured that the persisting cancer will continue to receive proper medical attention), and can "monitor" its progress, thus retaining a sense of control over the condition. (2) The substitute sensation is not particularly pleasant, so its presence may seem more plausible to the patient than a pleasurable sensation. (3) Because the patient does not lose financial and social incentives (because the pain still persists), this interim strategy may be a means for negotiating with the patient further treatment goals that might involve the loss of some or all such incentives.

Here follows an example of suggestions for sensory substitution:

> Those sharp sensations in your shoulder, the ones you describe as "like a knife blade," are very likely to begin to feel peculiarly different in a little while. I'm not sure exactly how they will begin to feel. It might seem, at first, as if the sharpness just becomes more and more dull … as if the sensation is less deep, maybe. Or, maybe you have already begun to notice that the steadiness of the sensations has begun to change … as if they seem to come in waves now … strange, not altogether pleasant waves of dull pressure.

Displacement of pain. Displacement of pain from one area of the body to another is yet another example of perceptual modulation. It can be useful both to render an intolerable pain more tolerable as well as to embolden a patient to experience fuller relief. Displacement may be particularly appropriate when the pain is well-localized and primarily intolerable because of its location. Midline pain, for instance, is usually less tolerable than pain located more peripherally.

You have probably already noticed that the pain moves, sometimes just a little, sometimes surprisingly … and you might begin to notice, as I talk with you, that the movement seems to become more noticeable … and that it moves in an almost circular way, like an outward spiral. Spiraling outward, always spiraling outward, sometimes so slowly that it's almost as if it isn't happening. If you pay attention to that movement, though, you might notice that the feeling seems to be moving out of the center of your belly, spiraling ever outward; almost as if it's reaching, reaching … so curious, so odd, yet farther and farther from the center of your belly.

Diminution of intensity and/or affect. Most of us have had the experience of being able, by using our imagination, to modulate a perceptual experience. Sometimes we feel a change in the intensity of the perception, sometimes we notice a change in how we feel about the perception, and sometimes our experience is that both components have changed.

The hypnotic experience greatly amplifies this phenomenon and makes it possible for an individual to modulate the sensation of pain, sometimes only a little, and sometimes to a dramatic degree. Here is an example of a suggestion that might be made to a patient in order to reduce the sensory component of pain:

You remember that you have rated the intensity of the painful feeling as a "7." Picture in your mind an image of that "7." Do you see it? That's fine. The number you see is the number you feel. And the number you feel is going to become smaller and smaller. Now, notice, as you watch that "7" very closely, watch how it begins to change. Notice how curiously the sharp angles of the "7" begin to soften, to become a gentle curve. Tell me when you begin to first notice that the "7" has become a "6." [The patient has reported seeing the "6."] That's fine. Now, as we continue, notice how the loop of the "6" begins to separate and, ever so slowly, becomes … what number do you see now? [The patient reports a "5."] That's fine. And tell me, now, do you feel the same or different than when we began?"

This conversation can proceed, with the clinician continuing to guide the patient to an experience of ever lower intensity of pain.

Alternatively, the same suggestions could focus upon the affective component, rather then the sensory. In this case, reduction of the sensory component is not an issue. All that matters is that the sensations are not perceived to be unpleasant or bothersome, and that the patient does not experience suffering. Essentially, the clinician is communicating the idea that, no matter what sensation the patient feels, it is not bothersome or unpleasant.

USE OF HYPNOSIS IN CHRONIC PAIN SYNDROMES

CANCER PAIN

Although some cancer patients experience pain of the disease itself, much of the pain associated with cancer is a result of clinical procedures (Syrjala et al. 1992). Such procedural pain can be treated as described above, under "Acute Pain."

The most significant feature of cancer pain that requires the clinician's awareness is the meaning of the pain to the patient. Cancer pain threatens the patient's sense of safety and security. Some patients report feeling a particular dread of "being eaten" by the cancer. The pain of cancer is usually a source of anxiety and fear. As with treatment of other syndromes, the amelioration of the pain associated with cancer requires that hypnotic suggestions encompass the patient's own sense of the pain. For instance, does the patient equate pain with death? Does the patient have a vivid sense that the cancer is consuming him or her? These questions can guide the clinician toward interventions that can alter the meaning of the pain—and the meaning of reducing the pain. Sometimes, patients are reluctant to become fully unaware of the pain of cancer because they experience it as a way to monitor the progress of the disease. The clinician will be more effective if the meaning of the pain is clear, however the patient may experience the pain.

HEADACHE

Although the etiology of headache is complex and varied, I will simplify the problem for purposes of this chapter by collapsing the many headache categories to the following few, which encompass most of the headaches likely to be treated by hypnotic methods: migraine headache, muscular tension headache, cluster headache, and post-traumatic headache.

Headache pain is often less easy for a patient to tolerate than pain located elsewhere because it is seems so central to awareness and to one's sense of self. It may be helpful, then, to "co-opt" the pain by incorporating it into the suggestions for hypnotic induction so that the patient does not have to struggle to resist the pain in order to pay attention to the clinician. Here is an example of suggestions that might be made when employing such a strategy:

> As you listen to the sound of my voice, notice that the sensations of aching [or pressure or whatever the patient experiences] can be almost at the very center of your awareness. You can hear my voice and pay attention to those sensations. As you do, nothing else seems to matter. Everything else just

fades away. You hear my voice, you understand my words, you feel the sensations in your head, and nothing else matters. And notice how curiously those sensations seem to change as I speak. You might notice that they seem to fade, momentarily, with each word. Or you might notice that they seem to move, almost in a spiral, each time I speak. I don't know exactly how you'll notice those sensations change, but I hope you can be interested and curious to notice.

Also, it may be helpful to treat the patient when the headache is not present, using posthypnotic suggestions to intervene when the pain subsequently recurs (see "Posthypnotic Suggestion," below). This strategy is crucial when treating migraine pain. Ordinarily, the pain of a migraine is sufficiently debilitating that a patient cannot tolerate hypnotic treatment during a migraine episode. Migraines are treated most effectively by posthypnotic treatment. When a patient is not in pain, hypnotic suggestions are given that utilize prodromal signs as posthypnotic cues that then result in the posthypnotic experience of aborting the headache before it begins. This strategy, in modified form, is also effective for patients whose migraines are not accompanied by an aura. For details of this technique, see Barber (1996).

NEUROPATHIC PAIN

The pain of facial neuropathy or of the various peripheral neuropathies can be approached in a number of ways, using the principles above. Here is an example of suggestions that might be given to a patient with facial neuropathic pain:

It is so curious that those painful feelings in your face are going to begin to change. I'd like you to be particularly alert to the ways they feel different in the future. For instance, you might notice that the instant you feel the sensation of electricity just below your eye, in the very next instant it will feel more like a strange sort of soft sensation … almost as if someone is moving a feather across your face. Or, you might notice that the painful sensation seems to "want to start," but just can't get started. As if those feelings are becoming weaker and weaker. And soon it will be very difficult to feel them at all. Or, you might notice that you have learned a kind of control over the painful feelings in your face. The next time you feel one, you can take a very deep breath, hold it for a moment, and then, as you let it all the way out, you notice that you are also letting the pain all the way out … almost as if you are breathing it out. And you can continue to breathe it out, with every breath, so that you feel better and better. And you can enjoy discovering just how much difference you can make to how well you feel.

MUSCULOSKELETAL PAIN

The most effective treatment of recurring musculoskeletal pain is likely to be medical: a combination of anti-inflammatory medication, physical therapy, and strengthening exercises. Except for the relief of acute pain, and perhaps to facilitate the patient's compliance with nonhypnotic treatment, it may be that there is no appropriate role for hypnotic treatment of musculoskeletal pain.

PHANTOM LIMB PAIN

This syndrome can be particularly vexing to both patient and clinician, both because its etiology remains mysterious and its treatment meets with variable success. Hypnotic treatment may contribute to the patient's pain relief (Siegel 1979; Willoch et al. 2000; Rosen et al. 2001; Oakley and Halligan 2002; Oakley et al. 2002), especially if, in addition to suggestions for analgesia, suggestions are also focused upon the patient's sense of loss and how to accommodate to loss—to make peace—with respect to the amputation. It can be especially effective to help the patient experience the phantom limb as comfortable (e.g., the limb is no longer twisted or crushed or otherwise in pain). Subsequently, suggestions may be given for lessening of any awareness of the limb.

STRATEGIES FOR EXTENDING PAIN RELIEF

Just as the temporary relief of a local anesthetic is likely to not be a satisfactory clinical result for the patient with recurring pain, so the relief a patient may feel only during the hypnotic treatment is also not sufficient. Once temporary relief has been achieved, then, it becomes necessary to extend the duration further, so the patient may feel more comfortable at work, at play, while awake, and while asleep.

POSTHYPNOTIC SUGGESTION

The unique and significant role played by posthypnotic suggestions in the effective management of pain has been explored in greater detail elsewhere (Barber 1998b). In this chapter, I describe the utility of posthypnotic suggestions and offer a model for their use in order to extend hypnotic pain relief, for it is through the application of posthypnotic suggestions that the practical and clinically meaningful relief of pain is most readily accomplished.

Although we await a satisfactory theory of action of posthypnotic analgesia, the following is an explanatory schema that serves as a first attempt:
(1) Hypnotic suggestions (and their subsequent repetition) result in the dissociation of noxious perceptions, reducing the sensory and/or affective components of pain. (2) Over time, this analgesia results in neural reorganization
(Flor et al. 1995) so that pain responses are replaced by new, nonpainful
responses that are developed in response to painful stimuli that no longer
produce suffering. (3) The hypnotic effect is greatly facilitated by the clinical relationship.

Every clinician knows that the reality of the therapeutic enterprise does
not break down neatly into the principles described above. However, in
formulating treatment from those principles—of promoting a trusting therapeutic relationship and an openness to new learning—two components may
be identified: the simultaneous communication to the patient of certain ideas
and the employment of posthypnotic suggestion. These ideas include: (1) an
initial empathic joining with the patient's hopelessness while suggesting a
paradoxical hopefulness and (2) an extension of the patient's usual experience of being controlled by the onset of pain by suggesting the subsequent
reduction of pain will also be out of the patient's control. An example might
be: "You've had such frustration, you must find it almost impossible to
believe that anything can help your pain. It must be very hard to believe that
I can help you. So it can be a very interesting, maybe very pleasant surprise
when you begin to notice that you really are feeling better." The attitude that
seems to be helpful in supporting therapeutic effect is similar to that associated with Twelve Step programs: Abandon your inflexible belief in total
personal control and relinquish your usual attitude of either unreasonable
hopelessness or hopefulness.

Occasional subsequent reversals in the course of the patient's life (e.g.,
emotional trauma, reinjury, and progression of disease) can markedly reduce
the patient's continued pain relief. However, if subsequent treatment takes
into account the meaning of the reversals, improvement may once again be
reestablished. Patients who successfully experience significant pain reduction tend to focus on those experiences and to minimize occasional failures,
partly by incorporating the clinician's own optimism and partly by virtue of
their own optimistic qualities. This optimism is supported by clinical success, which is why effective hypnotic treatment usually progresses stepwise,
built initially upon occasional noticeable differences in the pain, yet also
acknowledging occasions when the patient is unable to reduce the pain.

Using posthypnotic suggestion for analgesia uses the patient's experience of being unable to control the pain, of feeling hopeless, and yet of
wishing that pain would be relieved. The clinician hopes that this attitude

will facilitate the development of a therapeutic relationship that capitalizes on the patient's benign archaic memories—pleasant early memories of being well cared for—and needs for nurturing, thereby empowering the clinical intervention. Although suggestions must necessarily be highly idiosyncratic, responding to the patient's needs and expectations, the following suggestions may serve as illustrations:

> I wonder if you'll feel surprised, later today ... I don't know what time, later today, of course ... maybe at 10 minutes before 4 o'clock ... or maybe at 4 minutes after 10 o'clock ... I really don't know what time it will be ... that you will have the opportunity to suddenly notice that you're feeling better than you expected to feel. I don't know, though ... it might not actually be the time on the clock ... maybe it will have to do with what you are doing at the time ... maybe you'll be turning the pages of a magazine ... or sipping from a cup ... or turning to catch a glimpse of color going by ... I don't know what you'll be doing later today when you have the opportunity to suddenly notice that you're feeling better than you expected to feel.

SELF-HYPNOTIC MANAGEMENT

Another means for extending the duration of relief is by teaching the patient how to use self-hypnotic techniques (Fromm and Kahn 1990). Self-hypnosis requires the patient to take the initiative of taking time from his or her day to settle in comfortably, and to provide suggestions for inducing the hypnotic experience, followed by therapeutic suggestions. Most patients seem able to learn self-hypnotic techniques, although, as with most efforts toward personal development, this process may involve complications. A patient's interest in learning self-hypnotic techniques and willingness to use them provide a valuable index of his or her motivation for actively participating in recovery, as well as a means of assessing broader psychological issues, such as attitude toward pain and readiness for self-care. If not effectively assessed, passive or pessimistic attitudes may become an obstacle to therapeutic success.

It is sometimes the case that, even when experiencing hypnotic analgesia, some patients are resistant to initiating and maintaining such treatment for themselves. A common issue that emerges when such resistance is addressed is the patient's preference for being taken care of by the clinician, rather than initiating self-care. Most people enjoy being nurtured and cared for by someone else, and hypnotic treatment is likely to evoke this preference. For some, the pleasure of being nurtured can be threatened by what may be perceived as the clinician's demand for patient self-care. Exploration of a patient's reluctance to use self-hypnosis may reveal that: (1) Although hypnotic analgesia is a relief, self-hypnotic training and treatment may feel emotionally empty and, therefore, aversive. (2) Hypnotic treatment may recall a patient's earlier experiences of nurturing and care, so self-hypnotic training may feel like abandonment. (3) Hypnotic treatment feels virtually effortless, but self-hypnotic treatment may feel unpleasantly effortful.

A patient's experience of self-hypnotic training as effortful or as abandonment by the clinician may be sufficient to lead to avoidance of using self-hypnotic techniques. When a patient's motivation for learning self-hypnosis has been established, however, a number of techniques are available. One simple technique involves a posthypnotic suggestion. For example, the clinician might say:

> Whenever you want to feel this kind of comfort and well-being, all you have to do is rest back in a chair, a sofa, or a bed, and take a very deep, very satisfying breath ... and hold it, hold it. Then, as you let it all the way out, these feelings of comfort and well-being automatically come washing over you, just like water in a hot tub, with nothing to bother you and nothing to disturb you.

Self-hypnotic methods involve learning a skill; as with other skills, competence improves with practice. Sometimes it is helpful to make an audiotape for the patient to use at home as practice aid, although it is also helpful to emphasize to the patient that the development of this skill and the consequent increase in the duration of pain relief require a substantial commitment of time and effort.

As a patient's improving condition permits greater independence from treatment, less frequent treatments are necessary. At this point, clinical follow-up becomes increasingly important. Sometimes, substantial time passes during which a patient successfully maintains pain relief. Then, for a variety of reasons, he or she may find such pain management difficult. At such times, a "booster" treatment may be all that is necessary to return the patient to independent functioning. It may also be useful to help the patient identify the antecedents to the present difficulty in using self-hypnosis, so that future coping will be more effective. Sometimes, of course, with a worsening medical condition, more intensive treatment may become necessary.

OUTCOME

SELF-REPORTED PAIN

Hypnotic treatment can be expected to reduce both a patient's subjective report and experience of pain and suffering. Use of a visual analogue scale simplifies the patient's task of reliably reporting both the sensory-discriminative and the affective-motivational components of pain. There is tremendous variation in both the latency and degree of reported pain relief. Some patients report relief following the first treatment, while others do not report relief until undergoing several treatments. Similarly, the duration of relief may be initially highly variable. The clinician can help the patient to tolerate this initial variability in order to capitalize upon the improvement it represents and to develop more stable and durable pain relief.

FUNCTIONAL STATUS

The clinician's interventions need to be focused upon rehabilitation because return to function, not merely analgesia, is the clinical goal. Patients successfully treated for recurrent pain can be expected to return to good function, subject to the physical limitations of their condition. If a patient's pain is substantially reduced by hypnotic intervention, the patient can be expected to return to work. Patients whose coping strategies include self-hypnotic skills learn to integrate them into their daily work lives. Symptomatic relief is unlikely in patients for whom the opportunity to return to work presents unconscious conflict.

COMPLICATIONS

Hypnotic methods are not without risks. Though rare, complications may result from accelerated transference, acting out, disorientation, hysterical manifestations (e.g., paralysis), and memory contamination (Barber 1998a). As is evident from this list, these risks are more likely to be associated with the use of hypnotic methods in psychotherapy and are less likely in the context of pain management.

If the therapeutic goals are not aligned with the patient's perceived self-interest, then complications are likely to arise from any treatment, including hypnotic treatment. Although there is no evidence that the hypnotic experience is itself harmful, if the patient is severely depressed, psychotic, or has a severe personality disturbance, complications to hypnotic treatment may arise.

As was described earlier in the chapter, an adequate medical and psychological evaluation will be likely to alert the clinician to potential complications, and adequate clinical training will prepare the clinician for such complications.

CONCLUSIONS

Hypnotic intervention can be effective for the palliative treatment of a wide range of acute and recurring painful conditions. Medical treatment of pain is evolving, with an increasing understanding of the role of psychological processes in pain modulation. Hypnotic treatment is also evolving, with a greater emphasis on active participation by the patient, primarily through greater utilization of self-hypnosis and posthypnotic strategies. As research and clinical techniques develop further, the unscientific attitudes identified with the earlier history of hypnosis will become increasingly rare, and clinical effectiveness will becoming increasingly common.

ACKNOWLEDGMENTS

Mary Pepping, PhD, and Donald D. Price, PhD, were helpful in the revision of this chapter, for which I am grateful.

REFERENCES

Adams PC, Stenn PG. Liver biopsy under hypnosis. *J Clin Gastroenterol* 1992; 15:122–124.
Alman BM, Carney RE. Consequences of direct and indirect suggestions on success of post-hypnotic behavior. *Am J Clin Hypn* 1981; 213:112–118.
Arendt-Nielsen L, Zachariae R, Bjerring P. Quantitative evaluation of hypnotically suggested hyperaesthesia and analgesia by painful laser stimulation. *Pain* 1990; 42:243–251.
Barber J. Rapid induction analgesia: a clinical report. *Am J Clin Hypn* 1977; 19:138–147.
Barber J. Hypnosis and the unhypnotizable. *Am J Clin Hypn* 1980; 23:4–9.
Barber J. Incorporating hypnosis in the management of chronic pain. In: Barber J, Adrian C (Eds). *Psychological Approaches to the Management of Pain*. New York: Brunner/Mazel, 1982, pp 40–59.
Barber J. The locksmith model. In: Lynn SJ, Rhue JW (Eds). *Theories of Hypnosis: Current Models and Perspectives*. New York: Guilford Press, 1991, pp 241–274.
Barber J. *Hypnosis and Suggestion in the Treatment of Pain: A Clinical Guide*. New York: Norton, 1996.
Barber J. When hypnosis causes trouble. *Int J Clin Exp Hypn* 1998a, 46:157–170.
Barber J. The mysterious persistence of hypnotic analgesia. *Int J Clin Exp Hypn* 1998b; 46:28–43.
Barber J, Adrian C (Eds). *Psychological Approaches to the Management of Pain*. New York: Brunner/Mazel, 1982.

Barber J, Mayer DJ. Evaluation of the efficacy and neural mechanism of a hypnotic analgesia procedure in experimental and clinical dental pain. *Pain* 1977; 4:41–48.

Bejenke CJ. Painful medical procedures. In: Barber J (Ed). *Hypnosis and Suggestion in the Treatment of Pain: A Clinical Guide.* New York: Norton, 1996, pp 209–266.

Bernheim H. Suggestive therapeutics: a treatise on the nature and uses of hypnotism. Westport, CN: Associated Booksellers, 1957.

Bowers KS. Unconscious influences and hypnosis. In: Singer JL (Ed). *Repression and Dissociation: Defense Mechanisms and Personality Styles.* Chicago: University of Chicago Press, 1990, pp 143–179.

Bowers KS. Imagination and dissociation in hypnotic responding. *Int J Clin Exp Hyp* 1992; 40:253–275.

Bowers KS, Davidson TM. A neodissociation critique of Spanos's social-psychological model of hypnosis. In: Lynn SJ, Rhue JW (Eds). *Theories of Hypnosis: Current Models and Perspectives.* New York: Guilford, 1991, pp 105–143.

Brown DP, Fromm E. *Hypnotherapy and Hypnoanalysis.* Hillsdale, NJ: Erlbaum, 1986.

Crasilneck HB, Hall JA. *Clinical Hypnosis: Principles and Applications.* New York: Grune and Stratton, 1975.

Croft RJ, Williams JD, Haenschel C, Gruzeliera JH. Pain perception, hypnosis and 40 Hz oscillations. *Int J Psychophysiol* 2002; 46:101–108.

DeBenedittis G, Panerai AA, Villamira MA. Effects of hypnotic analgesia and hypnotizability on experimental ischemic pain. *Int J Clin Exp Hypn* 1989; 37:55–69.

Deltito JA. Hypnosis in the treatment of acute pain in the emergency department setting. *Postgrad Med J* 1984; 60:263–266.

De Pascalis V, Chiaradia V, Carotenuto C. The contribution of suggestibility and expectation to placebo analgesia phenomenon in an experimental setting. *Pain* 2002; 96:393–402.

Diamond MJ. It takes two to tango: the neglected importance of the hypnotic relationship. *Am J Clin Hypn* 1984; 26:1–13.

Eastwood JD, Gaskovski P, Bowers KS. The folly of effort: ironic effects in the mental control of pain. *Int J Clin Exp Hypn* 1998; 46:77–91.

Enqvist B. *Pre-surgical Hypnosis and Suggestions in Anesthesia.* Stockholm: Kongl Carolinska Medico Chirurgiska Institute, 1996.

Esdaile J. *Hypnosis in Medicine and Surgery.* New York: Julian, 1957.

Finer B, Terenius L. Endorphin involvements during hypnotic analgesia in chronic pain patients. *Pain* 1981; Suppl 1:S273.

Flor H, Elbert T, Knecht S, et al. Phantom-limb pain as a perceptual correlate of cortical reorganization following arm amputation. *Nature* 1995, 375:482–484.

Frankel FH. *Hypnosis: Trance as a Coping Mechanism.* New York: Plenum, 1976.

Fricton JR, Roth P. The effects of direct and indirect hypnotic suggestions for analgesia in high and low susceptible subjects. *Am J Clin Hypn* 1985: 27:226–231.

Friederich M, Trippe RH, Ozcan M, et al. Laser-evoked potentials to noxious stimulation during hypnotic analgesia and distraction of attention suggest different brain mechanisms of pain control. *Psychophysiology* 2001; 38:768–776.

Fromm E, Kahn S. *Self-hypnosis: The Chicago Paradigm.* New York: Guilford, 1990.

Fromm E, Nash MR (Eds). *Contemporary Hypnosis Research.* New York: Guilford, 1992.

Gfeller JD, Lynn SJ, Pribble WE. Enhancing hypnotic susceptibility: interpersonal and rapport factors. *J Pers Soc Psychol* 1987; 52:586–595.

Goldstein A, Hilgard ER. Lack of influence of the morphine antagonist naloxone on hypnotic analgesia. *Proc Natl Acad Sci USA* 1975; 72:2041–2043.

Haley J (Ed). *Advanced Techniques of Hypnosis and Therapy: Selected Papers of Milton H. Erickson, MD.* New York: Grune and Stratton, 1967.

Hall H, Chiarucci K, Berman B. Self-regulation and assessment approaches for vaso-occlusive pain management for pediatric sickle cell anemia patients. *Int J Psychosom* 1992; 39:28–33.

Hargadon R, Bowers KS, Woody EZ. Does counterpain imagery mediate hypnotic analgesia? *J Abnorm Psychol* 1995; 104:508–516.

Hilgard ER. Hypnosis. *Annu Rev Psychol* 1965a; 16:157–180.

Hilgard ER. *Hypnotic Susceptibility*. New York: Harcourt Brace Jovanovich, 1965b.

Hilgard ER. A quantitative study of pain and its reduction through hypnotic suggestion. *Proc Natl Acad Sci USA* 1967; 57:1581–1586.

Hilgard ER. Pain as a puzzle for psychology and physiology. *Am Psychol* 1969; 24:103–113.

Hilgard ER. A neodissociation interpretation of pain reduction in hypnosis. *Psychol Rev* 1973; 80:396–411.

Hilgard ER, Morgan AH. Heart rate and blood pressure in the study of laboratory pain in man under normal conditions and as influenced by hypnosis. *Acta Neurol Exp* 1975; 35:741–759.

Hilgard ER, Hilgard JR. *Hypnosis in the Relief of Pain,* revised ed. New York: Brunner/Mazel, 1994.

Hilgard ER, Morgan AH, MacDonald H. Pain and dissociation in the cold pressor test: a study of hypnotic analgesia with "hidden reports" through automatic key pressing and automatic talking. *J Abnorm Psychol* 1975; 87:17–31.

Hilgard JR. *Personality and Hypnosis: A Study of Imaginative Involvement,* revised ed. Chicago: University of Chicago Press, 1975.

Hilgard JR, LeBaron S. *Hypnotherapy of Pain in Children with Cancer*. Los Altos, CA: Wm. Kaufmann, 1984.

Janet P. *The Mental State of Hystericals* (Paul E, Paul C, Trans). New York: Putnam, 1901.

Jensen MP, Barber J. Hypnotic analgesia of spinal cord injury pain. *Aust J Clin Exp Hypn* 2000; 28:150–168.

Kiernan B, Dane J, Phillips L, Price D. Hypnotic analgesia reduces R-III nociceptive reflex: further evidence concerning the multifactorial nature of hypnotic analgesia. *Pain* 1995; 60:39–47.

Kihlstrom JF. Hypnosis: a sesquicentennial essay. *Int J Clin Exp Hypn* 1992; 50:301–314.

Kihlstrom JF. Dissociation and dissociation theory in hypnosis: comment on Kirsch and Lynn. *Psychol Bull* 1998; 123:186–191.

Kihlstrom JF. Mesmer, the Franklin commission, and hypnosis: a counterfactual essay. *Int J Clin Exp Hypn* 2002; 50:407–419.

Kirsch I. The social learning theory of hypnosis. In: Lynn SJ, Rhue JW (Eds). *Theories of Hypnosis: Current Models and Perspectives*. New York: Guilford, 1991, pp 439–466.

Kirsch I, Lynn S. Dissociation theories of hypnosis. *Psychol Bull* 1998; 123:100–115.

Lambert SA. The effects of hypnosis/guided imagery on the postoperative course of children. *J Dev Behav Pediatr* 1996; 17:307–310.

Lynn SJ, Rhue JW (Eds). *Theories of Hypnosis: Current Models and Perspectives*. New York: Guilford, 1991.

Mayer D, Price D, Barber J, Rafii A. Acupuncture analgesia: evidence for activation of a pain inhibitory mechanism of action. In: Bonica JJ, Albe-Fessard D (Eds). *Proceedings of the First World Congress on Pain,* Advances in Pain Research and Therapy, Vol. 1. New York: Raven Press, 1976, pp 751–754.

Meier W, Klucken M, Soyka D, Bromm B. Hypnotic hypo- and hyperalgesia: divergent effects on pain ratings and pain-related cerebral potentials. *Pain* 1993; 53:175–181.

Miller ME, Bowers KS. Hypnotic analgesia: dissociated experience or dissociated control? *J Abnorm Psychol* 1993; 102:29–38.

Mulligan R. Dental pain. In: Barber J (Ed). *Hypnosis and Suggestion in the Treatment of Pain: A Clinical Guide*. New York: Norton, 1996, pp 185–208.

Nahum LH. Dangers of hypnosis. *Conn Med* 1965; 767:771–781.

NIH Technology Assessment Panel on Integration of Behavioral and Relaxation Approaches into the Treatment of Chronic Pain and Insomnia. Integration of behavioral and relaxation approaches into the treatment of chronic pain and insomnia. *JAMA* 1996; 276:313–318.

Oakley DA, Halligan PW. Hypnotic mirrors and phantom pain: a single case study. *Contemp Hypn* 2002; 19:75–84.

Oakley DA, Whitman LG, Halligan PW. Hypnotic imagery as a treatment for phantom limb pain: two case reports and a review. *Clin Rehabil* 2002; 16:368–377.

Olness K, Gardner GG. *Hypnosis and Hypnotherapy with Children,* 2nd ed. New York: Grune and Stratton, 1988.

Orne MT. The nature of hypnosis: artifact and essence. *J Abnorm Psychol* 1959; 58:277–299.

Orne MT. On the social psychology of the psychological experiment: with particular reference to demand characteristics and their implications. *Am Psychol* 1962; 17:776–783.

Orne MT. Mechanisms of hypnotic pain control. In: Bonica JJ, Albe-Fessard D (Eds). *Proceedings of the First World Congress on Pain,* Advances in Pain Research and Therapy, Vol. 1. New York: Raven Press, 1976.

Orne MT. Hypnotic control of pain: toward a clarification of different psychological processes involved. In: Bonica JJ (Ed). *Pain.* New York: Raven Press, 1980.

Price DD. Hypnotic analgesia: psychological and neural mechanisms. In: Barber J (Ed). *Hypnosis and Suggestion in the Treatment of Pain: A Clinical Guide.* New York: Norton, 1996, pp 85–120.

Price DD, Barber J. A quantitative analysis of factors that contribute to the efficacy of hypnotic analgesia. *J Abnorm Psychol* 1987; 96:46–51.

Price DD, Barrell JJ. The structure of the hypnotic state: a self-directed experiential study. In: Barrell JJ (Ed). *The Experiential Method: Exploring the Human Experience.* Acton, MA: Copely, 1990, pp 85–97.

Rainville P, Duncan GH, Price DD, Carrier B, Bushnell MC. Pain affect encoded in human anterior cingulate but not somatosensory cortex. *Science* 1997; 277:968–971.

Rainville P, Hofbauer RK, Paus T, et al. Cerebral mechanisms of hypnotic induction and suggestion. *J Cogn Neurosci* 1999a; 11:110–125.

Rainville P, Carrier B, Hofbauer RK, Bushnell MC, Duncan GH. Dissociation of sensory and affective dimensions of pain using hypnotic modulation. *Pain* 1999b; 82:159–171.

Rainville P, Hofbauer RK, Bushnell MC, Duncan GH, Price DD. Hypnosis modulates activity in brain structures involved in the regulation of consciousness. *J Cogn Neurosci* 2002; 14:6:1–15.

Ray WJ, Keil A, Mikuteit A, Bongartz W, Elbert T. High resolution EEG indicators of pain responses in relation to hypnotic susceptibility and suggestion. *Pain* 2002; 60:17–36.

Rosen G, Willoch F, Bartenstein P, Berner N, Rosjo S. Neurophysiological processes underlying the phantom limb pain experience and the use of hypnosis in its clinical management: an intensive examination of two patients. *Int J Clin Exp Hypn* 2001; 49:38–55.

Sarbin TR, Coe WC. *Hypnosis: A Social Psychological Analysis of Influence Communication.* New York: Holt, Rinehart and Winston, 1972, p 65.

Sheehan PW, McConkey KM. *Hypnosis and Experience: The Exploration of Phenomena and Process.* Hillsdale, NJ: Lawrence Erlbaum Associates, 1982.

Siegel EF. Control of phantom limb pain by hypnosis. *Am J Clin Hypn* 1979; 21:285–286.

Spanos NP. A sociocognitive approach to hypnosis. In: Lynn SJ, Rhue JW (Eds). *Theories of Hypnosis: Current Models and Perspectives.* New York: Guilford, 1991, pp 324–361.

Sternbach RA. On strategies for identifying neurochemical correlates of hypnotic analgesia. *Int J Clin Exp Hypn* 1982; 30:251–256.

Syrjala KL, Cummings C, Donaldson GW. Hypnosis or cognitive behavioral training for the reduction of pain and nausea during cancer treatment: a controlled clinical trial. *Pain* 1992; 48:137–146.

Szechtman H, Woody E, Bowers KS, Nahmias C. Where the imaginal appears real: a positron emission tomography study of auditory hallucinations. *Proc Natl Acad Sci USA* 1998; 95:1956–1960.

Tellegen A, Atkinson G. Openness to absorbing and self-altering experiences ("absorption"), a trait related to hypnotic susceptibility. *J Abnorm Psychol* 1974; 83:268–277.

Weitzenhoffer AM, Hilgard ER. *Stanford Hypnotic Susceptibility Scale, Forms A and B*. Palo Alto, CA: Consulting Psychologists Press, 1959.

Wik G, Fischer H, Bragee B, Finer B, Fredrikson M. Functional anatomy of hypnotic analgesia: a PET study of patients with fibromyalgia. *Eur J Pain* 1999; 3(1):7–12.

Willoch F, Rosen G, Tolle TR, et al. Phantom limb pain in the human brain: unraveling neural circuitries of phantom limb sensations using positron emission tomography. *Ann Neurol* 2000; 48:842–849.

Woody EZ, Bowers KS. A frontal assault on dissociated control. In: Lynn SJ, Rhue JW (Eds). *Dissociation: Clinical and Theoretical Perspectives*. New York: Guilford, 1994, pp 52–79.

Woody EZ, Sadler P. On reintegrating dissociated theories: comment on Kirsch and Lynn. *Psychol Bull* 1998; 123:192–197.

Zachariae R, Andersen OK, Bjerring P, Jorgensen MM, Arendt-Nielsen L. Effects of an opioid antagonist on pain intensity and withdrawal reflexes during induction of hypnotic analgesia in high- and low-hypnotizable volunteers. *Eur J Pain* 1998; 2:25–34.

Zamansky HS, Ruehle BL. Making hypnosis happen: the involuntariness of the hypnotic experience. *Int J Clin Exp Hypn* 1995; 43:386–398.

Correspondence to: Joseph Barber, PhD, Department of Rehabilitation Medicine, University of Washington School of Medicine, Seattle, WA 98195, USA. Email: jbarber@u.washington.edu.

Index